HOLT

Decisions for Health

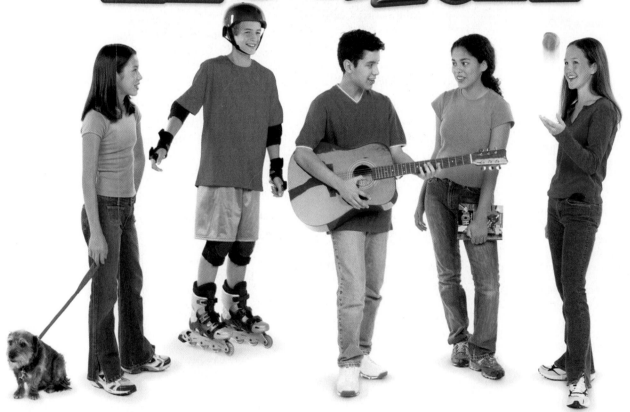

HOLT, RINEHART AND WINSTON

A Harcourt Education Company

Orlando • **Austin** • New York • San Diego • Toronto • London

Acknowledgments

Contributing Authors

Katy Z. Allen
Science Writer and Former Science Teacher
Wayland, Massachusetts

Balu H. Athreya, M.D.
Staff Physician
Alfred I. duPont Hospital
for Children
Wilmington, Delaware

Kate Cronan, M.D.
Chief, Division of Emergency Medicine
Alfred I. duPont Hospital
for Children
Wilmington, Delaware

Sharon Deutschlander
Department of Health and Physical Education
Indiana University of
Pennsylvania
Indiana, Pennsylvania

Efrain Garza Fuentes, Ed.D.
Director, Patient and Family Services
Childrens Hospital Los Angeles
Los Angeles, California

Keith S. García, M.D., Ph.D.
Instructor of Psychiatry
Washington University School
of Medicine
St. Louis, Missouri

Patricia J. Harned, Ph.D.
Director of Character Development and Research
Ethics Resource Center
Washington, D.C.

Craig P. Henderson, LCSW, MDIV
Therapist
Youth Services of Tulsa
Tulsa, Oklahoma
Trainer
National Resource Center
for Youth Services
Norman, Oklahoma

Jack E. Henningfield, Ph.D.
Associate Professor of Behavioral Biology
The Johns Hopkins University
School of Medicine
Baltimore, Maryland

Peter Katona, M.D., FACP
Associate Professor of Clinical Medicine, Infectious Disease Division, Department of Medicine
UCLA School of Medicine
Los Angeles, California

Linda Klingaman, Ph.D.
Professor
Indiana University
of Pennsylvania
Indiana, Pennsylvania

Joe S. McIlhaney, Jr., M.D.
President
The Medical Institute
for Sexual Health
Austin, Texas

Kweethai Chin Neill, Ph.D., C.H.E.S., FASHA
Assistant Professor, Department of Kinesiology, Health Promotion, and Recreation
University of North Texas
Denton, Texas

Christine Rose, M.S.
Project Director, Innovators Combating Substance Abuse
Robert Wood Johnson
Foundation
Pinney Associates
Bethesda, Maryland

Stephen E. Stork, Ed.D., C.H.E.S.
Assistant Professor
Department of Kinesiology,
Health Promotion, and
Recreation
University of North Texas
Denton, Texas

Richard Yoast, Ph.D.
Director, American Medical Association Office of Alcohol and Other Drug Abuse
Director, Robert Wood Johnson Foundation National Alcohol Program Offices
American Medical Association
Chicago, Illinois

2005 Printing

ISBN 0-03-066812-3

5 6 7   048   07 06 05

Contributing Writers

Presentation Series Development

Carol Badran, M.P.H.
Health Educator
San Francisco Department
of Public Health
San Francisco, California

Pirette McKamey
Teacher
Thurgood Marshall Academic
High School
San Francisco, California

Inclusion Specialists

Ellen McPeek Glisan
Special Needs Consultant
San Antonio, Texas

Joan A. Solorio
Special Education Director
Austin Independent
School District
Austin, Texas

Feature Development

Katy Z. Allen
Wayland, Massachusetts

Angela Berenstein
Princeton, New Jersey

Marilyn S. Chakroff
Christiansted, Virgin Islands

Mickey Coakley
Pennington, New Jersey

Allen Cobb
La Grange, Texas

Theresa Flynn-Nason
Voorhees, New Jersey

Chris Hess
Boise, Idaho

Charlotte W. Luongo
Austin, Texas

Eileen Nehme, M.P.H.
Austin, Texas

Clementina S. Randall
Quincy, Massachusetts

Answer Checking

Helen Schiller
Taylor, South Carolina

Medical Reviewers

David Ho, M.D.
Professor and Scientific Director
Aaron Diamond AIDS
Research Center
The Rockefeller University
New York, New York

Ichiro Kawachi, Ph.D., M.D.
*Associate Professor of Health
and Social Behavior*
School of Public Health
Harvard University
Boston, Massachusetts

Leland Lim, M.D., Ph.D.
Year II Resident
Department of Neurology
and Neurological Sciences
Stanford University School
of Medicine
Palo Alto, California

Iris F. Litt, M.D.
Professor
Department of Pediatrics
and Adolescent Medicine
School of Biomedical
and Biological Sciences
Stanford University
Palo Alto, California

Ronald Munson, M.D., F.A.A.S.P.
*Assistant Clinical Professor,
Family Practice*
Health Sciences Center
The University of Texas
San Antonio, Texas

Alexander V. Prokhorov, M.D., Ph.D.
*Associate Professor of
Behavioral Science*
M.D. Anderson Cancer Center
The University of Texas
Houston, Texas

Gregory A. Schmale, M.D.
Assistant Professor
Pediatrics and Adolescent
Sports Medicine
University of Washington
Seattle, Washington

Hans Steiner, M.D.
*Professor of Psychiatry and
Director of Training*
Division of Child Psychiatry
and Child Development
Department of Psychiatry
and Behavioral Sciences
Stanford University School
of Medicine
Palo Alto, California

Professional Reviewers

Nancy Daley, Ph.D., L.P.C., C.P.M.
Psychologist
Austin, Texas

Linda Gaul, Ph.D.
Epidemiologist
Texas Department of Health
Austin, Texas

Linda Jones, M.S.P.H.
*Manager of Systems
Development Unit*
Children with Special
Healthcare Needs Division
Texas Department of Health
Austin, Texas

William Joy
President
The Joy Group
Wheaton, Illinois

Edie Leonard, R.D., L.D.
Nutrition Educator
Portland, Oregon

Professional Reviewers
(continued)

JoAnn Cope Powell, Ph.D.
*Learning Specialist
and Licensed Psychologist*
Counseling, Learning and
Career Services
University of Texas
Learning Center
The University of Texas
Austin, Texas

Hal Resides
Safety Manager
Corpus Christi Naval Base
Corpus Christi, Texas

Eric Tiemann, E.M.T.
Emergency Medical Services
Hazardous Waste Division
Travis County Emergency
Medical Services
Austin, Texas

Lynne E. Whitt
Director
National Center for Health
Education
New York, New York

Academic Reviewers

Nigel Atkinson, Ph.D.
*Associate Professor of
Neurobiology*
Institute For Neuroscience
Institute for Cellular and
Molecular Biology
Waggoner Center for Alcohol
and Addiction Research
The University of Texas
Austin, Texas

John Caprio, Ph.D.
George C. Kent Professor
Department of Biological
Sciences
Louisiana State University
Baton Rouge, Louisiana

Joe Crim, Ph.D.
*Professor and Head, Biological
Sciences Department*
University of Georgia
Athens, Georgia

Susan B. Dickey, Ph.D., R.N.
*Associate Professor, Pediatric
Nursing*
College of Allied Health
Professionals
Temple University
Philadelphia, Pennsylvania

Stephen Dion
Associate Professor
Sport Fitness
Salem College
Salem, Massachusetts

Ronald Feldman, Ph.D.
*Ruth Harris Ottman Centennial
Professor for the
Advancement
of Social Work Education*
*Director, Center for the
Study of Social Work Practice*
Columbia University
New York, New York

William Guggino, Ph.D.
Professor of Physiology
The Johns Hopkins University
School of Medicine
Baltimore, Maryland

**Kathryn Hilgenkamp, Ed.D.,
C.H.E.S.**
*Assistant Professor, Community
Health and Nutrition*
University of Northern
Colorado
Greeley, Colorado

Cynthia Kuhn, Ph.D.
*Professor of Pharmacology and
Cancer Biology*
Duke University Medical Center
Duke University
Durham, North Carolina

**John B. Lowe, M.P.H., Dr. P.H.,
F.A.H.P.A.**
Professor and Head
Department of Community and
Behavioral Health
College of Public Health
The University of Iowa
Iowa City, Iowa

**Leslie Mayrand, Ph.D., R.N.,
C.N.S.**
Professor of Nursing
Pediatrics and Adolescent
Medicine
Angelo State University
San Angelo, Texas

Karen E. McConnell, Ph.D.
Assistant Professor
School of Physical Education
Pacific Lutheran University
Tacoma, Washington

Clyde B. McCoy, Ph.D.
Professor and Chair
Department of Epidemiology
and Public Health
University of Miami School of
Medicine
Miami, Florida

Hal Pickett, Psy.D.
*Assistant Professor of
Psychiatry*
Department of Psychiatry
University of Minnesota
Medical School
Minneapolis, Minnesota

Philip Posner, Ph.D.
*Professor and Scholar in
Physiology*
College of Medicine
Florida State University
Tallahassee, Florida

John Rohwer, Ph.D.
Professor
Department of Health Sciences
Bethel College
St. Paul, Minnesota

Susan R. Schmidt, Ph.D.
Postdoctoral Psychology Fellow
Center on Child Abuse and
Neglect
The University of Oklahoma
Health Sciences Center
Oklahoma City, Oklahoma

**Stephen B. Springer, Ed.D.,
L.P.C., C.P.M.**
*Director of Occupational
Education*
Southwest Texas State
University
San Marcos, Texas

Richard Storey, Ph.D.
Professor of Biology
Colorado College
Colorado Springs, Colorado

Acknowledgments continued on page 455.

Contents
in Brief

Chapters

Contents

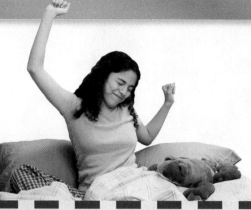

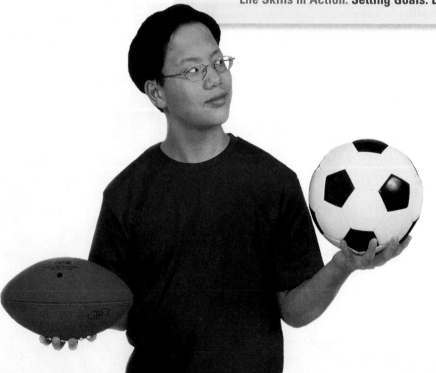

Myth & Fact

Myth: You get lung cancer only if you smoke.

Fact: Go to page 9 to get the facts.

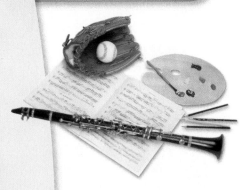

CHAPTER 2 Successful Decisions and Goals 20

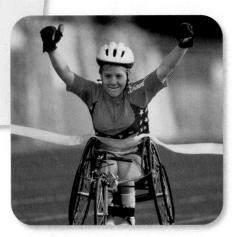

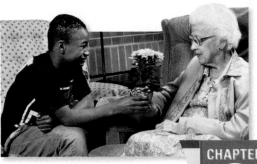

CHAPTER 3 Building Self-Esteem 48

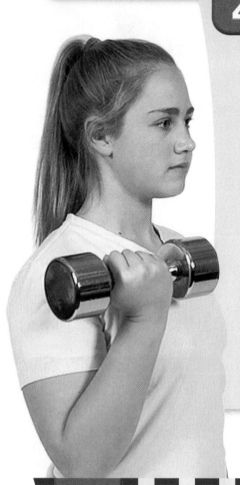

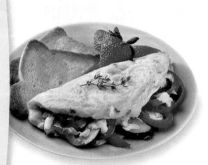

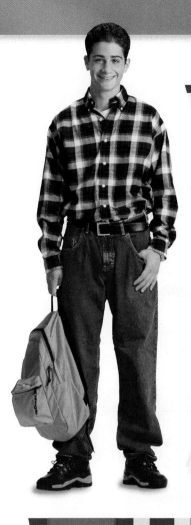

Myth & Fact

Myth: A person can tell if he or she is going to like or dislike another person the first time they meet.

Fact: Go to page 136 to get the facts.

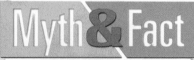

Myth: All stress is bad.

Fact: Go to page 159 to get the facts.

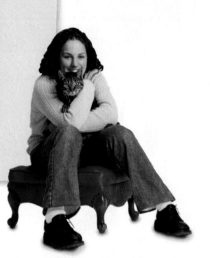

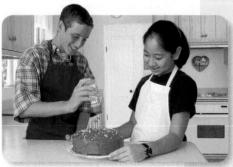

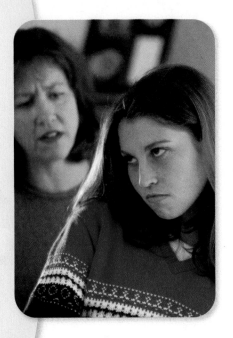

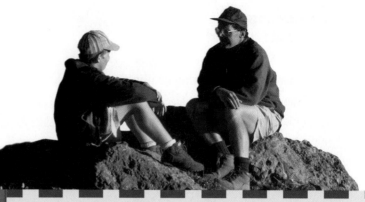

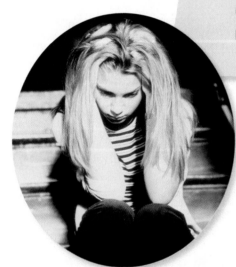

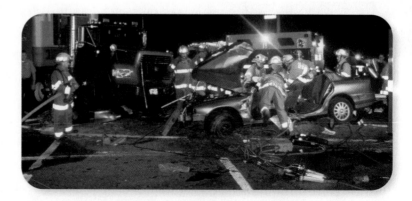

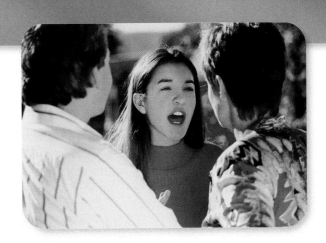

Myth & Fact

Myth: Using tobacco in the form of chewing tobacco or snuff is much safer than smoking.

Fact: Go to page 272 to get the facts.

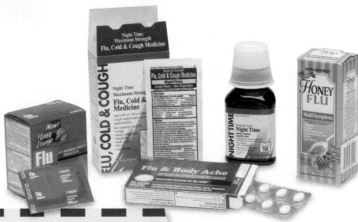

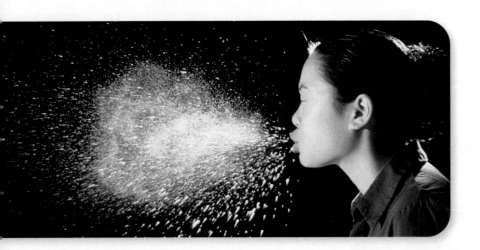
Myth & Fact

Myth: You catch a cold when you are out in cold or wet weather.

Fact: Go to page 307 to get the facts.

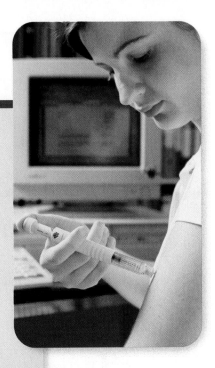

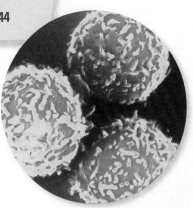

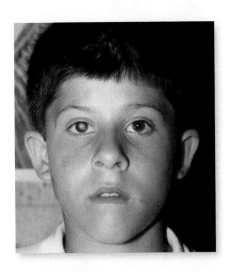

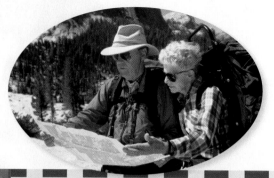

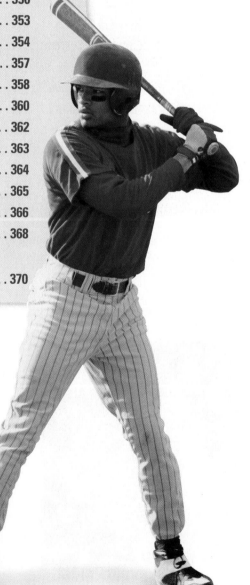

Myth & Fact

Myth: Ovulation always happens on the fourteenth day of the menstrual cycle.

Fact: Go to page 355 to get the facts.

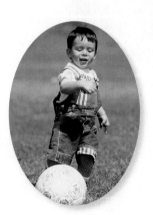

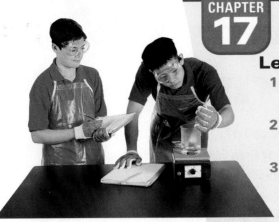

Myth & Fact

Myth: You should slap a choking person on the back.

Fact: Go to page 395 to get the facts.

Appendix

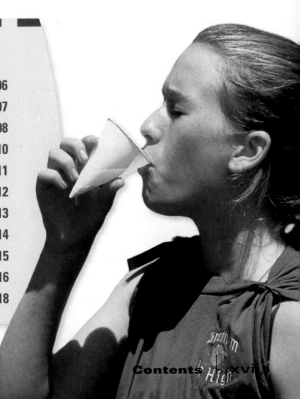

Activities

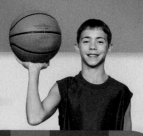

Hands-on ACTIVITY

LIFE SKILLS ACTIVITY

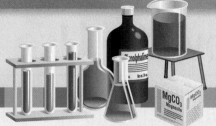

CROSS-DISCIPLINE ACTIVITY

Life Skills IN ACTION

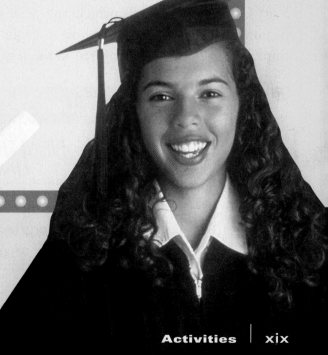

How to Use Your Textbook

Your Roadmap for Success with *Decisions for Health*

Read the Objectives

The objectives, which are listed under the **What You'll Do** head, tell you what you'll need to know.

STUDY TIP Reread the objectives when studying for a test to be sure you know the material.

Study the Key Terms

Key Terms are listed for each lesson under the **Terms to Learn** head. Learn the definitions of these terms because you will most likely be tested on them. Use the glossary to locate definitions quickly.

STUDY TIP If you don't understand a definition, reread the page where the term is introduced. The surrounding text should help make the definition easier to understand.

Start Off Write

Start Off Write questions, which appear at the beginning of each lesson, help you to begin thinking about the topic covered in the lesson.

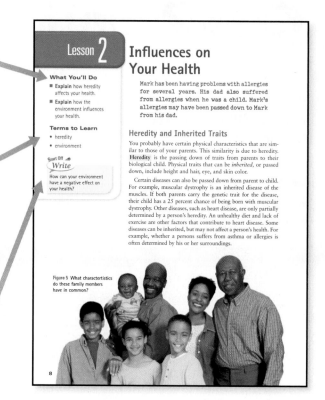

Take Notes and Get Organized

Keep a health notebook so that you are ready to take notes when your teacher reviews the material in class. Keep your assignments in this notebook so that you can review them when studying for the chapter test.

Be Resourceful, Use the Web

Internet Connect boxes in your textbook take you to resources that you can use for health projects, reports, and research papers. Go to **scilinks.org/health** and type in the HealthLinks code to get information on a topic.

HEALTH LINKSsm
Maintained by the National Science Teachers Association

Visit **go.hrw.com**
Find worksheets, *Current Health* magazine articles online, and other materials that go with your textbook at **go.hrw.com.** Click on the textbook icon and the table of contents to see all of the resources for each chapter.

go.hrw.com

Use the Illustrations and Photos

Art shows complex ideas and processes. Learn to analyze the art so that you better understand the material you read in the text.

Tables and graphs display important information in an organized way to help you see relationships.

A picture is worth a thousand words. Look at the photographs to see relevant examples of health concepts you are reading about.

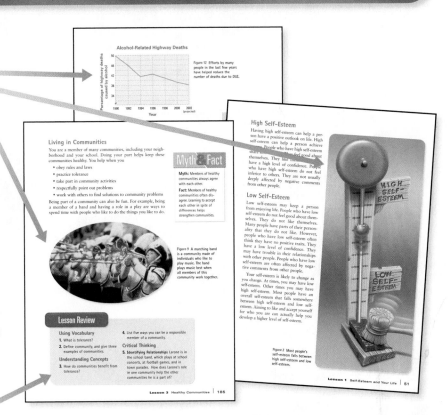

Answer the Lesson Reviews

Lesson Reviews test your knowledge over the main points of the lesson. Critical Thinking items challenge you to think about the material in greater depth and to find connections that you infer from the text.

STUDY TIP When you can't answer a question, reread the lesson. The answer is usually there.

Do Your Homework

Your teacher will assign Study Guide worksheets to help you understand and remember the material in the chapter.

STUDY TIP Answering the items in the Chapter Review will prepare you for the chapter test. Don't try to answer the questions without reading the text and reviewing your class notes. A little preparation up front will make your homework assignments a lot easier.

Visit Holt Online Learning
If your teacher gives you a special password to log onto the **Holt Online Learning** site, you'll find your complete textbook on the Web. In addition, you'll find some great learning tools and practice quizzes. You'll be able to see how well you know the material from your textbook.

Holt Online Learning
For more information go to:
www.hrw.com

Visit CNN Student News®
You'll find up-to-date events in science at **cnnstudentnews.com**.

Health and Wellness

Check out
Current Health
articles related to this chapter by
visiting go.hrw.com. Just type in
the keyword **HD4CH16**.

“ I belong to a lot of **school** groups, and I'm making pretty good **grades**. I have a lot of **friends**, too. I really like where I am **in my life** right now. **”**

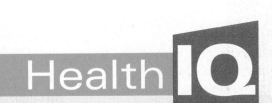

PRE-READING

Answer the following multiple-choice questions to find out what you already know about health and wellness. When you've finished this chapter, you'll have the opportunity to change your answers based on what you've learned.

1. **Which of the following characteristics is NOT hereditary?**
   a. the tendency to get certain diseases or conditions
   b. height
   c. eye color
   d. taste in music

2. **Brushing and flossing your teeth regularly is an example of**
   a. a healthy lifestyle.
   b. preventive healthcare.
   c. good hygiene.
   d. All of the above

3. **Which of the following behaviors is an example of good hygiene?**
   a. eating a balanced diet
   b. avoiding harmful substances
   c. washing your hands
   d. getting plenty of exercise

4. **Your social health is made up of all of the following EXCEPT**
   a. being a team player.
   b. exercising.
   c. sharing your true feelings with your friends.
   d. being considerate of others.

5. **Telling someone that you do not want to do something is an example of**
   a. using refusal skills.
   b. practicing wellness.
   c. coping.
   d. making good decisions.

6. **Being able to express yourself clearly to avoid misunderstandings describes which of the following skills?**
   a. communicating effectively
   b. practicing wellness
   c. coping
   d. emotional health

ANSWERS: 1. d; 2. d; 3. c; 4. b; 5. a; 6. a

Being Healthy and Well

Mary and Chris have been helping to plan the seventh-grade dance. They have been juggling these duties with their schoolwork and responsibilities at home. Now both girls are feeling tense and tired. And they miss seeing their other friends.

What You'll Do

- **Identify** the four parts of health.
- **Explain** the difference between health and wellness.

Terms to Learn

- health
- wellness

Start Off
Write

Write down three things that you can do daily to improve your physical health.

Mary and Chris have a lot going on in their lives. The stress of their many activities is affecting their overall health. **Health** is the condition of physical, emotional, mental, and social well-being. To be healthy, you need to balance your physical, emotional, mental, and social health. In this lesson, you will learn ways that you can maintain each part of your health to stay healthy.

Physical Health

The part of health that deals with the body is *physical health*. The following are habits you should practice to have good physical health:

- Eat a balanced diet.
- Participate in plenty of physical activities.
- Get 8 hours of sleep every night.
- Avoid drugs, alcohol, and tobacco.
- Practice safety by wearing protective sports gear and selt belts whenever you are in a moving vehicle.
- Practice good hygiene. *Hygiene* is the practice of keeping clean to prevent the spread of disease.
- Visit your doctor and dentist regularly.

Remember that today's choices will affect your physical health for years to come. And the choices you make now are going to be tomorrow's habits. So, make them good habits!

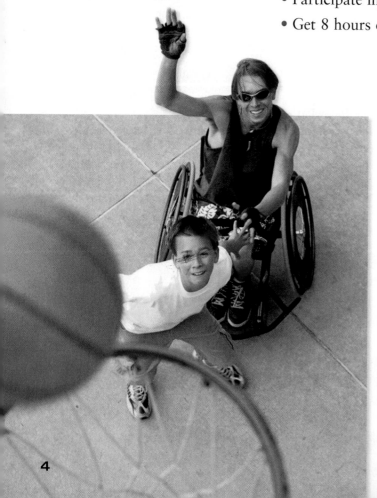

Figure 1 Playing sports is not only fun, but it is a good way to keep yourself physically fit.

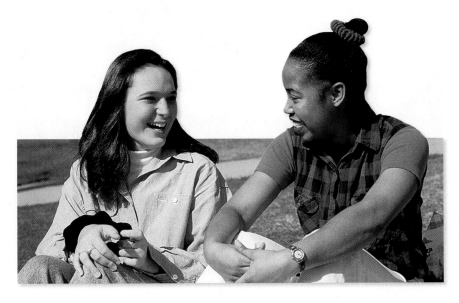

Figure 2 It's great to have friends you can talk to about your problems.

Emotional Health

Your emotional health can affect how you feel about yourself and how you treat other people. *Emotional health* is the way you recognize and deal with your feelings. An emotionally healthy person has the ability to

- express emotions in calm and healthy ways
- deal with sadness and get help for depression
- accept his or her strengths and weaknesses

During adolescence, you experience some major life changes. Your body is changing and you also have more responsibilities both at home and at school. As a result, you may become more emotional than you once were. Although having emotional ups and downs isn't pleasant, this experience is a normal part of growing up. Talk to your parents if you have concerns about controlling your emotions or if you are worried about being depressed.

Mental Health

Being able to easily adjust to change is a sign of good mental health. *Mental health* is the way that you cope with the demands of daily life. Having good mental health means that you can

- solve problems with little trouble
- deal with stress effectively
- accept new ideas

Your mental health can be affected by many of the same things that affect your physical health. For example, lack of sleep hurts your mental alertness and your ability to deal with stress. Good judgment comes more easily after a good night's sleep.

Health Journal

Write a few lines in your Health Journal about a time when one of your friends helped you work through a difficult problem.

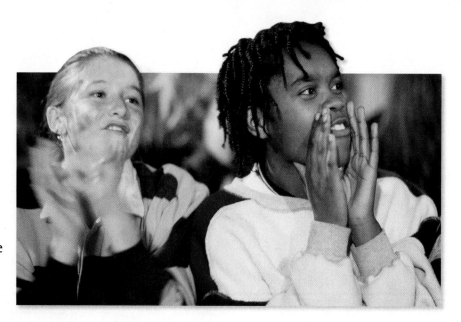

Figure 3 Spending time with your friends is important for your social health.

Social Health

Good social skills help you get along better with people. The way you interact with other people describes your *social health*. You can build good social skills in the following ways:

- Be considerate of other people. Treat others the way that you would like to be treated.
- Show respect for other people.
- Share your true feelings with your friends.
- Be dependable.
- Volunteer to do things for your community.
- Be supportive of your friends when they make the right choice.

Having friends and being close to your family give you a sense of belonging. You know that these people care about you. And when you know that your friends and family care about you and want the best for you, you feel even better about yourself. As a result, you want to be a better person and do things for your friends and family.

LIFE SKILLS ACTIVITY

MAKING GOOD DECISIONS

A new student has joined your class. Some of the popular students in the class are making fun of her when the teacher's back is turned. What will you do? Will you join these students so you can be part of their crowd? If not, what are some things that you could do to let these students know that you don't approve of their actions? How do you think you would feel if you were this new student?

Wellness

Your overall wellness is affected by each of the four parts of your health. **Wellness** is a state of good health that is achieved by balancing your physical, emotional, mental, and social health. For example, if you are physically, emotionally, and mentally healthy but have ignored the social part of your health, you can't achieve total wellness.

If you are not sure of your level of wellness, take a health assessment. A *health assessment* is a set of questions that rates your overall health. The following are examples of questions that you should ask yourself:

- Do I get at least 8 hours of sleep each night?

- Do I eat balanced meals?

- Is talking openly with my friends an important part of my day?

- Do I have a trusted adult, such as a parent, who is a main source of support for me?

- Do I deal well with stress?

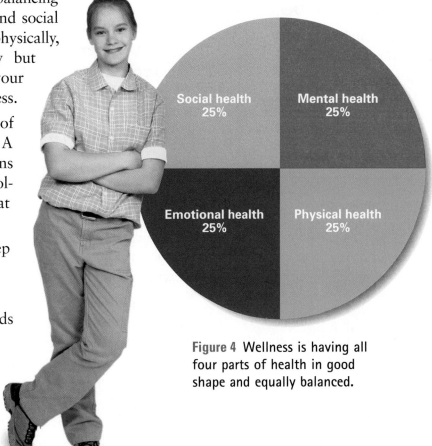

Figure 4 Wellness is having all four parts of health in good shape and equally balanced.

Lesson Review

Using Vocabulary

1. Distinguish between health and wellness.

Understanding Concepts

2. Identify the four parts of health. Write a sentence describing each part.

3. Explain why you must balance all four parts of health to achieve wellness.

4. Why is hygiene important for good physical health?

5. Explain what a health assessment is and how it can help you rate your overall health.

Critical Thinking

6. Analyzing Ideas Your friend is sad because she thinks none of her friends care about her. What part of her health is out of balance? Explain.

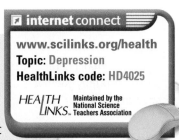

internet connect

www.scilinks.org/health
Topic: Depression
HealthLinks code: HD4025

HEALTH
LINKS. Maintained by the National Science Teachers Association

Influences on Your Health

Mark has been having problems with allergies for several years. His dad also suffered from allergies when he was a child. Mark's allergies may have been passed down to Mark from his dad.

What You'll Do

- **Explain** how heredity affects your health.
- **Explain** how the environment influences your health.

Terms to Learn

- heredity
- environment

Start Off *Write*

How can your environment have a negative effect on your health?

Heredity and Inherited Traits

You probably have certain physical characteristics that are similar to those of your parents. This similarity is due to heredity. **Heredity** is the passing down of traits from parents to their biological child. Physical traits that can be *inherited,* or passed down, include height and hair, eye, and skin color.

Certain diseases can also be passed down from parent to child. For example, muscular dystrophy is an inherited disease of the muscles. If both parents carry the genetic trait for the disease, their child has a 25 percent chance of being born with muscular dystrophy. Other diseases, such as heart disease, are only partially determined by a person's heredity. An unhealthy diet and lack of exercise are other factors that contribute to heart disease. Some diseases can be inherited, but may not always affect a person's health. For example, whether a persons suffers from asthma or allergies is often determined by his or her surroundings.

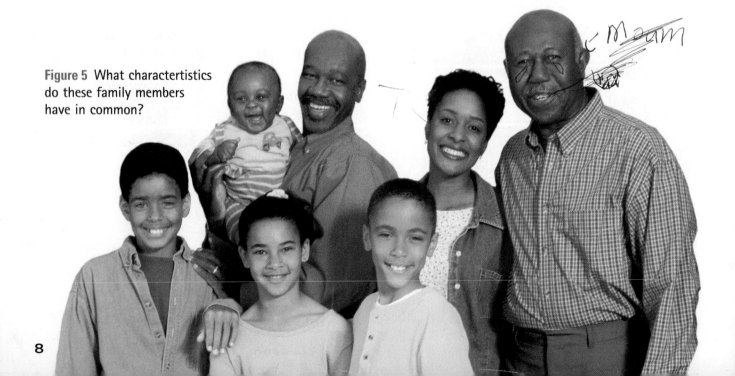

Figure 5 What charactertistics do these family members have in common?

(handwritten in margin: I hate my Life From At the Tits)

Your Environment

Some disease can be triggered by your environment. Your **environment** includes all of the living and nonliving things around you. Asthma attacks are one such example of the way in which the environment can affect your health. Environmental factors that may bring on an asthma attack include things such as air pollution, tobacco smoke, and pollen. Emotional stress has also been known to trigger asthma attacks.

Your environment can affect more than just your physical health. For example, your emotional and mental health can suffer from noise pollution around your home or school. Loud or constant noise disturbs your ability to concentrate, thereby causing you stress. Your emotional health can even be affected by the amount of daylight you receive. Seasonal affective disorder, or SAD, causes depression in some people if they do not get enough sunlight. Most of the time, people suffer from SAD during the winter months, when there are fewer daylight hours. SAD is treated by having the patient sit in front of a light box for a certain period of time.

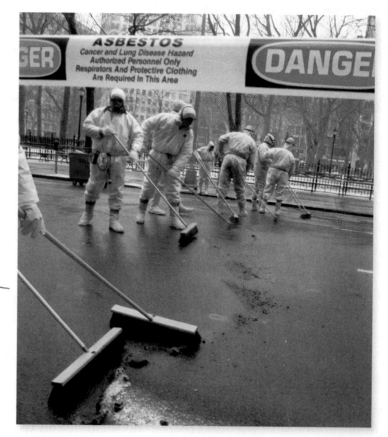

Figure 6 Years ago, asbestos was used as fireproof insulation in buildings. Today, we know that asbestos is an environmental hazard because it damages your lungs.

Myth & Fact

Myth: You get lung cancer only if you smoke.

Fact: It is possible to get lung cancer from second-hand smoke as well as other kinds of air pollutants.

Lesson Review

Using Vocabulary

1. Define the term *heredity*.

Understanding Concepts

2. Explain how heredity influences your health.

3. What are ways that the environment can affect your health?

Critical Thinking

4. Making Inferences What can you do to reduce health hazards such as air and water pollution?

5. Identifying Relationships Poor air quality is an environmental factor that can trigger asthma attacks. What kind of environment would be healthy for a person with asthma? Explain your answer.

internet connect
www.scilinks.org/health
Topic: Genes and Traits

HealthLinks code: HD4045

HEALTH LINKS Maintained by the National Science Teachers Association

Making Good Health Choices

What You'll Do

■ **Describe** the relationship between your lifestyle and your health.

■ **Identify** four things that you can do to have a healthy lifestyle.

■ **Explain** how your attitude affects your health.

■ **Explain** what you can do to take responsibility for your healthcare.

Terms to Learn

• lifestyle

• attitude

• preventive healthcare

Start Off
Write

Describe ways that you can have a healthier lifestyle.

Taitia was entering a new school and decided that this was a good time to make some changes. Taitia wanted to learn how to make better choices about things that influence her health and life.

At some point, you may decide to make some major changes in your life just as Taitia did. In this lesson, you'll learn how you can take responsibility for your health by making good choices.

Living Healthily

Every day, you make choices that influence your health. For example, you choose what to eat for lunch, when to study, what to do for fun, and whom to have as your friends. These choices determine your lifestyle. A **lifestyle** is a set of behaviors that you live by. To maintain a healthy lifestyle, you will want to develop a good attitude about your health. Your **attitude** is a way of acting, thinking, or feeling that causes you to make one choice over another. A good attitude will allow you to listen to advice about healthy living. It will also help you avoid things that will harm you, such as tobacco, alcohol, and drugs. A good attitude puts you in charge of your health.

Taking Control of Your Health

How can you take charge of your health? Like Taitia, you must first decide to improve your lifestyle. Next, you should decide which part of health you want to work on. For example, you may want to focus on your physical health by starting an exercise routine. But don't forget your emotional, mental, and social health, too. If you are not exactly sure how to improve a certain part of your health, talk to your parents or another trusted adult.

Figure 7 Choosing which sport to play is a decision that you can make to improve your physical health.

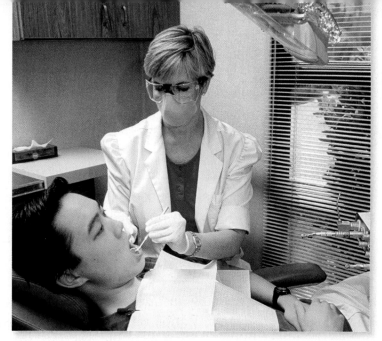

Figure 8 Having a dental exam every year is a good way to find and fill cavities before they get very large.

Healthcare and Personal Responsibility

What responsibilities do you have? You may answer that you are responsible for cleaning your room and feeding your dog. But what is your responsibility for your healthcare. How often do you

- brush and floss your teeth?
- eat healthy food, exercise, and sleep for 8 hours every night?
- wear safety equipment when you play sports?
- buckle your seat belt?
- avoid behavior that will get you in trouble?

If you do these things regularly, you are being responsible for your health by practicing preventive healthcare. **Preventive healthcare** is taking steps to help prevent illness and accidents. These steps include regular visits to your doctors and dentist as well as regular vaccinations. Finding health problems early can prevent serious illness.

LIFE SKILLS ACTIVITY

ASSESSING YOUR HEALTH

Work in a group so that you can share ideas. Draw two columns on a piece of paper. In the first column, write the ways that you already practice preventive healthcare. In the other column, write things that you could start doing to prevent illness or accidents.

internet connect

www.scilinks.org/health
Topic: Physical Fitness

HealthLinks code: HD4076

HEALTH LINKS. Maintained by the National Science Teachers Association

Lesson Review

Using Vocabulary

1. Define the term *lifestyle*.

2. Identify three ways to practice preventive healthcare.

Understanding Concepts

3. List four health choices that you make every day.

4. How does your attitude influence the decisions that you make about your health?

Critical Thinking

5. Identifying Relationships How can breaking bad habits improve your lifestyle?

Nine Life Skills for Better Health

What You'll Do

- **Identify** the nine life skills that can improve your life and health.
- **Describe** how practicing the life skills can help you master them.
- **Explain** how you can assess your progress in learning the life skills.
- **Describe** why the life skills should be a part of your daily life.

Terms to Learn

- life skills

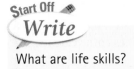

Start Off Write

What are life skills?

Stephanie and her sister, Shannon, are always arguing about things that seem unimportant. They both want to get along better with each other, but they are not sure what to do to improve their relationship.

Stephanie and Shannon probably just need to learn how to communicate better. Good communication is one of the nine life skills you will learn about in this lesson. **Life skills** are skills that will help you deal with the many kinds of situations that you will face throughout your life.

The Nine Life Skills

Using life skills can help you maintain a healthy lifestyle. They can help you solve both simple problems and more complicated health problems. Table 1, on the next page, lists and briefly explains each life skill. As you read through this textbook, you will become more familiar with these life skills. In each chapter, you will have several opportunities to practice using the life skills.

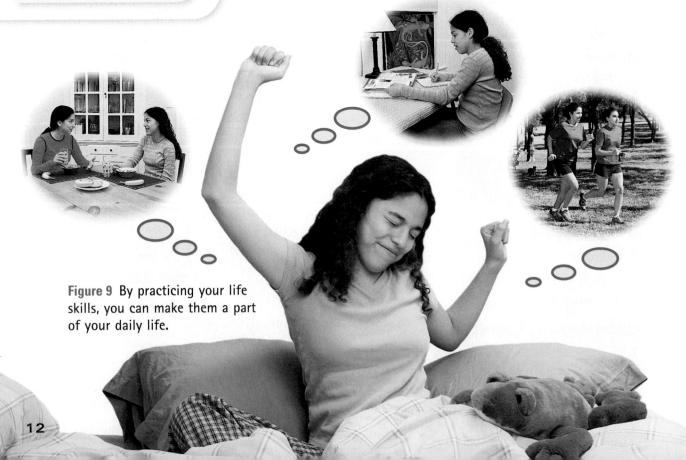

Figure 9 By practicing your life skills, you can make them a part of your daily life.

TABLE 1 The Nine Life Skills

Life skill	Definition
Assessing your health	evaluating each of the four parts of your health and assessing your health behaviors
Making good decisions	making choices that are healthy and responsible
Setting goals	deciding to do things that will give you a sense of accomplishment, such as breaking bad habits and planning your future
Using refusal skills	saying no to things that you don't want to do and avoiding dangerous situations
Communicating effectively	avoiding misunderstandings by expressing your feelings in a healthy way
Coping	dealing with problems and emotions in an effective way
Evaluating media messages	judging the accuracy of advertising and other media messages
Practicing wellness	practicing good habits, such as getting plenty of sleep and eating healthy foods
Being a wise consumer	comparing products and services based on value and quality

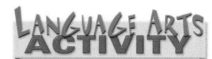

LANGUAGE ARTS ACTIVITY

Select three life skills from the table on this page, and write a story about a student who improved his or her lifestyle by using these three life skills.

Hands-on ACTIVITY

GENERIC VERSUS BRAND-NAME PRODUCTS

1. Your teacher will provide you with at least two items that are the same type of product but different brands. One item will be a generic, or store brand, and the other item will be a brand-name product. You will compare these products.

2. Look at the items' packaging. Note which package is more attractive.

3. Compare the price of each item.

4. Compare the ingredients on the label of each item.

5. With your teacher's permission, test both the generic and brand-name products.

Analysis

1. Make a chart that has two rows. In each of the rows, write the name of one of the items. Make five columns, and title the columns "Packaging," "Price," "Ingredients," "Quality," and "Overall rating."

2. Fill in each column with an analysis of your findings. You may analyze your findings by answering the following questions:

- Would you buy one product instead of the other based on the appearance of the package?
- What is the difference in the prices of the two items?
- Is there a difference in the kinds of ingredients?
- Did you notice any difference in the quality of the products?

3. Summarize your findings by writing a paragraph about whether brand-name products are worth the extra money.

Practice Makes Perfect

You may find that using certain life skills is difficult or awkward at first. But that is true of any new skill that you are trying to learn. Remember that the best way to master any skill is to practice it. Try practicing one of the life skills that you think you may have trouble with. First, think of a situation in which you may need this skill and play out the situation in your mind. For example, what would you do if you said no to a friend but that person wouldn't take no for an answer? Would you stand your ground or give in to your friend? Remember that if you prepare yourself for these kinds of situations, you will have less trouble when you face the real thing. Practice these skills, and you will soon find them easier to use.

Assessing Your Progress

You may already be familiar with some of the life skills, while other life skills may be new to you. But, you will want to assess the progress that you are making in using all of these skills. To assess your progress, ask yourself questions such as the following:

- Which skills do I use most often?
- Which skills do I rarely use but should use more often?
- Are there skills that I don't feel comfortable using?
- Am I having problems with a specific skill?
- How can I improve my use of life skills?

Some skills are more difficult to master than others are. So, spend time practicing the skills that you have trouble with. It may help to role-play a life skill with a friend or family member. And remember that you can always talk to your parents or another trusted adult to get advice on how best to use certain life skills.

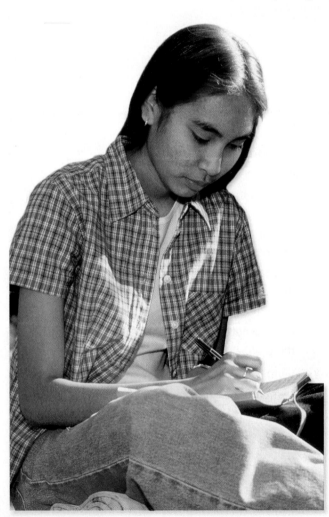

Figure 10 Keep a record of daily events in your life. This record will show you how well you are using the life skills.

Maintaining a Healthy Lifestyle

Life skills will help you make good choices both now and in the future. Remember that you want to maintain the four parts of your health to achieve wellness. The following examples describe ways that you can keep your health balanced:

- Spending quality time with parents and friends can improve your social health.
- Talking openly about problems and expressing yourself in healthy ways can improve your emotional health.
- Opening your mind to new ideas and new ways of doing things can improve your mental health.
- Eating properly, getting rest, and engaging in physical activity regularly can improve your physical health.

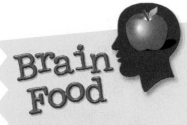

Brain Food

The risk of cancer can be reduced by eating at least five servings of fruits and vegetables every day and by decreasing the fat in your diet.

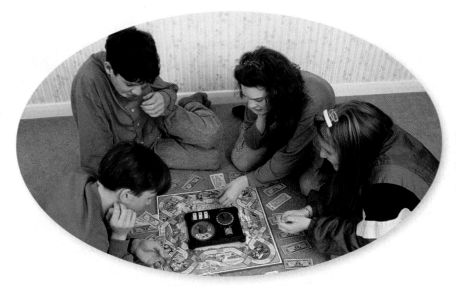

Figure 11 What life skills would you possibly use when playing a game with your friends?

Lesson Review

Using Vocabulary

1. Define the term *life skill*, and briefly describe each life skill.

Understanding Concepts

2. Explain how you can assess your progress in using the life skills.

3. Describe why life skills should be a part of your everyday life.

4. How does practicing the life skills help you master them?

Critical Thinking

5. **Making Inferences** Which life skill would you use in each of the following situations?

- You and your brother argued, and now you aren't talking to each other.
- Two brands of shampoo are advertised as being the best.
- Your friend wants to copy your homework.

Chapter Summary

■ The four parts of your health are physical, emotional, social, and mental health. ■ A balanced diet, exercise, and 8 hours of sleep each night are needed for good physical health. ■ Expressing your feelings in a healthy way is a sign of good emotional health. ■ Having good mental health helps you deal with problems effectively. ■ Getting along well with other people is a sign of good social health. ■ Wellness is having all parts of your health balanced. ■ Your heredity and environment can influence your health. ■ Your lifestyle and attitude affect your health. ■ Life skills help you deal with problems that can affect your health, and these skills should be used in your everyday life.

Using Vocabulary

For each sentence, fill in the blank with the proper word from the word bank provided below.

hygiene	heredity
environment	life skills
preventive healthcare	health
lifestyle	attitude
health assessment	wellness

❶ The passing of traits from a parent to his or her offspring is ___.

❷ Taking care of yourself before you have an accident or get an illness is ___.

❸ The set of behaviors by which you live is your ___.

❹ The ___ is everything around you, including the air.

❺ Someone who is always clean and well groomed is said to have good ___.

❻ Your ___ includes a state of mind that affects the decisions you make.

❼ Your ___ is based on balanced physical, mental, emotional, and social well-being.

Understanding Concepts

❽ Name the four parts of your health.

❾ How does the term *wellness* differ from the term *health*?

❿ What seven things can you do to contribute to good physical health?

⓫ How does heredity influence your health?

⓬ How can the environment affect your health?

⓭ What four choices can you make to ensure a healthy lifestyle?

⓮ What are five things you can do to practice preventive healthcare?

⓯ List the nine life skills.

⓰ What five questions can you ask yourself to assess your life skills?

⓱ What is the relationship between having a good attitude and living a healthy lifestyle?

Critical Thinking

Applying Concepts

18 You've had infectious mononucleosis for a month, and your physical health isn't as good as it should be. Does your poor physical health have any effect on the other parts of your health? Explain your answer.

19 Your friend has learned that her father has an inherited medical condition. She is afraid that she may get it, too. How can your friend become informed about this medical condition? What information could you give her that would help her?

Making Good Decisions

20 Your friend told you that he has not been feeling well and doesn't have the energy to do anything. He said that some of his other friends suggested taking over-the-counter pills that would help him stay awake. Do you think that these pills are safe because they are sold over the counter? What could you say to your friend to help him?

21 Your friend's grandfather died a few months ago. Your friend has been quiet and doesn't want to hang out with anyone anymore. He finally tells you that he feels guilty because during his grandfather's illness, he spent more time with his friends than with his grandfather. What can you tell your friend to help him with his feelings?

22 Your friend has not been making good grades lately. She says that she prefers doing other things to studying. What life skills would you suggest to your friend to improve her grades?

Interpreting Graphics

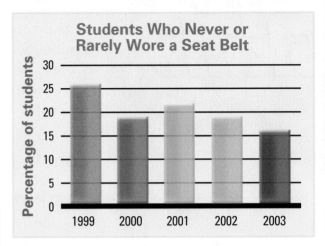

Students Who Never or Rarely Wore a Seat Belt

Use the figure above to answer questions 23–27.

23 What percentage of students never or rarely wore seat belts in 1999? in 2003?

24 According to this graph, what is the trend in the number of students who wear seat belts?

25 What percentage of students never or rarely wore seat belts in 2001?

26 What greater percentage of students wore seat belts in 2003 than in 2001?

27 What is one reason that you can give to explain why students are being more responsible in later years?

Reading Checkup

Take a minute to review your answers to the Health IQ questions at the beginning of this chapter. How has reading this chapter improved your Health IQ?

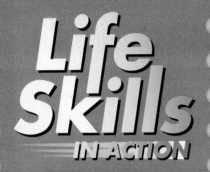

Setting Goals

A goal is something that you work toward and hope to achieve. Setting goals is important because goals give you a sense of purpose and achieving goals improves your self-esteem. Complete the following activity to learn how to set and achieve goals.

Lonely Logan

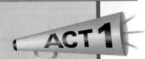

Setting the Scene

Logan's family moved to a new city over the summer. He started 7th grade in his new school a few weeks ago. Since then, Logan has met a lot of people but doesn't feel like he has any friends. Logan's older sister, Amy, isn't having any problems making new friends. Logan doesn't want to feel lonely forever, so he asks Amy for advice.

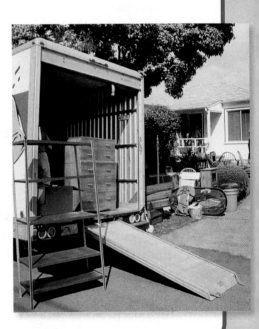

The 5 Steps of Setting Goals

1. Consider your interests and values.
2. Choose goals that include your interests and values.
3. If necessary, break down long-term goals into several short-term goals.
4. Measure your progress.
5. Reward your success.

Guided Practice

Practice with a Friend

Form a group of three. Have one person play the role of Logan and another person play the role of Amy. Have the third person be an observer. Walking through each of the five steps of setting goals, role-play Logan setting and working toward his goal of making new friends. Amy may give him advice and support when necessary. The observer will take notes, which will include observations about what the person playing Logan did well and suggestions of ways to improve. Stop after each step to evaluate the process.

Independent Practice

Check Yourself

After you have completed the guided practice, go through Act 1 again without stopping at each step. Answer the questions below to review what you did.

1. What interests and values could Logan consider before setting his goal?

2. Logan's long-term goal is to make new friends. What short-term goals could help him to meet his long-term goal?

3. How does Logan's goal relate to the four parts of his health?

4. What is one of your long-term goals? On which part of your health does your goal focus?

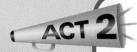

On Your Own

After several weeks, Logan has made many new friends. Two of his friends are reporters for the school newspaper. Logan thinks it would be fun to be a reporter and knows that working on the newspaper will allow him to spend more time with his friends. His friends tell him that he has to apply for a position as a reporter and write a sample newspaper article. Make a poster that shows how Logan could use the five steps of setting goals to work toward his goal of being a reporter.

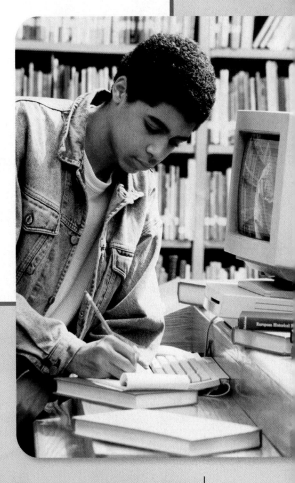

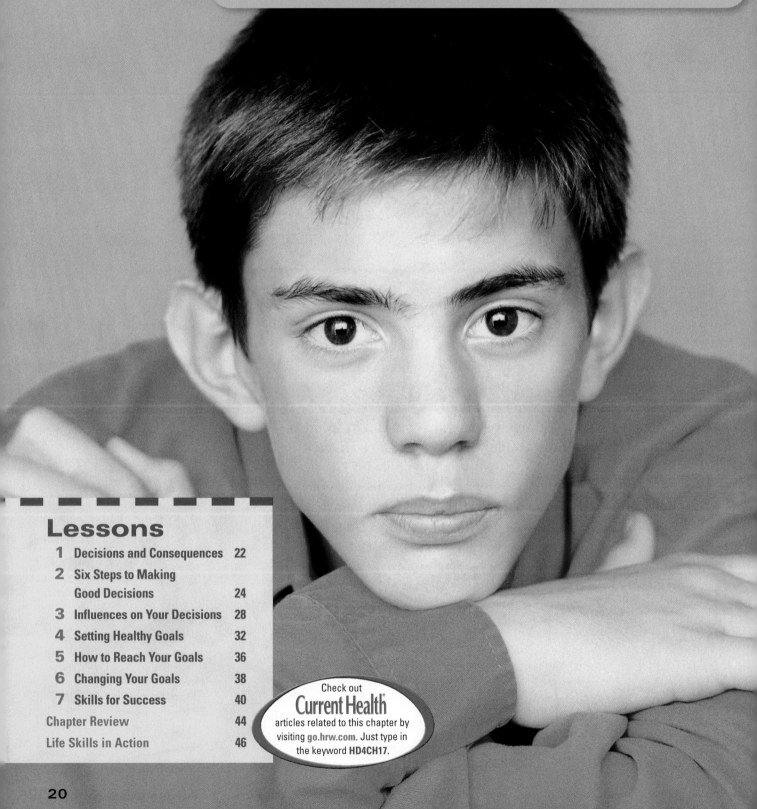

CHAPTER 2

Successful Decisions and Goals

Check out
Current Health®
articles related to this chapter by
visiting **go.hrw.com**. Just type in
the keyword **HD4CH17**.

"My friends kept **bugging** me to go to this **party.** I didn't know **anyone** that was going to be there, so I **didn't want to go.**

But my friends just kept pushing me. Finally, I had to put my foot down and tell them to quit bothering me. I must have gotten through to them, because after that they left me alone.**"**

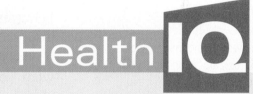

PRE-READING

Answer the following multiple-choice questions to find out what you already know about making decisions. When you've finished this chapter, you'll have the opportunity to change your answers based on what you've learned.

1. Which of the following is an example of peer pressure?

a. You have power over your actions.

b. An adult has power over your actions.

c. Your friend has power over your actions.

d. The media has power over your actions.

2. Choose the correct statement about values.

a. Values are beliefs that are important to you.

b. Values change as goals change.

c. Values change depending on your situation.

d. Values are the beliefs you get from your friends.

3. Which of the following statements about interests is true?

a. Interests never change.

b. Interests change easily.

c. Interests are steps to reaching your goal.

d. Interests always lead to a career.

4. Success can best be defined by

a. making good decisions.

b. defining your values.

c. becoming famous.

d. reaching your goals.

5. What may cause you to change your action plan?

a. a change in interests

b. a change in goals

c. a setback

d. all of the above

6. When you make a good decision, you

a. do what other people tell you to do.

b. make a lot of money.

c. carefully consider your options.

d. make others happy.

ANSWERS: 1. c; 2. a; 3. b; 4. d; 5. d; 6. c

Decisions and Consequences

What You'll Do

- **Explain** how a good decision is a responsible decision.
- **Explain** the different types of consequences that decisions have.

Terms to Learn

- good decision
- consequence

Start Off *Write*

What was the consequence of the last decision that you made?

What are three decisions you've made since you woke up this morning? You make decisions every day, from what clothes to wear to what lunch to eat. You control what happens to you. And each day is shaped by your decisions.

Most teenagers think they don't have much control over their life. But you probably have more control than you realize! In this lesson, you'll learn more about what you can control and how your decisions affect you.

You Are in Control

Being in control means that you can make your own choices. You make choices every day. You don't have to do what your friends tell you to do. You make choices about how you will act, what you will do, and who your friends are. A *decision* is a choice that you make and act upon. But how do you know if you are making a good decision? A **good decision** is a decision in which you have carefully considered the outcome of each choice. A good decision is a responsible decision. To be responsible, you must think through each decision to select the best choice possible. A responsible person knows right from wrong and makes wise choices.

Figure 1 Even decisions about what to do on a Friday night can be difficult to make.

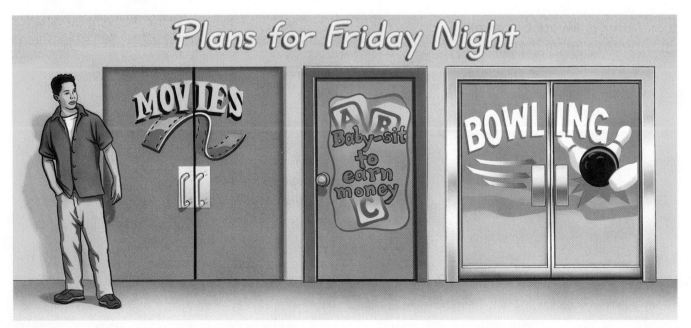

Your Decisions Have Consequences

Whenever you make a decision, something happens. For example, if you decide to turn on a light, the room you are in fills with light. Your decision to turn on a light had a consequence. A **consequence** is the result of a decision. Every decision has consequences. Even a decision to do nothing has consequences. For example, if it's time to sign up for electives at school and you do nothing, what happens? You won't get the classes you want, and you may have to take a class you don't want to take.

Consequences of your decisions not only affect you but also affect the people around you. There are three types of consequences:

- *Positive consequences* help you or others.
- *Negative consequences* do harm to you or to others.
- *Neutral consequences* are neither helpful nor harmful.

What consequences occur if a player on the soccer team shown in Figure 2 decides to quit? A positive consequence is that the player will have more free time. A negative consequence is that the team will lose an experienced player. The player's decision affects her and the people around her.

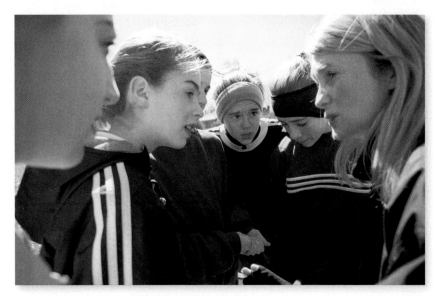

Figure 2 If a player quits, the entire team will suffer the consequences!

Lesson Review

Using Vocabulary

1. Use an example to explain what a good decision is.

2. What is a consequence?

Understanding Concepts

3. What is the difference between positive, negative, and neutral consequences?

4. How does a responsible person make good decisions?

Critical Thinking

5. Making Predictions What consequences would your decision to join the track team have for your family? for your friends?

Six Steps to Making Good Decisions

Emma really isn't sure what to do. Elizabeth, her friend, asked her to go to the movies on the same night that Bobby asked her to his party. She doesn't want to hurt anyone's feelings. How can she decide what to do?

Whether you're choosing what you will do Friday night or what career you want to have someday, making decisions is tough! In this lesson, you'll learn six steps that you can follow to make good decisions. You'll see how your values influence your choices. You will also learn how to make the best choices possible.

Identify the Problem

The first step in making a decision is to identify the problem. For example, what would you do if your friends dared you to cut class with them? At first, you may think that the problem is taking the dare. You might take the dare just because they asked you to. However, the real problem is to decide if missing class is okay. If you thought about that problem, your decision might be very different. Problems can be hard to identify. Asking a parent or trusted friend for advice may help you.

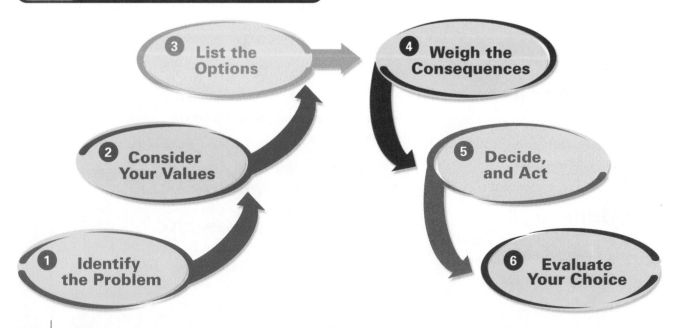

Figure 3 Steps to Making Good Decisions

3 List the Options
4 Weigh the Consequences
2 Consider Your Values
5 Decide, and Act
1 Identify the Problem
6 Evaluate Your Choice

Consider Your Values

Knowing your values will help you make good decisions. **Values** are the beliefs that you consider to be of great importance. Some good values are honesty, kindness, and generosity. It's important to know your values before you face problems. Your values influence your decisions by guiding you when problems arise. For example, if you value being responsible, you won't skip class. How do you determine your values? Think about what kind of person you want to be. In other words, think about your character. *Character* is the way a person thinks, feels, and acts. Your character is a reflection of your values. Character based on good values will help you make good decisions.

List the Options

After you consider your values, the next step is to list your options. **Options** are different choices that you can make. The best way to identify your options is by brainstorming with several other people. **Brainstorming** is thinking of all the possible ways to carry out your decision. If possible, you should write down your ideas. A written list will allow you to quickly compare your options. For example, when you are deciding if you will cut class, one option is to tell your friends no. A second option is to agree with your friends' idea and cut class together. Another possibility is to suggest that you all go to class but do something fun after school. There is always more than one option for you to choose from.

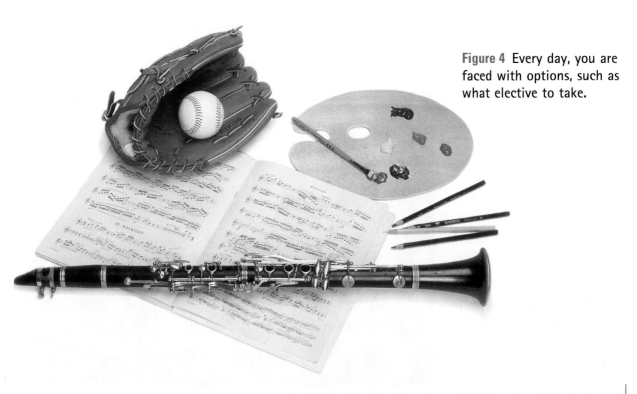

Figure 4 Every day, you are faced with options, such as what elective to take.

Weigh the Consequences

When you weigh the consequences of a possible decision, you compare the benefits and risks of your options. Every option will have risks and benefits to consider. Start by making two columns. Label one column "Benefits" and the other column "Risks." Consider the example of cutting class again. One benefit of deciding to skip class is that your friends wouldn't be angry with you. Another benefit is not having to sit through your least favorite class. But what are the risks? First, cutting class would get you in serious trouble with the school. Second, you would miss the lesson and get behind, which could cause your grade to suffer. Another, more serious risk is that your parents might lose trust in you. Now, look at your list. Do the benefits outweigh the risks? Whenever you have to make a decision, weigh the benefits and risks of each option very carefully. Doing so will help you make good decisions.

Decide, and Act

You have done your best to think about your options. Now you are ready to act on your decision. Think hard. Some decisions can be made only once. When you make your choice, take action! For example, you decide that getting in trouble with your parents and the school is not worth cutting class. In this case, the risks of cutting class certainly outweigh the benefits. So, you decide to tell your friends that you aren't cutting class with them. When they try to change your mind, you stay firm. You make a decision, and you follow through with it. Making a choice and acting on your decision are important in decision making.

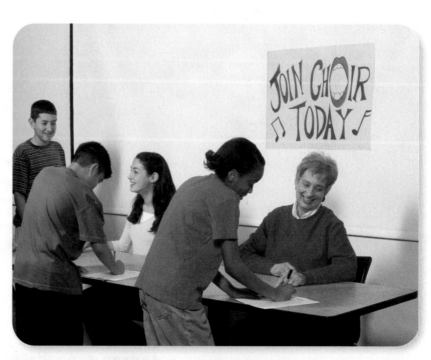

Figure 5 These teens have decided to join choir. By signing up for choir, they are following through with their decision.

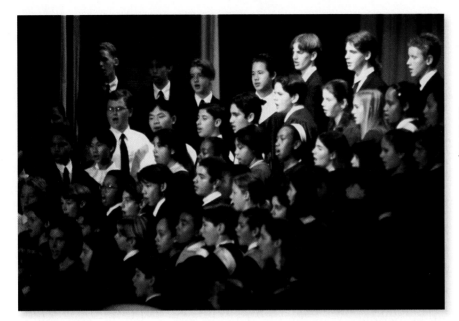

Figure 6 These teens appear happy with their decision to join the choir.

Evaluate Your Choice

You made your decision, and you carried it out. But you aren't finished yet. You may face this problem again, so it is important to look back at your decision. If you answer yes to one or more of the following questions, you may want to choose a different option in the future.

- Did your decision harm anyone?

- Were you unhappy with the result?

- Would another option have had a better consequence?

By evaluating your choices, you learn which options work for you and which don't. Using this procedure takes practice. But the more you use it, the easier it gets!

LIFE SKILLS ACTIVITY

MAKING GOOD DECISIONS

In a small group, think of a situation in which a decision is needed. Write your scenario on a card, and swap cards with another group. In your group, brainstorm ways to solve the problem. Remember to use the six-step method for making decisions. What was your group's decision? Each group will evaluate the other group's decision.

Lesson Review

Using Vocabulary

1. Define the term *values* in your own words. How do your values influence your decisions?

2. What is an option?

3. Explain what you do when you brainstorm.

Understanding Concepts

4. Why should you weigh the risks and benefits of your options?

5. Why is it important to evaluate your choices?

Critical Thinking

6. Making Good Decisions Imagine a situation in which you are having trouble making a decision. Write down each of the six decision-making steps. Then apply each step to the situation that you imagined.

internet connect

www.scilinks.org/health
Topic: Smoking and Health
HealthLinks code: HD4090

HEALTH LINKS. Maintained by the National Science Teachers Association

Influences on Your Decisions

What You'll Do

- **Describe** how family and cultural traditions influence your decisions.
- **Explain** how peer pressure affects the decisions that you make.
- **Identify** the media as a major influence in your decision making.
- **Explain** how your decisions change based on new information.

Terms to Learn

- peer pressure

Start Off Write

Who influences most of your major decisions? Why is this person so influential?

Marcus is trying to decide what CD to buy. His friend is telling him to get the newest rock release. But he really wants to buy a new rap CD. At the same time, he knows that his parents would like him to develop an interest in **classical music**.

Like Marcus's choices, many of your choices are influenced by other people. Your family, friends, other people, and things around you all have an influence on your decisions.

Your Family

Your family is the most important influence in your life. Every family has values, cultural beliefs, and traditions. How often you have to help out at home reflects your family value of responsibility. What your parents say about dating reflects their cultural beliefs. What your family does on holidays reflects your family's traditions. These values, beliefs, and traditions are a part of your character. You are aware of them whenever you make decisions. Therefore, they influence your decisions.

Your family also affects your decisions about your health practices. Decisions you make about how much you exercise, what food you eat, and how you react to stress probably reflect your family's habits.

Figure 7 Your family is one of the biggest influences on your decisions.

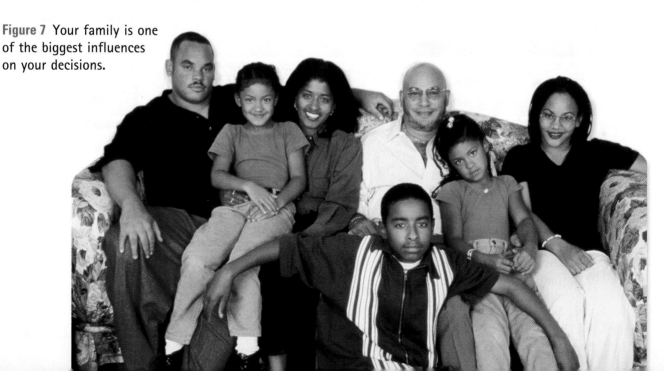

28

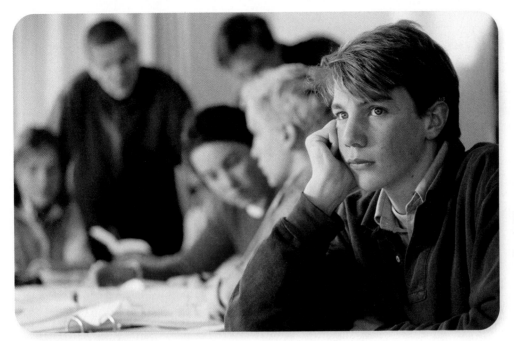

Figure 8 Convincing your friends to ask the new student to join your group is an example of positive peer pressure.

Peer Pressure

Your peers are another important influence in your life. A *peer* is someone who is about the same age as you are and with whom you interact. Sometimes, you get pressure from your peers to do something. This pressure is called peer pressure. **Peer pressure** is a feeling that you should do something that your friends want you to do. Peer pressure can come from one friend or from a group of friends. Groups can have a powerful influence on teens. A group expects certain behaviors from its members. Think about a certain group at your school. Do the members of the group dress alike? Do they enjoy most of the same activities? Peer pressure from a group can be particularly powerful. It is hard to say no to a group of people who are your friends.

Most teens face peer pressure related to drinking alcohol, smoking, cheating, or gossiping. In these situations, your friends may tell you that everyone else is doing these things. By telling you that, your friends put pressure on you to go along with them. But everyone else is probably not doing the things that your friends are suggesting. This kind of peer pressure is negative. *Negative peer pressure* is pressure to do things that could harm you or others. But not all peer pressure is negative. *Positive peer pressure* influences you to do something that will benefit you or someone else. For example, if your friends are studying together for a big math test, you may join in and study, too. This kind of peer pressure makes you feel good about yourself and your friends.

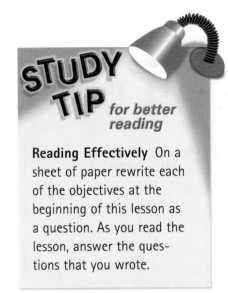

STUDY TIP *for better reading*

Reading Effectively On a sheet of paper rewrite each of the objectives at the beginning of this lesson as a question. As you read the lesson, answer the questions that you wrote.

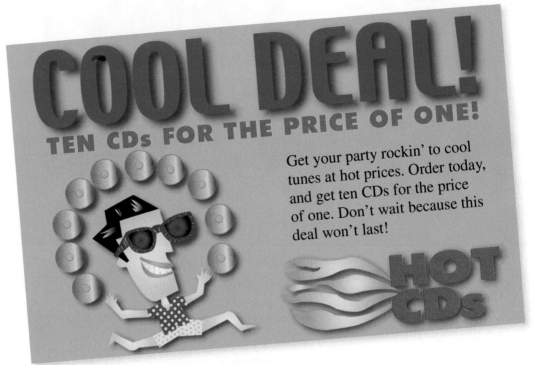

Figure 9 How are you influenced by ads like the one shown above?

Other Influences in Your Life

Your family and friends are not the only influences in your life. Some of the most powerful messages that you hear come from the media. The media includes TV, radio, the Internet, movies, magazines, music, and news reports. The media tells you what is going on in the world. The media gives you messages about what is important, what is good, and what is bad. But not all of the information you receive is correct. Commercials can be an example of misinformation.

Some of the products advertised on TV don't do what advertisers claim. Advertisers want you to identify with their products. So, they try to make you believe that you will become more popular or feel better about yourself if you use the products. But most products won't make you be popular or feel better about yourself. Yet it is hard not to believe the messages, at least a little. You want to believe that you can feel better, have more friends, and change things that you don't like about yourself. As a result, you might decide to buy some of the products after hearing these messages from the media.

Learn the truth about advertising. There are many good sources of information. Seek out accurate information about products. Talk with your parents. You will discover how much the media really influences you.

When Things Change

New information causes people to change their minds and to make new decisions. For example, from the 1950s to the 1970s, cigarette ads on TV made smoking seem cool. The ads influenced many people to start smoking. At that time, nobody knew that smoking was harmful. Scientific studies later showed that cigarettes are dangerous and addictive and can cause lung diseases. Studies also found that smoking affects not only smokers but also the people around the smoking. Some health organizations started to make commercials explaining the dangers of smoking. People started to quit after learning that smoking was a dangerous habit.

When you receive new information, stop and think. First, make sure you can trust the information to be true. Then, think about how the information affects you. You may have to make new decisions based on the information. You also may have to rethink decisions you made in the past. If you do, remember to follow the six steps to making good decisions!

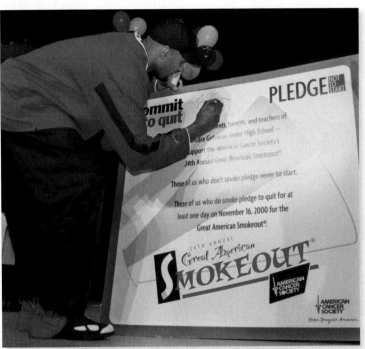

Figure 10 The Great American Smokeout is one of many campaigns against smoking.

Lesson Review

Using Vocabulary

1. What is peer pressure?

Understanding Concepts

2. Describe how your family influences your decisions.

3. Explain how peer pressure affects the decisions that you make.

4. What is the media? How does it influence your choices?

Critical Thinking

5. **Analyzing Ideas** Describe a time when you had to rethink a decision because something changed.

6. **Applying Concepts** You see a commercial that says a product will make you lose weight without dieting or exercising. Should you believe this claim? Explain.

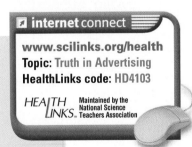

internet connect

www.scilinks.org/health
Topic: Truth in Advertising
HealthLinks code: HD4103

HEALTH LINKS Maintained by the National Science Teachers Association

Setting Healthy Goals

Jim and Parag are good friends and have known each other since they were 4 years old. Jim has always wanted to become a great judge. Parag wants to be a famous surgeon when he grows up.

What You'll Do

■ **Explain** why goals are important.

■ **Identify** two influences on your goals.

■ **Compare** short-term goals and long-term goals.

■ **Describe** how goals can help build healthy relationships.

Terms to Learn

● goal
● self-esteem
● interest

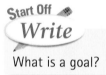

Start Off
Write

What is a goal?

Jim and Parag are good friends. But like most friends, they don't always like the same things. They also have different goals. A **goal** is something that you work toward and hope to achieve. In this lesson, you will learn why goals are important. You will also learn how to set goals.

Why Are Goals Important?

Goals are an important part of growing up. They give you a sense of purpose and direction. As you accomplish your goals, your self-esteem grows. **Self-esteem** is the way you value, respect, and feel confident about yourself. For example, suppose you set a goal of earning an A in math. You study and do your homework every day. Many days, you see a tutor. When you get your report card and see that you earned an A, you are very proud of yourself. When you set and reach goals, you always feel good about your achievement and yourself.

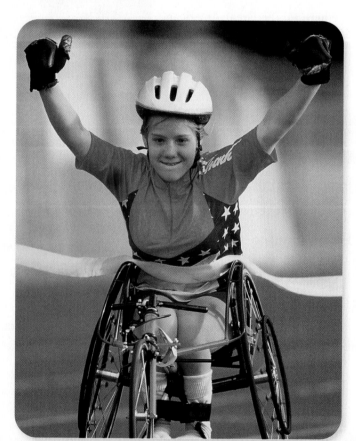

Figure 11 Accomplishing goals builds self-esteem.

TABLE 1 The Relationship Between Values, Interests, and Goals		
Value	**Interest**	**Possible goal**
Self-expression	public speaking	to act in a play
Helping others	woodworking	to help elderly people with household projects
Self-discipline	running	to run a 10-kilometer race
Honesty	current events	to join the newspaper staff

Examining Your Values

Your values influence the goals that you set. Remember that a value is an important belief. It is a reflection of the kind of person you want to be. Think about your values when you set goals. You are more likely to reach goals that are based on your values. In the example at the beginning of the lesson, both Jim and Parag value helping other people. But Jim wants to become a judge, while Parag wants to become a surgeon.

Your personal values develop over time and are based on your experiences. Not everyone has the same values, although there are certain values that most people believe in. For example, most people believe in honesty and responsibility. When you know your values, setting goals for yourself is easier.

Health Journal

Using Table 1 as an example, write down one thing that you value and one thing that interests you. How would you combine your value and your interest to set a possible goal?

Defining Your Interests

You also have interests. An **interest** is something that you enjoy and want to learn more about. You can have an interest in things such as art, athletics, music, or science. Like your values, your interests influence your goals. But unlike values, which develop over a long period of time, interests can start quickly and can end just as fast. You may have an interest in tennis for several months. But soon you may find that your interest has changed to basketball. Values usually do not change this rapidly. If you value honesty now, you will probably value it later in life, too. Your values reflect your character. Your interests reflect your personality and tastes.

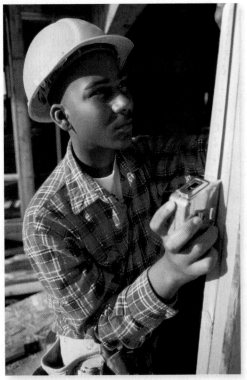

Figure 12 This teen is using his interest in carpentry to help build houses for the homeless.

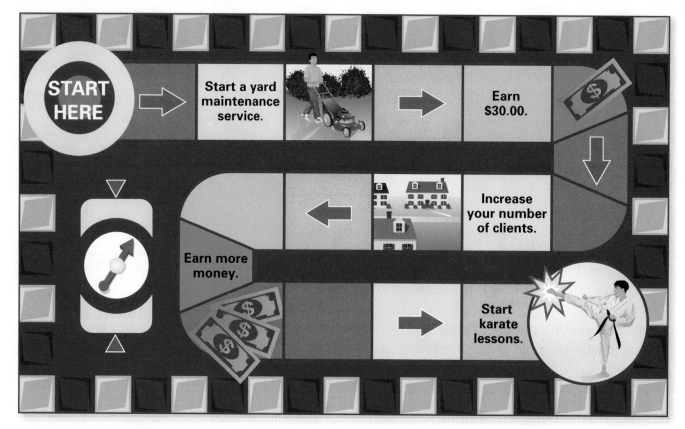

Figure 13 For Jeff to reach his long-term goal of taking karate lessons, he must first accomplish several short-term goals.

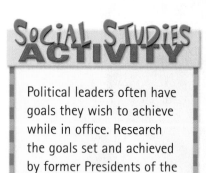

SOCIAL STUDIES ACTIVITY

Political leaders often have goals they wish to achieve while in office. Research the goals set and achieved by former Presidents of the United States.

Short-Term Goals and Long-Term Goals

After you have determined your values and interests, you are ready to identify your goals. There are two kinds of goals: short-term goals and long-term goals. *Short-term goals* are tasks that you can accomplish in hours, days, or weeks. For example, making a good grade on a test is a short-term goal. Finishing your chores in time to watch a TV show is a short-term goal.

Long-term goals may take months or even years to reach. Usually, long-term goals are made up of several short-term goals and even other long-term goals. For example, suppose you set a long-term goal of going to college. What goals would help you reach your final goal? One goal would be to make good grades in your classes so that you can graduate. Another might be to save money to help pay for your tuition. Getting accepted into college is another goal. Each goal builds on the other to help you reach your long-term goal. The key to reaching a long-term goal is to identify all of the other goals that make up that goal. Then, you must work through all of your goals. If you don't accomplish one goal along the way, don't give up! Think about what you can do to get back on track. You may need to change one of your short-term goals. Or you may need to add a goal to your plans. There is more than one way to reach your final goal.

Goals Build Healthy Relationships

Goals not only help you in your activities and at school but also can help you build healthy relationships. A healthy relationship begins when you and a friend or family member work toward goals together. For example, many people around you can help you reach your goal of going to college. Your parents help by giving you support every day. They may also teach you how to save money and may work with you to fill out college applications. Your friends help you reach your goal by studying with you so that you will earn good grades. Your teachers also help you reach your goal. Teachers can help you choose classes that will prepare you for college and can teach you good study habits. Working with others to reach a goal strengthens your relationships with them.

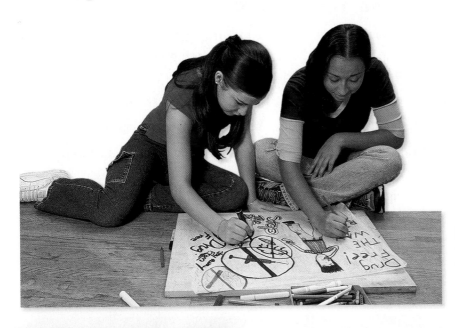

Figure 14 Working with others to achieve a goal helps build healthy relationships.

Lesson Review

Using Vocabulary

1. Define the term *interest*.

2. What is the relationship between having self-esteem and achieving goals?

Understanding Concepts

3. Explain the importance of interests and values in setting your goals.

4. How do short-term goals and long-term goals differ?

5. How do goals build healthy relationships?

Critical Thinking

6. **Making Inferences** Alan enjoyed fishing a few years ago. Now, he prefers to go hiking. Did his interests change, his values change, or did both change? Explain.

internet connect

www.scilinks.org/health
Topic: Building a Healthy
Self-Esteem
HealthLinks code: HD4020

HEALTH LINKS Maintained by the National Science Teachers Association

How to Reach Your Goals

What You'll Do

- **Explain** the relationship between goals and success.
- **Describe** how you can learn from your mistakes.

Terms to Learn

- success
- persistence

Start Off Write

Why must you learn from your mistakes to reach your goals?

Elena daydreams about making the winning basket for her team. She practices shooting baskets every day. Elena's goal is to become a professional basketball player.

No matter what your goal is, you will need to make many decisions along the way. In this lesson, you will learn how to use the six steps to making good decisions to reach your goals.

Reaching Your Goals

Success is the achievement of your goals. You can follow the six steps to making good decisions to reach goals. For example, let's say you set a goal to get in shape.

- **Identify the problem.** How do you get in shape?
- **Consider your values.** You value being physically fit.
- **List the options.** Your options are to ride a stationary bike or jog.
- **Weigh the consequences.** If the weather is bad, you won't be able to run. The bike is indoors.
- **Decide, and act.** You decide to ride the bike.
- **Evaluate your choice.** You ride for an hour every day. You are getting in shape! You reached your goal.

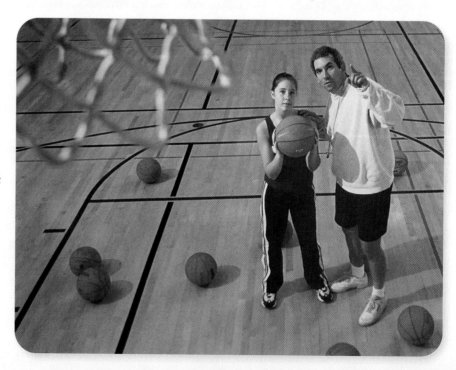

Figure 15 Many goals require a lot of practice.

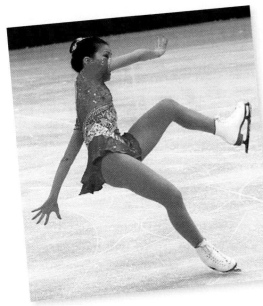

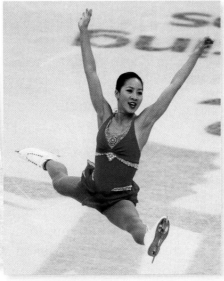

Figure 16 Mistakes can be valuable learning tools. They make you think about how you can improve.

Learning from Your Mistakes

The most important thing to remember about goals is that it takes time, energy, and determination to reach them. Success rarely comes easily, so persistence is important. **Persistence** is the commitment to keep working toward your goal even when things that make you want to quit happen. Sometimes, it will be hard to stay focused. And you will make mistakes along the way. Everyone who sets goals sometimes makes a bad decision when trying to reach his or her goal. To be successful, you must learn from your mistakes. Take time to think about what you did. What can you do differently next time? Making a mistake might have gotten you off track temporarily, but do not let it stop you from reaching your goal. You can get back on track again. Tell yourself that making a mistake is OK. You must convince yourself to stay positive and keep going.

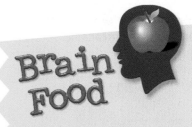

The greatest challenge Thomas Edison faced while inventing the light bulb was to find a material that would glow without burning. Edison tried more than 1,600 materials before he found the right one.

Lesson Review

Using Vocabulary

1. In your own words, define success.

2. What is persistence?

Understanding Concepts

3. Explain the relationship between goals and success.

4. Explain how a mistake can be a valuable learning tool.

Critical Thinking

5. Applying Concepts Using the six steps to making decisions, outline a plan for reaching one of your goals.

Changing Your Goals

What You'll Do

- **Explain** the importance of measuring your progress when pursuing a goal.

- **Explain** why changing your plans is sometimes part of reaching your goals.

Terms to Learn

- coping

Start Off
Write

How do you measure your progress when reaching a goal?

Manuel did not make the tennis team the first time he tried out. At first, he wasn't sure whether to try out for the team again or to try something new. Manuel decided that being on the tennis team was important enough to him to try out again.

Like Manuel, when things don't go as planned, you may be disappointed, but you do not have to give up on your dreams. In this lesson, you'll look at ways to measure your progress as you work toward a goal. You will also see how to make changes to meet your goal.

Measuring Your Progress

Your goal is to run the mile faster and to break your old record. After a month, how can you tell if you are running faster? You can time yourself. When you are trying to reach a goal, it is important to measure your progress. By measuring your progress, you can see if you are on the right track. And the only way to be sure that you have progressed is to check your results. Scores, grades, and measurements are ways that you can track your progress. You can also make charts or keep a journal. Reviewing results is just as important as working on the goal itself. When you see how far you've come, you will feel great. And you will want to work even harder to reach your goal.

Figure 17 This athlete measures her time whenever she swims.

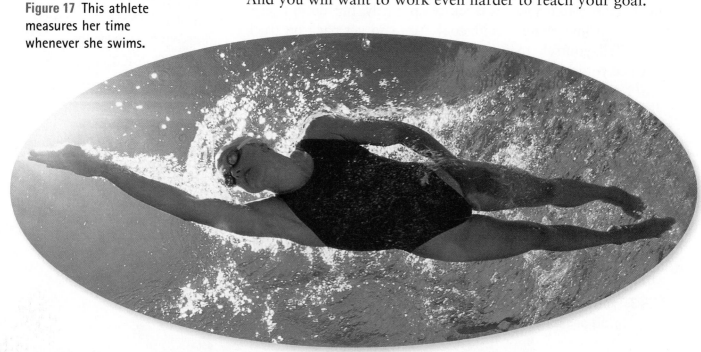

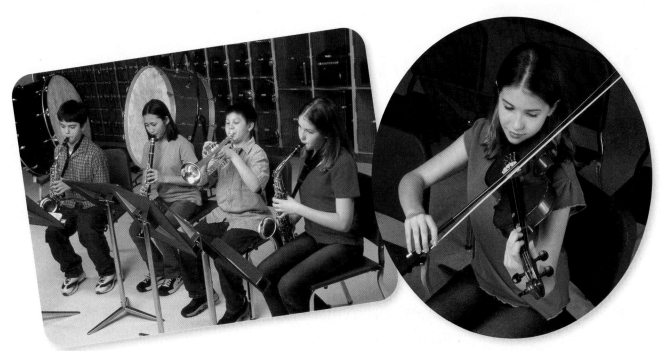

Figure 18 Goals sometimes change because our interests change.

Changing Your Plan

Sailors chart a course on a map to show where they want to go. Even with the best boat and the best skills, they still have to change course sometimes. You face the same situation when you try to reach a goal. You may have all of the desire and skill in the world, but sometimes you will have to change your direction. You will occasionally have to cope with setbacks. **Coping** is dealing with problems in an effective way. When things don't go as planned, try a different path. You may find new energy to keep working toward your original goal. You might even find that your new direction inspires you to work toward a new goal. Remember that goals worth achieving are not easy to reach. Such goals are rarely reached on the first try.

Lesson Review

Using Vocabulary

1. Define the term *coping*.

Understanding Concepts

2. Why is it important to measure your progress as you work toward a goal?

3. Explain why changes must sometimes be made when you work toward a goal.

Critical Thinking

4. **Applying Concepts** Why is it important to learn to cope with disappointments at an early age? How do you think your ability to cope with disappointments will help you as you get older?

5. **Making Inferences** Identify three reasons why a plan for reaching a goal may need to be changed.

Skills for Success

What You'll Do

■ **Explain** why communication is important.

■ **Identify** four skills that you need to be a good listener.

■ **Identify** five refusal skills.

Terms to Learn

● communication

● refusal skill

Start Off
Write

What do you do to let people know that you are listening to them?

Keesha hates it when her friend Maren doesn't listen to her. Sometimes, Keesha will be talking about something really important when she realizes that Maren hasn't heard a word that she has said.

Keesha wishes that Maren had better listening skills. In this lesson, you'll learn how to communicate so that people will listen to you. You will also learn listening skills.

Communication

Sometimes, it is difficult to get your ideas across. To do so, you need to be able to communicate. **Communication** is the ability to exchange information and the ability to express your thoughts and feelings clearly. The ability to communicate is an important skill, especially when you are trying to reach a goal. This skill allows you to let others know exactly what you want or expect so that no misunderstandings take place. Someone can offer good advice to you only if he or she knows your intentions. When you express your ideas, be open, but choose your words carefully. Good communication can mean the difference between getting the information you need to reach a goal or not.

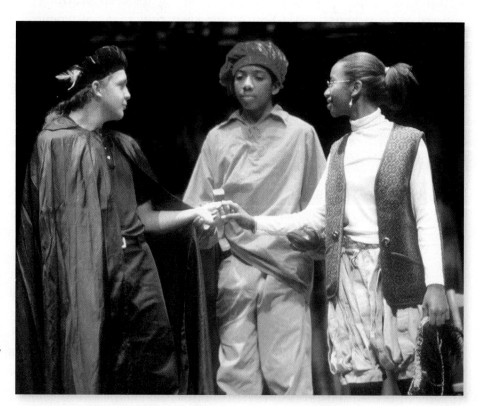

Figure 19 Good communication skills are important here as well as in everyday life.

Listening Skills

Having good listening skills is as important to reaching your goal as communicating clearly is. To develop good listening skills, follow these suggestions:

- **Pay attention to the person who is speaking.** Facing a person shows that you are interested in what the person is saying.

- **Make eye contact.** Looking around makes people think that you are not listening to them.

- **Nod when you understand.**

- **Ask questions when you don't understand.** Try to ask open-ended questions. *Open-ended questions* call for an answer other than yes or no. Ask questions such as, "What do you think about that?"

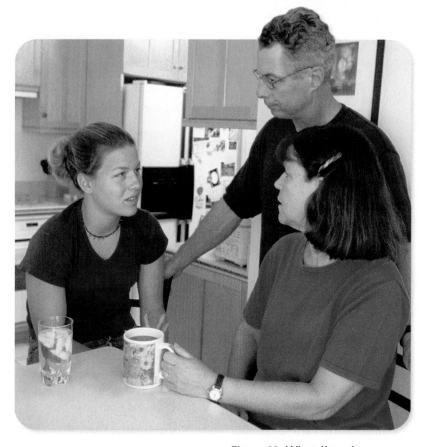

Figure 20 What listening skills are this teen's parents exhibiting?

How do good listening skills help you reach your goals? Very few people reach their goals without help from others. To get this help, you need to listen to the person who is giving you advice. People can point you in the right direction and can give you tips to save you time and energy. But you must listen!

Hands-on ACTIVITY

LISTENING LAB

1. Go to a place where students spend time talking together.

2. Find a place where you can observe some people without disturbing them. Be sure to take a pencil and a piece of paper with you.

3. What do you observe about the way that students talk and listen to each other?

Note the following things in your observations:
- body position
- facial expressions
- tone of voice
- hand movements
- eye contact

Analysis

1. Describe your observations. For example, could you tell if the people were friends or if they were casual acquaintances? Were they happy, sad, or angry with each other? Explain.

Figure 21 Using Refusal Skills

You and a friend have just finished watching a movie at the theater. Your friend wants you to sneak into one of the other movies with him. You can use any of the following refusal skills in this situation.

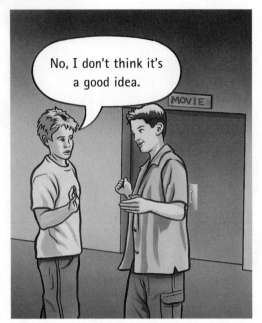

Say no.

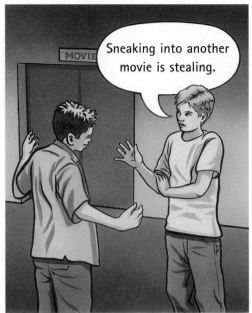

Stay focused on the issue.

Refusal Skills

Sometimes, saying no when you are faced with peer pressure is difficult. But remembering your values and goals will give you the strength to say no. How do you say no? You use refusal skills. **Refusal skills** are strategies to avoid doing something you don't want to do. There are five ways to deal with negative peer pressure.

- **Avoid dangerous situations.** You won't have to say no if you avoid situations that you know will be a problem.
- **Say, "No."** Use a tone of voice that shows that you mean no.
- **Stay focused on the problem.** Picture what is wrong with the situation. Point out the problem if your friends argue with you.
- **Stand your ground.** Don't give in when your friends give you a hard time.
- **Walk away.** If your friends won't accept a simple no, walking away may be the best thing to do.

Using refusal skills will help you stay focused on your goals. Friends may use negative peer pressure to try to get you to do things that are not good for you. These kinds of things never help you reach your goals. They distract you and get you off track. Using refusal skills help you throughout your life. Begin practicing these skills now to keep your goals in sight.

Health Journal

Write a journal entry about a time when you were faced with negative peer pressure. Describe how you handled the situation.

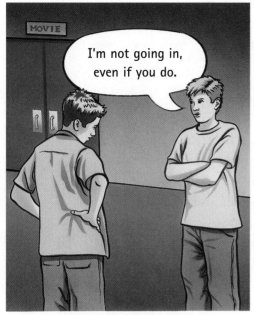

I'm not going in, even if you do.

Stand your ground.

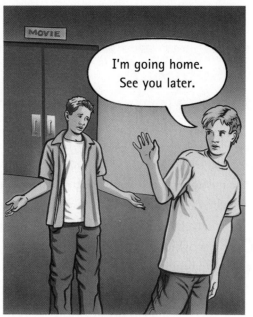

I'm going home. See you later.

Walk away.

Putting It All Together

Suppose you are helping your dad build a room onto your house. When you need a certain tool, you reach into the toolbox and pull out the tool that is best suited for the job. Think of the skills in this lesson as tools in a toolbox. Each skill is a tool that you can use to solve a certain problem. If you need information to reach a goal, use good communication to express what you want to know. When getting advice, use your listening skills to get the information you need. If you find yourself in a situation in which you need to say no, use one or more of your refusal skills. These skills can help you in everyday life as well as in problem situations. Remember these skills, and use them often!

Lesson Review

Using Vocabulary

1. Define the term *communication*.

2. What are refusal skills?

Understanding Concepts

3. Why are communication and listening skills important? What four things make you a good listener?

Critical Thinking

4. **Analyzing Ideas** List the five refusal skills. Which refusal skill do you use the most? Which skill is the most difficult for you to use? Explain why.

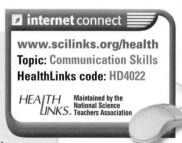

internet connect

www.scilinks.org/health
Topic: Communication Skills
HealthLinks code: HD4022

HEALTH LINKS™ Maintained by the National Science Teachers Association

Chapter Summary

■ A good decision has a positive outcome. ■ A consequence is the result of a decision. ■ There are six steps to making good decisions. ■ Values are beliefs that you consider to be of great importance. ■ Brainstorming can help you identify options when making a decision. ■ Your decisions are influenced by your family, your friends, and the media. ■ Peer pressure can be negative or positive. ■ Your values and interests influence your goals. ■ There are short-term goals and long-term goals. ■ Success is the achievement of your goals. ■ You should measure your progress and be persistent when working toward a goal. ■ Communication and listening skills are important when working toward a goal. ■ Refusal skills are ways to avoid doing something that you don't want to do.

Using Vocabulary

For each sentence, fill in the blank with the proper word from the word bank provided below.

brainstorming   goal
refusal skills   persistence
interest   self-esteem
values   consequence
options   coping
good decision

1. When making a decision, ___ are the possible choices you can make.

2. Planning to save $100 to buy something you want is called a(n) ___.

3. Actions that mean "no" are called ___.

4. Your ___ are made up of all of the beliefs that you consider important.

5. Wanting to know more about stamp collecting would be a(n) ___.

6. A(n) ___ is one that is responsible.

7. If you value and respect yourself you have high ___.

8. Sometimes, plans do not go as expected, but ___ is the ability to move beyond the problems.

Understanding Concepts

9. What are the four skills of being a good listener?

10. What are the six steps to making good decisions?

11. How do your decisions change based on new information?

12. Why are goals important?

13. How does making mistakes contribute to success?

14. What should you do if you don't understand someone?

15. List five different strategies that indicate refusal.

16. Give an example of a positive consequence and an example of a negative consequence.

Critical Thinking

Analyzing Ideas

17 You are trying to tell a friend about a problem that you have. He doesn't seem to be listening to you. What nonverbal communication clues might tell you that he isn't listening? What could you tell your friend about good listening skills?

18 You see a commercial on television that shows athletes wearing a certain kind of shoe. Do you think that you need those shoes to be an athlete? Why do you think that advertisers use sports heroes to sell their products? Explain your answer.

Using Refusal Skills

19 You are taking a test in class, and you see one of your friends cheating. When she sees that you realize what is going on, she asks you if you want the answers, too. What refusal skills would you use in this situation?

20 Imagine that all your friends have started wearing a certain type of shirt. They are all telling you that you need to wear the same type of shirt as them. You don't like the style of the shirt. What refusal skills would you use?

21 A friend dares you to shoplift an item from a store. Your friend says that you are a coward if you don't do it. You think about it. List some of the consequences of not shoplifting the item. Describe how you can use refusal skills in this situation.

Interpreting Graphics

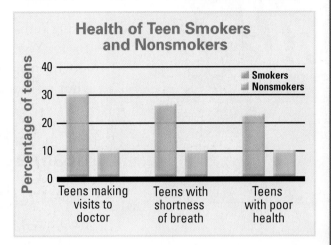

Use the figure above to answer questions 22–25.

22 Overall, do you think smokers or non-smokers are healthier? Explain your answer.

23 The number of smokers who visit the doctor is greater than the number of students who report poor health. Why do you think this happens?

24 Athletes depend on being healthy and being able to breathe easily while exercising. Do you think many athletes smoke? Explain.

25 If your friend wanted to start smoking, how would you use the chart above to convince him otherwise?

Reading Checkup

Take a minute to review your answers to the Health IQ questions at the beginning of this chapter. How has reading this chapter improved your Health IQ?

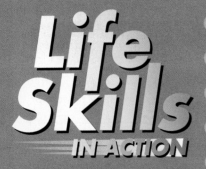

Life Skills IN ACTION

ACT 1

Using Refusal Skills

Using refusal skills is saying no to things you don't want to do. You can also use refusal skills to avoid dangerous situations. Complete the following activity to develop your refusal skills.

Reanna's Refusal

Setting the Scene

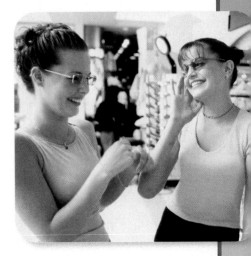

Reanna and her best friend Kelsey are shopping at the mall. Near the end of their shopping trip, Reanna sees a bracelet that she likes a lot. Unfortunately, she cannot buy the bracelet because she has already spent all of her money. Kelsey tells Reanna that she should just take the bracelet. "It's small," Kelsey says, "No one will ever notice that it is missing."

The 5 Steps of Using Refusal Skills

1. Avoid dangerous situations.
2. Say "No."
3. Stand your ground.
4. Stay focused on the issue.
5. Walk away.

Guided Practice

Practice with a Friend

Form a group of three. Have one person play the role of Reanna and another person play the role of Kelsey. Have the third person be an observer. Walking through each of the five steps of using refusal skills, role-play Reanna responding to Kelsey. Kelsey should try to convince Reanna to shoplift the bracelet. The observer will take notes, which will include observations about what the person playing Reanna did well and suggestions of ways to improve. Stop after each step to evaluate the process.

Independent Practice

Check Yourself

After you have completed the guided practice, go through Act 1 again without stopping at each step. Answer the questions below to review what you did.

1. To stand her ground, what could Reanna say to Kelsey?

2. What could Reanna say to convince Kelsey that shoplifting is wrong?

3. How could Reanna avoid dangerous situations similar to this one in the future?

4. Think about a time when you had to say no to a good friend. Why was it difficult to say no?

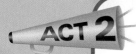

On Your Own

At school the next day, Kelsey hands Reanna a present. Reanna opens it and finds the bracelet that Kelsey tried to convince her to steal. Reanna asks Kelsey if she paid for the bracelet. Kelsey admits that she didn't and tells Reanna not to say anything about it. Reanna tries to give the bracelet back to Kelsey, but Kelsey insists that she keep it. Draw a comic strip that shows how Reanna could use the five steps of using refusal skills in this situation.

Building Self-Esteem

Lessons

Check out
Current Health
articles related to this chapter by
visiting **go.hrw.com**. Just type in
the keyword **HD4CH18**.

> **"** I was **upset** when I found out that I **didn't** have any classes **with my friends** this year.
>
> But a few weeks after school started, I began to meet some of my new classmates. I wasn't afraid to make new friends, and now I'm not so sad about going to school. **"**

Health IQ

PRE-READING

Answer the following multiple-choice questions to find out what you already know about self-esteem. When you've finished this chapter, you'll have the opportunity to change your answers based on what you've learned.

1. Self-esteem is
a. a measure of how well you get along with others.
b. a measure of how much you value and respect yourself.
c. the way you see yourself.
d. a measure of how popular you are.

2. Which of the following is a characteristic of a person who has low self-esteem?
a. accepts himself or herself
b. has integrity
c. has little confidence in himself or herself
d. is not affected deeply by negative comments

3. What is self-concept?
a. the way you see or imagine yourself as a person
b. the way you choose to deal with a person who teases you
c. how you handle your relationships
d. how much you value yourself as a person

4. Being assertive means that you
a. take responsibility for your actions.
b. act on your thoughts and values without hurting others.
c. are trustworthy.
d. refuse to take part in activities that you know are wrong.

5. Which of the following might help you build healthy self-esteem?
a. volunteering your time
b. setting a goal
c. accepting yourself
d. all of the above

ANSWERS: 1. b; 2. c; 3. a; 4. b; 5. d

Self-Esteem and Your Life

It is Jessie's first day at her new school. She is nervous because she doesn't know anyone. She doesn't know her way around. Before she leaves the house, she looks in the mirror and says to herself, "I can do this!"

Have you ever been nervous when faced with a new situation? Even though Jessie is nervous about going to a new school, she is confident about herself. Jessie has high self-esteem.

What Is Self-Esteem?

You may not realize that your self-esteem has a big impact on your life. **Self-esteem** is a measure of how much you value, respect, and feel confident about yourself. Your level of self-esteem determines how you face new challenges. Your level of self-esteem affects your relationships with others. It also affects how you make decisions. Finally, your self-esteem affects your success in anything you choose to do. If you have high self-esteem, you will be more likely to succeed at the new things you try. There will be times when you don't succeed. Having high self-esteem will help you deal with a disappointment better than if you have low self-esteem.

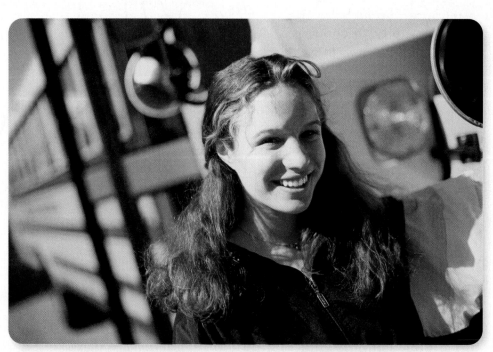

Figure 1 Jessie has high self-esteem. This helps her feel confident about her first day at school.

High Self-Esteem

Having high self-esteem can help a person have a positive outlook on life. High self-esteem can help a person achieve success. People who have high self-esteem share similar traits. They feel good about themselves. They like themselves. They have a high level of confidence. People who have high self-esteem do not feel inferior to others. They are not usually deeply affected by negative comments from other people.

Low Self-Esteem

Low self-esteem may keep a person from enjoying life. People who have low self-esteem do not feel good about themselves. They do not like themselves. Many people have parts of their personality that they do not like. However, people who have low self-esteem often think they have no positive traits. They have a low level of confidence. They may have trouble in their relationships with other people. People who have low self-esteem are often affected by negative comments from other people.

Your self-esteem is likely to change as you change. At times, you may have low self-esteem. Other times you may have high self-esteem. Most people have an overall self-esteem that falls somewhere between high self-esteem and low self-esteem. Aiming to like and accept yourself for who you are can actually help you develop a higher level of self-esteem.

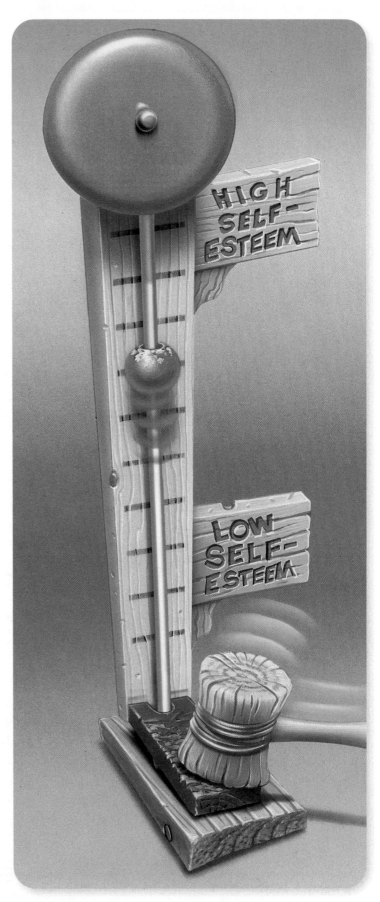

Figure 2 Most people's self-esteem falls between high self-esteem and low self-esteem.

Figure 3 | What Influences Your Self-Esteem?

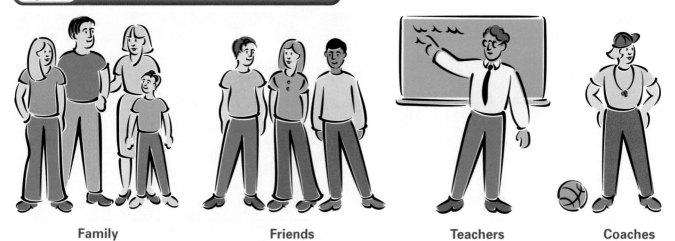

Family   Friends   Teachers   Coaches

Who Can Affect Your Self-Esteem?

Your level of self-esteem is influenced by the people around you. These people include your family, your friends, and people at school. Every person in your life can have a positive or negative effect on your self-esteem.

People who encourage you and give you support will help you feel good about yourself. They will help you develop confidence. People who do not support you may lead you to develop low self-esteem. These people may tease you, or make negative comments about you.

The most important person who influences your self-esteem is you. You can choose to value and like yourself. You can choose to focus on the positive influences on your self-esteem. Similarly, you can choose to deal with negative influences in a positive way.

Hands-on ACTIVITY

SELF-ESTEEM BOOSTER

1. Work in groups of four or five. Each person needs two sheets of paper. On the first sheet of paper, list three positive qualites about yourself. On the second sheet, write your name.

2. Keep the page on which you listed your three qualities. Then, give the sheet with your name on it to a person from your group. On the sheet that another person gives you, list two positive qualities about that person under his or her name.

3. Continue to exchange papers until everyone in the group has had a chance to write under each person's name. Then read your new list.

Analysis

1. How did the list of positive qualities that your classmates wrote compare with the qualities that you listed about yourself?

2. How will you use this list of qualities to boost your self-esteem?

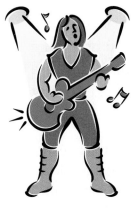
Music videos

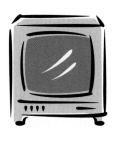
TV

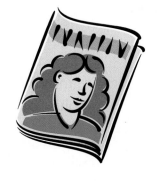
Magazines

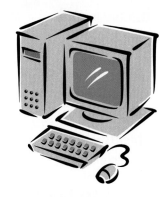
Internet

The Media and Your Self-Esteem

Did you know that the media can influence your self-esteem? The media includes TV, magazines, movies, and music videos. The media tends to show only people who are very successful or glamorous. The media also tends to show only people who are unusually thin or muscular. Some people may compare themselves to the people they see in the media. This comparison can cause a person to develop an unhealthy body image. **Body image** is the way you see and imagine your body. Your body image can affect your self-esteem. If you are uncomfortable with your body, you probably won't feel good about yourself. Therefore, if you have an unhealthy body image, you may develop low self-esteem. But having a healthy body image can boost your self-esteem. If you feel good about your body, you will probably feel good about yourself.

Health Journal

Write a paragraph describing which forms of media you think influence teens the most.

Lesson Review

Using Vocabulary

1. In your own words, describe the term *self-esteem*.

Understanding Concepts

2. Describe how self-esteem affects your life.

3. Describe the characteristics of a person who has high self-esteem.

4. Identify five influences on your self-esteem.

Critical Thinking

5. Analyzing Ideas Explain how having an unhealthy body image can affect your self-esteem. How would having a healthy body image affect your self-esteem?

Lesson 2

What You'll Do

- **Describe** how self-concept and self-esteem are different.

- **Identify** three areas of self-concept.

Terms to Learn

- self-concept

Start Off
Write

What is your self-concept?

Your Self-Concept

Steven tried out for the track team last week. Today he found out that he did not make the team. Steven felt disappointed, but he knows he's good at music. He decided to try out for the band too.

Steven did not let the fact that he didn't make the track team affect his self-esteem. In fact, Steven sees himself more as a musician than a track star. This helped him overcome his disappointment.

Self-Concept and Self-Esteem

Self-concept is a building block of self-esteem. **Self-concept** is the way you see and imagine yourself as a person. Self-concept is different from self-esteem. Self-esteem is the way you value and respect yourself. To find out more about your self-concept, ask yourself the following question: How would you describe yourself to a stranger? Perhaps you see yourself as an athlete. And you see yourself as a good student. Some people may describe themselves as a nice person who makes friends easily.

Imagine that you see yourself as an artist because you like to draw. This image of yourself is your self-concept. However, sometimes you may not feel confident around the people at school. This feeling is your self-esteem. Your self-concept can affect your self-esteem. Because you see yourself as an artist, you may choose to think to yourself, I like to draw, and I am good at it. This makes me feel more confident about myself.

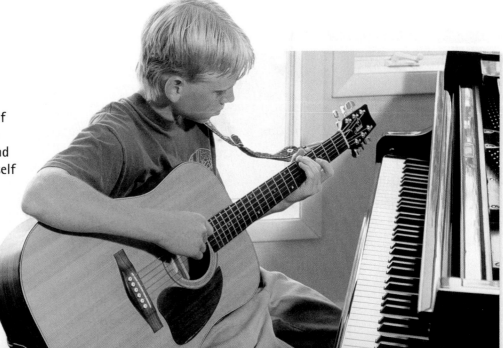

Figure 4 Andy sees himself as a musician because he likes to play the guitar and piano. This image of himself is his self-concept.

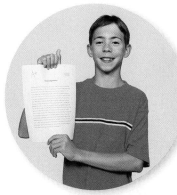
Academic

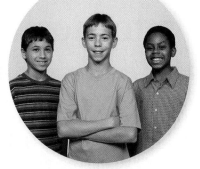
Social

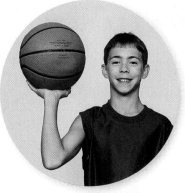
Physical

How Self-Concept Develops

Your self-concept can develop from many areas. Three very important areas are your academic self-concept, your physical self-concept, and your social self-concept.

Your academic self-concept is the way you see yourself as a student. You may see yourself as a good student. Or you may see yourself as an average student.

Your physical self-concept is the way you see your physical abilities. Some people see themselves as good athletes. Other people don't see themselves as athletes, but they are comfortable with their abilities.

Your social self-concept is the way you see yourself in your relationships. Some people see themselves as being very friendly, and they may have a lot of friends. Other people may see themselves as shy. They may have only a few close friends.

These three areas of self-concept contribute to your overall self-concept. As you get to know yourself better, your self-concept will change. In turn, your level of self-esteem may change, too. The way you see yourself in these three areas can help you find your positive traits. Finding your positive traits can boost your self-esteem.

Figure 5 How you see yourself academically, physically, and socially affects your overall self-concept.

Lesson Review

Using Vocabulary

1. What is self-concept?

Understanding Concepts

2. How is self-concept different from self-esteem?

3. What are three areas of self-concept?

Critical Thinking

4. **Making Inferences** Claudia sees herself as a good student who has a lot of friends. However, she does not feel that she is good at sports. Claudia does not let this feeling bother her. Instead she focuses on her strengths. What is Claudia's self-concept? What level of self-esteem does she have?

Keys to Healthy Self-Esteem

What You'll Do

- **Describe** three keys to healthy self-esteem.

- **Identify** eight strategies for building healthy self-esteem.

Start Off
Write

What can you do to boost your self-esteem?

Nicole got mad and yelled at her best friend. Nicole felt very sorry later and apologized to her friend. She asked her best friend for help in thinking of ways to behave when she gets mad in the future.

Everybody makes mistakes. It is easy to apologize, but it takes a healthy attitude to do something about the behavior so that it does not happen again. Doing the right thing helps build healthy self-esteem.

Three Keys to Healthy Self-Esteem

Your actions and behaviors affect the way you feel about yourself. You can have healthy self-esteem by building good character. The first step to developing good character and self-esteem is to have integrity (in TEG ruh tee). Your integrity is your honesty to yourself and others. Integrity is also your ability to take responsibility for your actions. If you are honest and you take responsibility for your actions, you will have a positive image of yourself. Also, the people in your life will be able to trust you.

Second, you must respect yourself to have a healthy self-esteem. Respecting yourself means knowing what is right for you and what is wrong for you. You are respecting yourself if you refuse to join in an activity that you know is wrong, even if it is the popular thing to do.

Third, being assertive can help you build a healthy self-esteem. Being assertive means acting on your thoughts and values in a firm but positive way. You are being assertive when you communicate your feelings clearly and with respect. For example, your friend may ask you to ride bikes one afternoon. But you need to study for a quiz. You can be assertive by telling your friend that you can't ride bikes because you have to study.

Figure 6 When you have healthy self-esteem, other people see you in a positive way and trust you.

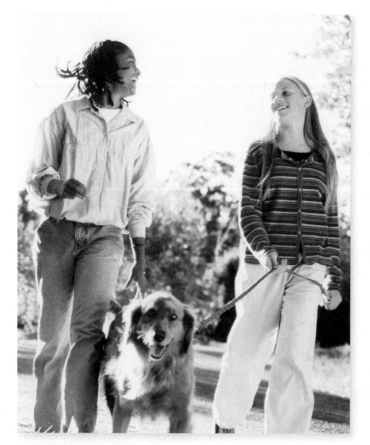

Eight Ways to Build Self-Esteem

You know what self-esteem is and how it affects your life. So, how do you build healthy self-esteem? Eight ways to build a healthier level of self-esteem are listed below.

Get to know yourself. Getting to know yourself sounds simple. Do you know yourself simply because you are you? One of the best things to do to improve your self-esteem is to understand who you are. This includes knowing what types of things you like and what things you don't like. For example, you may like to read scary stories. But, you may not like science fiction stories. Getting to know yourself also means knowing what your strengths and weaknesses are. What are you good at? What things could you improve on? You may be really good at math. However, sometimes you get really angry at your little brother, and you would like to improve your behavior towards him. Once you know who you are, it will be easier to know what is right for you and what isn't.

Learn to like yourself. Another step to building healthy self-esteem is learning to like yourself. You need to focus on what you like best about yourself. Imagine that a friend told you that you are a good listener. You like yourself for being a good listener. Liking yourself for your positive qualities helps you be assertive and confident. Liking yourself also means accepting all of your qualities, whether they are good or bad. Accepting and liking yourself helps you build high self-esteem.

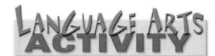

Write a story about a teen who chooses to do one of the items listed in this lesson to build self-esteem. In your story, describe what your character decided to do and how it helped your character improve his or her self-esteem.

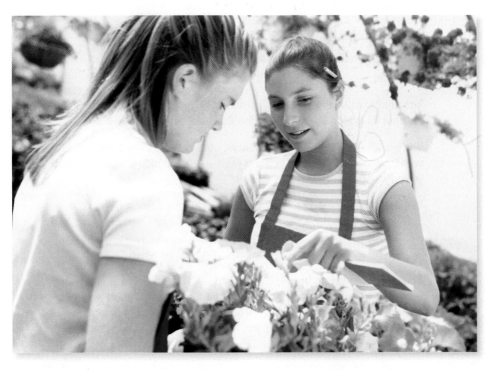

Figure 7 Jen knows that gardening is one of her strengths. This makes her feel good about herself.

Be good at something. One way to feel good about yourself is to be good at something. Find something you enjoy doing. It could be a hobby, a sport, an activity at school, or anything. In your free time, focus your efforts on the activity you choose. If you really enjoy what you are doing, you can try to become better at your activity. You will develop more confidence and higher self-esteem if you know you are good at something.

Set a goal. Setting goals helps you build self-esteem because reaching goals gives you a sense of accomplishment. When you try hard to reach a goal, you feel good about yourself. Once you reach your goal, you will feel successful. Start by setting small goals. When you feel more confident about setting and reaching goals, you can try to set higher goals. When you set a higher goal, you will have to stretch yourself to reach it. In turn, you will grow as a person. You will also discover your hidden strengths.

Be positive. Did you know that just believing in yourself can help you build self-esteem? Thinking positive thoughts when you are feeling unsure of yourself can help you be more confident in many situations. You can use positive self-talk to be your own cheerleader. Positive self-talk is a way of encouraging yourself by saying or thinking positive statements to yourself. The table below shows you some examples of positive self-talk. The next time you feel nervous in a situation, try using positive self-talk to give yourself a boost of confidence.

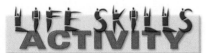

LIFE SKILLS ACTIVITY

USING REFUSAL SKILLS

Imagine a classmate approached you before math class. He asked if he could borrow your homework because he didn't do his homework. What will you tell your classmate? How will your actions affect your self-esteem?

TABLE 1 Positive Self–Talk	
Situation	**Positive self-talk**
You are nervous that you may not do well on a test.	"I studied for this test, and I know that I can do well. I know I can do it!"
You are afraid that you won't make any friends at your new school.	"Making friends takes time. I just have to be myself and be confident that I will meet people."
You don't like your new haircut.	"I don't like how my haircut turned out. But my hair will grow, and I can get it cut differently next time. Maybe if I try styling it a different way, I won't feel so bad about it."
Some of your classmates teased you about the way you run in gym class.	"I feel bad because they tease me when I run. But I know that I'm better at other things. I am very good at swimming, so I don't feel bad if I can't run as fast as everyone else."

Find a mentor. A mentor is someone who can give you support and encouragment. Often, a mentor is older than you. A mentor should have qualities that you would like to have. This person can be your role model. A mentor can help you set goals and discover your abilities. In this way, a mentor can help you build self-esteem.

Do something for others. Helping people who are less fortunate than you is a great way to build your self-esteem. It also gives you a chance to share your abilities with other people. Try volunteering at your local charity organization, such as a soup kitchen. Or participate in a food and clothing drive.

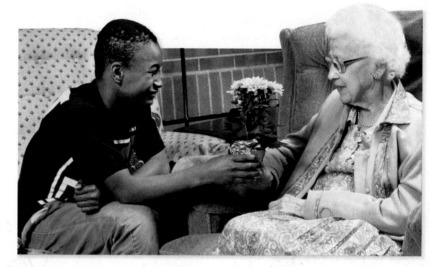

Figure 8 Participating in volunteer activities is a great way to boost your self-esteem.

Have a sense of humor. People who have a high level of self-esteem are not usually deeply affected by negative comments from others. In fact, people who have high self-esteem are able to laugh at themselves. Having a sense of humor means you are able to laugh at yourself. Having a sense of humor helps you accept some of your weaknesses. For example, suppose you are not a great basketball player. But when you play basketball, you have a sense of humor about yourself. You have a good time no matter what your abilities are. Approaching life with a sense of humor is a great way to build healthy self-esteem.

Lesson Review

Understanding Concepts

1. Describe three keys to self-esteem.

2. How can having a mentor help you build self-esteem?

3. How can volunteer work help you build self-esteem? List three volunteer activities you would like to try.

4. Name an activity that you enjoy. What steps can you take to become better at this activity? How can being better at the activity help your self-esteem?

Critical Thinking

5. **Making Inferences** How does having integrity, respecting yourself, and being assertive help you to have high self-esteem?

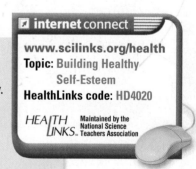

Chapter Summary

■ Self-esteem is the way you value, respect, and feel about yourself. ■ Self-esteem affects your relationships with other people and how you face new situations. ■ Influences on your self-esteem include family, friends, teachers, coaches, and the media. ■ Self-concept is how you see yourself as a person. ■ There are three areas of self-concept: academic self-concept, social self-concept, and physical self-concept. ■ Three keys to healthy self-esteem include having integrity, respecting yourself, and being assertive.

Using Vocabulary

For each pair of terms, describe how the meanings of the terms differ.

1. self-esteem/self-concept
2. self-esteem/body image

For each sentence, fill in the blank with the proper word from the word bank provided below.

> self-concept   body image
> self-esteem

3. How you feel about yourself as a person is your ___.
4. Your ___ is the way you see and imagine your body.
5. How you see yourself as a person is called your ___.

Understanding Concepts

6. What are the characteristics of a person who has low self-esteem?
7. What does being assertive mean?
8. Name three influences on your self-esteem.

9. How can the following actions help you build a healthy self-esteem?
   a. accepting yourself
   b. setting a goal
   c. being positive
   d. knowing yourself
   e. having a sense of humor
10. What is academic self-concept?
11. How do integrity, self-respect, and assertiveness help you have healthy self-esteem?
12. Give an example of how you would use positive self-talk to boost your self-esteem.
13. Discovering your strengths and weaknesses can help you build healthy self-esteem. Explain why this may be true.
14. What does having integrity mean?
15. What is a mentor?
16. List eight things you can do to boost your self-esteem.
17. What is physical self-concept?

Analyzing Ideas

18 Can the media affect a person's self-esteem? Explain your answer.

19 Why is it healthier to have high self-esteem rather than low self-esteem?

20 Explain how a classmate who teases you may affect your self-esteem.

21 How does your overall self-concept develop?

22 Why do you think you are the most important influence on your self-esteem?

Making Good Decisions

23 Use what you have learned in this chapter to set a personal goal. Write your goal, and make an action plan by using the Health Behavior Contract for building healthy self-esteem. You can find the Health Behavior Contract at go.hrw.com. Just type in the keyword HD4HBC05.

Name _____ Class _____ Date _____
(Health Behavior Contract)
Building Self-Esteem _____

My Goals: I, _____, will accomplish one or more of the following goals:
I will build a higher level of self-esteem.
I will make the three keys of self-esteem part of my character.
I will concentrate on my strengths and make a plan to overcome my weaknesses.
Other: _____

My Reasons: By improving my self-esteem, I will improve my overall character and attitude. I will feel good about myself as a person, and I will have more confidence.
Other: _____

My Values: Personal values that will help me meet my goals are
_____
_____
_____

My Plan: The actions I will take to meet my goals are
_____
_____
_____

Evaluation: I will use my Health Journal to keep a log of actions I took to fulfill this contract. After 1 month, I will evaluate my goals. I will adjust my plan if my goals are not being met. If my goals are being met, I will consider setting additional goals.
Signed _____
Date _____

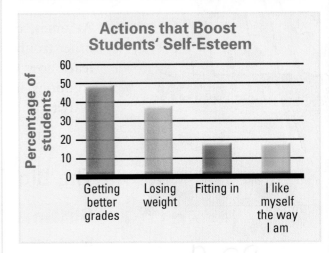

Actions that Boost Students' Self-Esteem

Use the figure above to answer questions 24–26.

24 Several teenagers were interviewed for a survey. The graph above shows the results of the survey. According to the graph, what percentage of teens like themselves as they are?

25 Which of the actions above would make the most teens feel better about themselves?

26 If 200,000 teens were interviewed for this survey, how many students feel that losing weight will help them feel better about themselves?

Reading Checkup

Take a minute to review your answers to the Health IQ questions at the beginning of this chapter. How has reading this chapter improved your Health IQ?

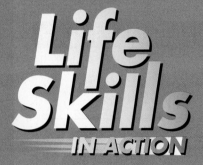

Coping

At times, everyone faces setbacks, disappointments, or other troubles. To deal with these problems, you have to learn how to cope. Coping is dealing with problems and emotions in an effective way. Complete the following activity to develop your coping skills.

The Big Test

Setting the Scene

Brent has never been a great student in science, but he always works hard enough to get a passing grade. This year, however, Brent is enjoying his science class and is determined to earn a B or better in it. He had his first big test in the class on Friday, and he studied very hard for it. Unfortunately, when Brent gets his test back, he learns that he failed it and is crushed. Brent decides to discuss his grade with his science teacher after school.

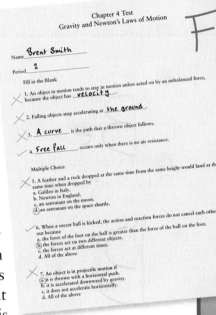

ACT 1

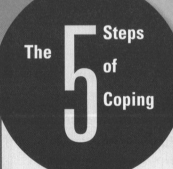

The 5 Steps of Coping

1. Identify the problem.
2. Identify your emotions.
3. Use positive self-talk.
4. Find ways to resolve the problem.
5. Talk to others to receive support.

Guided Practice

Practice with a Friend

Form a group of three. Have one person play the role of Brent and another person play the role of Brent's science teacher. Have the third person be an observer. Walking through each of the five steps of coping, role-play Brent dealing with his failing test grade. Brent can talk to his teacher to receive support. The observer will take notes, which will include observations about what the person playing Brent did well and suggestions of ways to improve. Stop after each step to evaluate the process.

Check Yourself

After you have completed the guided practice, go through Act 1 again without stopping at each step. Answer the questions below to review what you did.

1. What emotions could Brent have after learning what his grade on the test was?

2. What positive self-talk could Brent use to help him cope with his emotions?

3. What are some ways that Brent can resolve his problem?

4. How do you cope when you don't do as well as you had hoped on a test?

ACT 2

On Your Own

With the help of some study tips from his teacher, Brent is able to do better in science. However, to raise his grade, Brent has to spend a lot of time studying. Brent's friends are unhappy because he doesn't spend much time with them anymore. Some of his friends have started calling him a nerd and a teacher's pet. Brent doesn't like the teasing, but his friends won't leave him alone. Write a skit in which Brent uses the five steps of coping to deal with the teasing and name-calling.

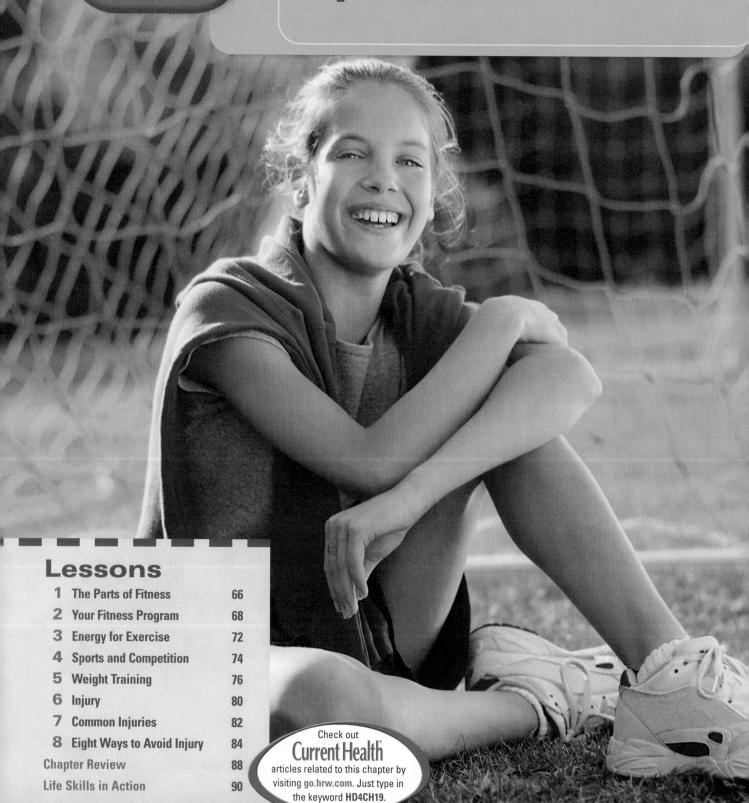

CHAPTER 4

Physical Fitness

Check out **Current Health** articles related to this chapter by visiting **go.hrw.com**. Just type in the keyword **HD4CH19**.

> " I thought I was **pretty fit** until my gym teacher had me do some **fitness tests.** I found out that I **wasn't as fit** as I thought!
>
> My teacher helped me make a fitness plan. It can be hard to stick to sometimes. But I can already tell that I'm getting healthier! "

Health IQ

PRE-READING

Answer the following multiple-choice questions to find out what you already know about physical fitness. When you've finished this chapter, you'll have an opportunity to change your answers based on what you've learned.

1. Which of the following best describes physical fitness?
   a. the ability to do everyday tasks without feeling tired
   b. any physical activity that improves your ability to complete tasks
   c. the way that your body adapts to the stress of exercise
   d. none of the above

2. Which of the following is a component of physical fitness?
   a. strength
   b. body composition
   c. flexibility
   d. all of the above

3. When you get regular exercise, your resting heart rate
   a. increases.
   b. stays the same.
   c. decreases.
   d. None of the above

4. ___ helps you stay safe when you lift weights.
   a. Using machines
   b. Being a spotter
   c. Using proper form
   d. Lifting alone

5. A ____ helps you if you can't finish a lift.
   a. bodybuilder
   b. spotter
   c. weight lifter
   d. good sport

6. Which of the following is NOT a warning sign of injury?
   a. achiness that goes away when you warm up
   b. tenderness in a single area
   c. muscle weakness
   d. numbness or tingling

7. All of the following are weight-training exercises EXCEPT
   a. bench press.
   b. hamstring curl.
   c. sit and reach.
   d. lunge.

ANSWERS: 1. a; 2. d; 3. c; 4. c; 5. b; 6. a; 7. c

The Parts of Fitness

What You'll Do

- **Describe** four parts of physical fitness.

Terms to Learn

- physical fitness
- strength
- endurance
- flexibility

Start Off
Write

How do you know when you are physically fit?

Sasha thought dance class would be easy. The class is actually a lot of work. But Sasha knows that she is stronger and more flexible since she started taking the class.

Dance is one of many activities that can improve physical fitness. **Physical fitness** is the ability to do everyday activities without becoming short of breath, sore, or tired. Four parts of fitness are strength, endurance (en DOOR uhns), flexibility (FLEKS uh BIL uh tee), and body composition (KAHM puh ZISH uhn).

Strength

The amount of force that muscles apply when they are used is called **strength.** Strength can be measured by the amount of weight you can lift. You use strength when you lift boxes or push a lawn mower. Strong muscles support bones and joints. Strength also helps prevent injury. Strength can help your body deal with accidents, such as falls.

Endurance

The ability to do activities for more than a few minutes is called **endurance.** There are two types of endurance. Muscular endurance is the ability of your muscles to keep working over time. The ability of your heart and lungs to work efficiently during physical activity is the other type of endurance. Heart and lung endurance keeps you from becoming short of breath.

Figure 1 Paddling a boat uses both strength and endurance.

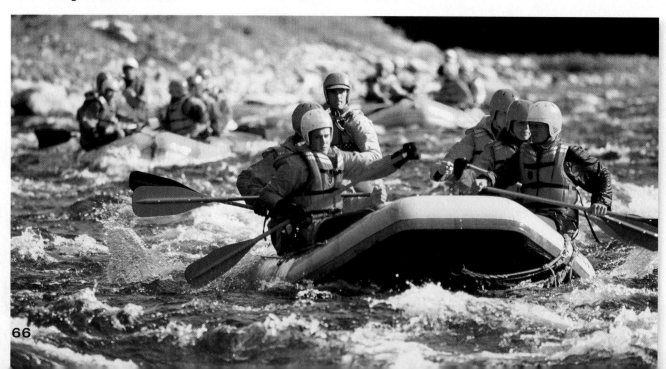

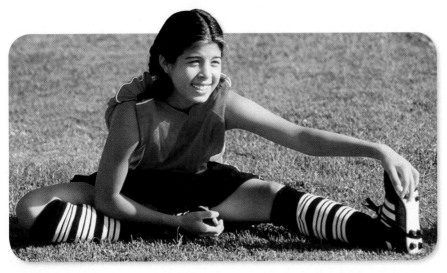

Figure 2 Stretching prevents injury by improving flexibility.

Flexibility

The ability to bend and twist joints easily is called **flexibility.** You use flexibility when you bend down, twist your body, or reach for something. If you are flexible, you are less likely to get hurt during physical activities. To improve your flexibility, you can stretch regularly. *Stretching* is any activity that loosens muscles and joints.

Body Composition

Fat plays an important role in how your body works. However, too much fat may lead to disease. It can also make improving your physical fitness harder. *Body composition* compares the weight of your fat to the weight of your muscles, bones, and organs. Physical activity can improve body composition. It helps your body burn fat.

Myth & Fact

Myth: If you are thin, you are fit.

Fact: Body composition is only one part of physical fitness. If you are thin but do not have good strength, endurance, or flexibility, you are not fit.

Lesson Review

Using Vocabulary

1. Use each of the following terms in a separate sentence: *physical fitness, strength, endurance,* and *flexibility.*

Understanding Concepts

2. What are two types of endurance?

3. What does body composition compare?

4. What part of fitness are you using when you stretch? when you carry your books?

Critical Thinking

5. Applying Concepts Josh plays basketball with his friends almost every day. He can run for most of the game. But he can't touch his toes. What part of fitness does Josh need to improve?

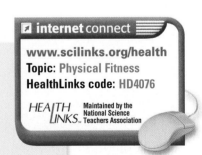

internet connect

www.scilinks.org/health
Topic: Physical Fitness
HealthLinks code: HD4076

HEALTH LINKS. Maintained by the National Science Teachers Association

Your Fitness Program

Henry has a friend who gets tired walking up a flight of stairs. When they get to the top, Henry has to wait while his friend catches his breath. His friend isn't overweight, but Henry knows that he doesn't go outside much.

Walking up a flight of stairs may not seem like hard work. But for people with poor physical fitness, it can be difficult. In this lesson, you'll learn how you can stay fit.

Why Should You Exercise?

It's pretty easy to spend a lot of time watching TV or using a computer. However, if you spend too much time doing these activities, your fitness could suffer. Regular exercise is important. **Exercise** is any physical activity that maintains or improves fitness. Exercise isn't just jumping jacks and push-ups. The sports you play for fun are also exercise.

Lack of exercise can make doing everyday tasks hard. You might become short of breath easily. Poor fitness can also make dealing with stress more difficult. People who don't get regular exercise increase their chances of diseases such as heart disease, diabetes, and obesity. So, people who don't exercise enough may not live as long.

What You'll Do

- **Explain** why you should exercise.
- **List** healthy fitness standards for your age group.
- **List** five things that affect your fitness goals.
- **Describe** how increasing frequency, intensity, and time of exercise affects fitness.
- **Estimate** your target heart rate zone.

Terms to Learn

- exercise
- resting heart rate (RHR)
- recovery time

Start Off *Write*

Why is it important for you to exercise regularly?

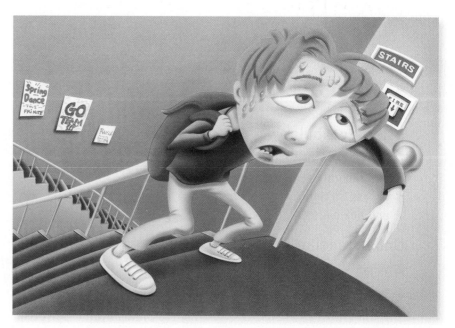

Figure 3 Regular exercise can help prevent shortness of breath.

Testing Your Fitness

When you take a test, you find out how well you know what you were taught. A test can tell you what your strengths and weaknesses are. Then, you can work on your weaknesses to get better. There are also ways to test your physical fitness. Knowing your fitness weaknesses can help you plan to improve your fitness.

There are simple tests for each part of fitness. For example, pull-ups and curl-ups test strength and muscular endurance. The 1-mile run tests heart and lung endurance. The sit-and-reach test measures flexibility.

The table below lists healthy fitness zones for your age group. You should try to meet these fitness standards. If you can meet the lower standard for each zone, then you are doing pretty well. If you meet the higher standard, then your fitness is great! People who are interested in playing sports usually need to reach the higher end of each fitness zone. If you are having trouble meeting any of the fitness standards, talk to your teacher or to your parents. They can help you come up with a plan to improve your fitness.

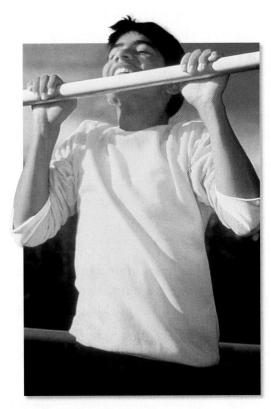

Figure 4 Pull-ups test your strength and muscular endurance.

TABLE 1 Healthy Fitness Zones for Ages 12 to 14				
Activity		**12**	**13**	**14**
Pull-ups	Boys	1–3	1–4	2–5
	Girls	1–2	1–2	1–2
Curl-ups	Boys	18–36	21–40	24–45
	Girls	18–32	18–32	18–32
1-mile run (minutes and seconds)	Boys	10:30–8:00	10:00–7:30	9:30–7:00
	Girls	12:00–9:00	11:30–9:00	11:00–8:30
Sit and reach (inches)	Boys	8	8	8
	Girls	10	10	10

Your Fitness Goals

Even if you meet healthy fitness standards, it is a good idea to set fitness goals. Setting short-term goals can help you meet a long-term goal.

The activities that you enjoy, your abilities, and the amount of work you want to do can influence your fitness goals. Your goals will also be influenced by how important fitness is to you and the people around you. Finally, there's always a chance you might get hurt during exercise. As you set goals, you need to balance risks against benefits.

A good place to start is to see a doctor. The doctor can make sure it is safe for you to exercise. Also, the doctor may be able to help you with your fitness goals.

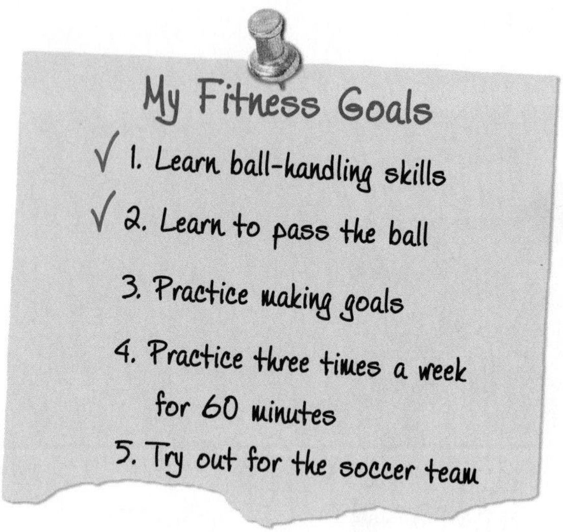

My Fitness Goals

✓ 1. Learn ball-handling skills

✓ 2. Learn to pass the ball

3. Practice making goals

4. Practice three times a week for 60 minutes

5. Try out for the soccer team

Figure 5 Setting short-term goals can make reaching a long-term goal easier.

FIT

Exercise improves your fitness. However, unless you exercise more over time, your fitness will stop improving. You can influence how quickly your fitness improves by changing three things:

- Frequency refers to how often you exercise. If you exercise more often, your fitness can improve faster.
- Intensity refers to how hard you exercise. Exercising harder can make you stronger. It can also improve endurance.
- Time is how long you exercise. If you spend more time exercising, your fitness can improve.

One way to remember frequency, intensity, and time is to remember that the first letters of the words spell *FIT*. To avoid injury, don't increase more than one part of FIT at a time. Also, don't increase any one part of FIT too much. Your teacher or parents can help you change parts of FIT safely.

LIFE SKILLS ACTIVITY

PRACTICING WELLNESS

Some people keep a fitness log when they exercise. They write down what activity they did, how long they did it, and how they felt during their activity. Try keeping a fitness log for 2 weeks. What are your goals? Do you think you are exercising often enough, hard enough, and long enough to improve your fitness? What parts of FIT do you think you need to change to meet your fitness goals?

Monitoring Your Heart Rate

One way to see how hard you are exercising is to check your heart rate. Heart rate is the number of times your heart beats per minute. The easiest places to check your heart rate are on your neck and wrist. Use your index and middle fingers to find your heartbeat. Count heartbeats for 10 seconds. Multiply by 6 to find your heart rate.

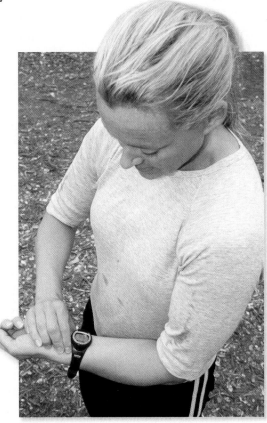

Figure 6 Monitoring your heart rate can help you meet your fitness goals.

If you exercise hard enough to improve fitness, you will be in your target heart rate zone. The *target heart rate zone* is 60 percent to 85 percent of your maximum heart rate. *Maximum heart rate (MHR)* is the largest number of times your heart can beat per minute while you exercise. You can use the following equations to estimate your target heart rate zone:

$$MHR = 220 - age$$
$$60\% \text{ of } MHR = MHR \times 0.6$$
$$85\% \text{ of } MHR = MHR \times 0.85$$

For example, a 13-year-old's target heart rate zone is about 124 to 176 beats per minute.

The number of times your heart beats per minute when you are not exercising is called your **resting heart rate (RHR).** RHR decreases as you become more fit. RHR decreases because your heart is stronger. **Recovery time** is the amount of time your heart takes to return to its RHR after exercising. As your fitness improves, your recovery time gets shorter.

Lesson Review

Using Vocabulary

1. What is exercise?

Understanding Concepts

2. List healthy fitness standards for a 12-year-old girl.

3. Name five things that affect your fitness goals.

4. Calculate your target heart rate zone.

Critical Thinking

5. **Making Predictions** If Tanya joins the track team, what may happen to her resting heart rate? to her recovery time?

6. **Applying Concepts** Alejandro isn't doing as well at basketball as he wants. If Alejandro wants to run faster and longer during basketball games, how can he use FIT to do so?

Energy for Exercise

A world-champion sprinter can run 100 meters in less than 10 seconds. But can a sprinter run a marathon in an hour?

What You'll Do

- **Compare** aerobic and anaerobic exercise.
- **Describe** when the body uses aerobic and anaerobic energy.

Terms to Learn

- aerobic
- anaerobic

Start Off
Write

Why can't a sprinter keep up his or her pace for an entire marathon?

A sprinter can't run a marathon in an hour. The sprinter would run out of energy before he or she could finish. Sprinters and marathon runners use different energy systems when they run.

With and Without Oxygen

Your body gets energy from the food you eat. The sugars in foods, such as fruit and bread, are changed into a sugar called *glucose* (GLOO KOHS). Your body uses oxygen to get energy from glucose. When your body uses oxygen to get energy, the process is *aerobic* (er OH bik). **Aerobic exercise** is exercise that uses oxygen to get energy. Endurance exercises, such as long-distance running and swimming, are aerobic exercises.

Glycogen (GLIE kuh juhn) is another sugar made from the food you eat. Your body releases energy from glycogen without using oxygen. A process that doesn't use oxygen is *anaerobic* (AN uhr OH bik). Exercise that is fueled without using oxygen is **anaerobic exercise.** Activities that use strength in short bursts, such as sprinting, are anaerobic exercises. A small amount of glycogen is stored in your muscles. When glycogen runs out, you won't be able to keep going at the same pace. So, a sprinter can't run a marathon in an hour. The sprinter runs out of glycogen and has to slow down.

Figure 7 Sprinters use anaerobic energy, while marathon runners use aerobic energy.

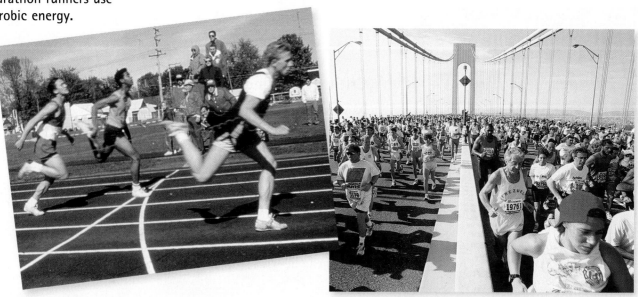

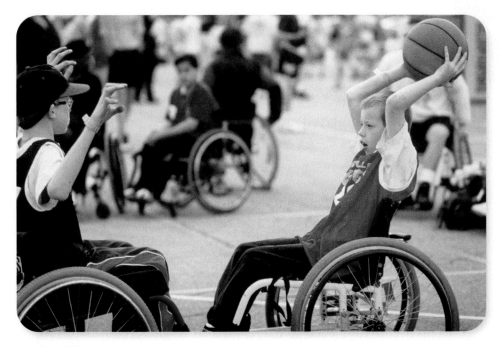

Figure 8 Many sports, such as basketball, require steady aerobic exercise with bursts of anaerobic exercise.

Working Together

How your body uses aerobic and anaerobic energy depends on what you do. For many activities, your body uses both types of energy. For example, tennis players use short bursts of strength when they serve or return a ball. So, they use anaerobic energy. But they also need to be able to play long games. Their bodies use aerobic energy to keep playing.

Fitness improves best if you do both aerobic and anaerobic exercise. Even if you want to do an aerobic exercise, such as distance running, anaerobic exercise can help you improve. Anaerobic exercises, such as sprinting and weight lifting, can improve your strength. Many people who do anaerobic exercise also do aerobic exercise. For example, a sprinter sometimes runs longer distances. This aerobic exercise helps a sprinter practice longer and more efficiently.

> **Health Journal**
>
> Make a list of 10 physical activities. Identify which activities rely on aerobic energy and which rely on anaerobic energy. If an activity uses both types of energy, identify when it uses each.

Lesson Review

Using Vocabulary

1. Compare aerobic and anaerobic exercise.

Understanding Concepts

2. Why can't a sprinter run a marathon in an hour?

Critical Thinking

3. **Identifying Relationships** Theo's track coach wants Theo to run a couple of miles during practice. Theo doesn't know why. He is usually a sprinter. Why would Theo's coach want him to run long distances?

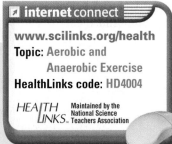

internet connect

www.scilinks.org/health
Topic: Aerobic and
    Anaerobic Exercise
HealthLinks code: HD4004

HEALTH LINKS. Maintained by the National Science Teachers Association

Sports and Competition

Rob likes to race on his bicycle. He hasn't won a race, but he still has fun. Rob has even started riding his bike more often. He knows that if he improves his fitness, he might do better at a race.

What You'll Do

■ **Describe** five characteristics of someone who is a good sport.

■ **List** two places to start playing sports.

Terms to Learn

• competition

• sportsmanship

Start Off
Write

What is a good sport?

A bicycle race is a competition. A **competition** is a contest between two or more people or teams. For people like Rob, competition can help them improve fitness. But Rob knows that winning isn't everything. Competition should also be fun!

Competition and Sportsmanship

Have you ever seen a player yell at a game official during a game? Or, have you seen a fight take place at a game? These people weren't practicing sportsmanship. **Sportsmanship** is the ability to treat all players, officials, and fans fairly during competition. Someone who practices sportsmanship is called a *good sport*. A good sports always plays his or her best. A good sport follows the rules of the game. He or she also considers the safety of the other players. A good sport congratulates players for a good job, even if they are on a different team. Finally, a good sport is polite if he or she loses and modest if he or she wins. Sportsmanship makes competition more fun for players, fans, and officials.

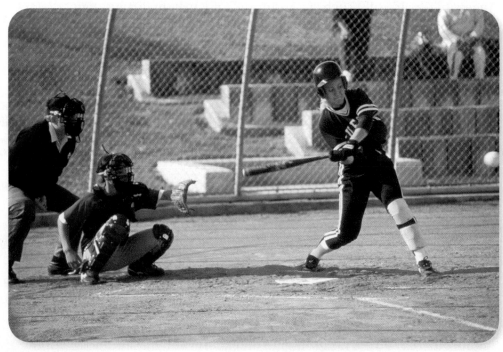

Figure 9 Competition can push you to get fitter and better at your sport.

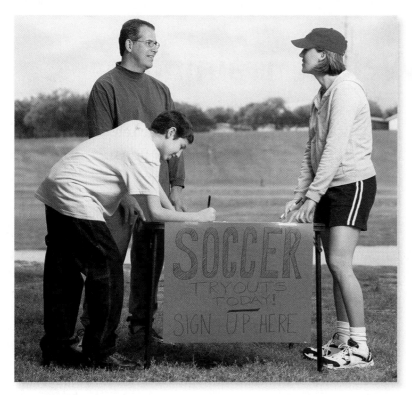

Figure 10 Community organizations sponsor many youth sports.

Getting Started in Sports

You may try several sports in the next few years. You'll probably pick sports that are interesting and fun. Try several sports before deciding which you like most. You may find a new sport that you really like.

Schools and community organizations often have sports teams and clubs. These teams give you a chance to get in shape or to compete against other people. Teams also provide a lot of the equipment you'll need to play your sport. Players are usually organized by age and skill level. Some sports teams may ask you to visit a doctor. A doctor can tell you if it's safe for you to play. Check with your school or local parks and recreation department to find out how you can start playing sports.

Myth & Fact

Myth: Winning isn't everything. It's the only thing.

Fact: This myth comes from misquoting Vince Lombardi, a famous football coach. What Coach Lombardi actually said was that winning isn't everything but that wanting to win is. He believed that we should always do our best.

Lesson Review

Using Vocabulary

1. What is competition?

Understanding Concepts

2. What are five characteristics of a good sport?

3. List two places to start playing sports.

Critical Thinking

4. Using Refusal Skills Katya has a friend who plays roughly and knocks people down during soccer games. Katya's friend wants Katya to do the same thing. How should Katya handle the situation?

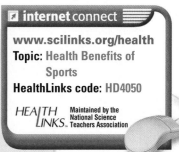

internet connect

www.scilinks.org/health
Topic: Health Benefits of Sports
HealthLinks code: HD4050

HEALTH
LINKS Maintained by the National Science Teachers Association

Weight Training

Todd wants to lift weights to get in shape. But he doesn't want huge muscles. His coach said that lifting weights doesn't always build big muscles.

What You'll Do

■ **Describe** two types of weight training.

■ **Compare** free weights and machines.

■ **List** seven safety tips for lifting weights.

■ **Describe** four weight-training exercises.

Terms to Learn

• weight training

Start Off
Write

Does everyone who lifts weights develop big muscles? Why or why not?

Sometimes, people lift weights to get bigger muscles. But Todd's coach is right. Weight training can improve strength without making muscles bigger. **Weight training** is the use of weight to make muscles stronger or bigger. Weight training improves strength and muscular endurance.

Types of Weight Training

There are two basic kinds of weight training: strength development and bodybuilding. How you lift weights depends on your fitness goals. Some people, like Todd, want to strengthen their muscles without making them bigger. Other people spend a lot of time making their bodies stronger and their muscles bigger. These people are bodybuilders. A bodybuilder usually lifts more weight, does fewer repetitions, and does a different number of sets than someone who doesn't want big muscles. *Repetitions* are the number of times you do an exercise. A *set* is a group of repetitions.

For some people, it doesn't matter how much they lift weights. They will have a hard time getting big muscles. For other people, developing big muscles is very easy. In fact, increasing muscle size is usually easier for boys than it is for girls. To get bigger muscles, female bodybuilders follow very specific weight-training programs.

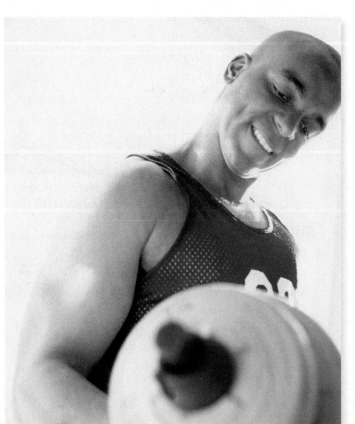

Figure 11 Biceps curls are one way to strengthen the upper arm.

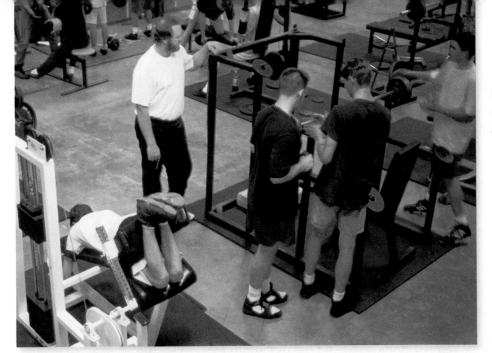

Figure 12 A variety of machines and free weights are used in weight training.

Equipment

There are two types of weight-training equipment: free weights and machines. Free weights include dumbbells, barbells, and curl bars. To use free weights, you add weight to an empty bar and secure the weight with a collar. You can usually do a greater variety of exercises with free weights than with machines. Machines use a system of pulleys to let you control the weight as you lift it. Machines are designed for a specific muscle group. The number of exercises you can do with a machine is often limited. But a machine ensures that a specific muscle group is exercised correctly.

Safety

Safety is very important. To lift weights safely, you should follow several simple rules:

- Use a spotter. A spotter is someone who can take weight away if you can't finish a lift.

- Lift weights in pairs or in small groups. Take turns to rest.

- Make sure that free weights are secured to the bar.

- Make sure you understand how a machine works. Adjust machines to your size.

- Lift only as much weight as you can lift with the correct form.

- Exercise both sides of a joint to prevent injury. For example, if you exercise your chest, you should exercise your shoulders.

- Always use correct form. If necessary, use a weight belt to support your back. But a weight belt is never a substitute for good form.

SCIENCE ACTIVITY

Weight training can be divided into three types of exercises: *isotonic* (IE soh TAHN ik), *isometric* (IE soh MET rik), and *isokinetic* (IE soh ki NET ik). Research the three types of weight-training exercises. Create a poster defining each type and describing how each type affects muscles.

Figure 13 Some Weight-Training Exercises

Bench press

1 Don't start lifting until your spotter is ready. Lift the bar from the supports until your hands are above your shoulders. Keep a very slight bend in your elbows.

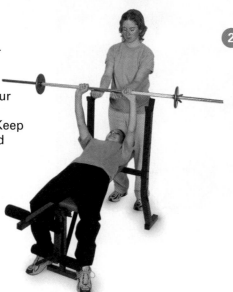

2 Lower the bar until it barely touches your chest. Push it back up to the start position, and lower it again until you finish your repetitions. Don't lock your elbows. This exercise works your chest muscles.

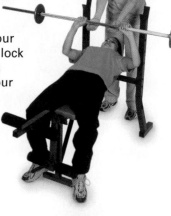

Biceps curl

1 With your hands about shoulder-width apart, start with your arm slightly bent or at a 90° angle. Be sure not to lock your elbow.

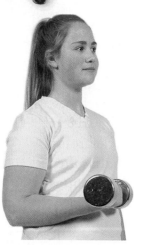

2 Curl up your arm toward your shoulder. Lower the dumbbell, and repeat the curl-up. Exercise both arms. This exercise works the biceps muscle in the front of your upper arm.

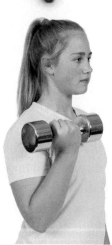

Getting Started

It is important to lift weights correctly. If your form is wrong, you can hurt yourself. You may also make it less likely for your muscles to get stronger. To ensure that you're lifting correctly, ask someone who knows. Ask a physical education teacher, coach, or fitness trainer. Any of these people can show you how to do the exercises correctly. They can also help you set goals for your training. And they can tell you which exercises will help you reach those goals. They may also suggest that you talk to your doctor first. Visiting your doctor before starting an exercise program is a good idea.

Weight training often starts with exercises that use body weight to make muscles stronger. These exercises include push-ups, pull-ups, and curl-ups. These exercises get your body ready to use free weights and machines.

Lunge

1 Start with your feet shoulder-width apart. Hold dumbbells at your sides.

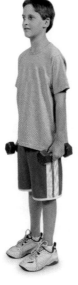

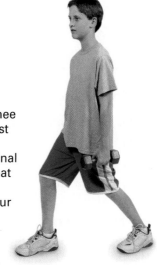

2 Step forward. Make sure your knee doesn't extend past your ankle. Step back into the original position, and repeat the lunge. This exercise works your thigh muscles.

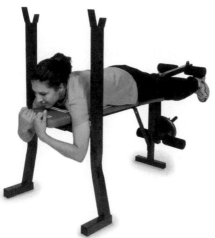

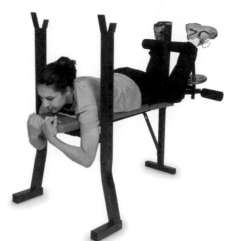

Hamstring curl

1 Make sure the bench is adjusted for your size. Put your ankles under the padded bar, and hold onto the bench for support.

2 Bending at the knee, pull up your feet. Then, lower your legs. Keep movements slow and controlled for the best workout. This exercise works the hamstrings, the muscles in the back of your leg.

Lesson Review

Using Vocabulary

1. What is weight training?

Understanding Concepts

2. How do free weights and machines differ?

3. What are seven safety tips for lifting weights?

4. Describe four weight-training exercises.

Critical Thinking

5. Making Inferences Georgia wants to start lifting weights. She wants to get stronger so that she can do better on the swim team. She really wants to focus on her arms and shoulders but worries about getting big muscles. Should she worry? Explain your answer.

Injury

What You'll Do

- **Describe** six warning signs of injury.
- **List** five signs of overtraining.

Terms to Learn

- overtraining

Start Off Write

How can you tell if you have a sports injury?

Kelly twisted her ankle during practice. She didn't want to tell her coach. But the ankle became swollen and bruised. She didn't want to stop playing, but the ankle was too painful.

There is a chance of injury whenever you exercise. Your chances of injury increase if you exercise often. You should watch for warning signs of injury. Swelling, bruising, and pain were signs that Kelly was hurt. So, she should stop playing.

Warning Signs of Injury

You should not experience pain when you exercise. Pain is an indication of injury. Six common warning signs of injury are

- sharp pain
- tenderness in a single area
- swelling
- a reduced range of motion around a joint
- muscle weakness
- numbness or tingling

Don't mistake muscle soreness for an injury. *Muscle soreness* is achiness that happens a day or two after hard exercise. It is normal. Muscle soreness usually goes away the next time you exercise. However, pay attention to muscle soreness that turns into sharp pain. If you experience any of the warning signs of injury, tell your parents or teacher. You may need to see a doctor.

Health Journal

Write about a time when you were injured or thought you were injured. Describe what you did to treat the injury.

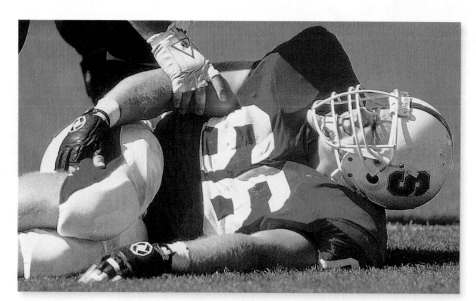

Figure 14 Pain is one sign of injury.

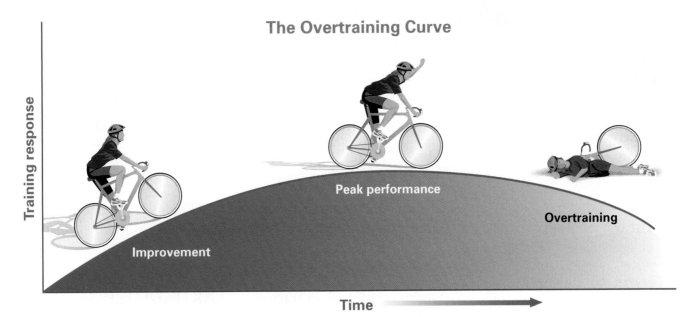

The Overtraining Curve

Training response

Peak performance

Overtraining

Improvement

Time

Overtraining

Most people need to exercise only three to four times a week. However, some people exercise too much. **Overtraining** is a condition that happens when you exercise too much. To recover from overtraining, people need to take a break from exercise. The following are signs of overtraining:

- You feel tired all the time.
- You aren't doing as well during games and practice.
- You are less interested in the activity. You start making excuses to avoid practice.
- Your resting heart rate increases.
- You may get hurt more often. Your body hasn't had a chance to heal from past injuries.

Figure 15 Once you have trained to your peak performance, more training may lead to overtraining.

Lesson Review

Using Vocabulary

1. What is overtraining?

Understanding Concepts

2. What are six warning signs of injury, and how do they compare with muscle soreness?

3. Why does someone who has overtrained experience more injuries?

Critical Thinking

4. Making Good Decisions Connie has been playing soccer 6 days a week. She has had some injuries in the past, but doesn't have any right now. However, she feels tired a lot. She is also not playing as well as she usually does. What do you think she should do?

Common Injuries

Li hurt a muscle in his thigh during a volleyball game. The injury was really painful, and he had trouble using his leg. He told his mom. She made him stop playing until the muscle healed.

Li suffered from an acute (uh KYOOT) injury. An **acute injury** is an injury that happens suddenly.

Acute Injuries

Strains, sprains, and fractures (FRAK churz) are three types of acute injuries. A *strain* happens when a muscle or tendon is overstretched or torn. A tendon is tissue that attaches a muscle to a bone. Strains are painful. The injured area may feel weak. *Sprains* happen when a joint is twisted suddenly. The ligaments (LIG uh muhnts) that connect the bones in the joint are stretched or torn. Sprains are painful and usually cause swelling. A *fracture* is a cracked or broken bone. A fracture is painful. The injured area can feel weak, can swell, and can bruise.

You should report an acute injury to your parents or teacher right away. You may need to see a doctor. First aid includes rest, ice, compression, and elevation. These steps reduce swelling and pain. You rest the injured limb. Then, you put ice on it. You compress the injury by wrapping it in bandages. Finally, you elevate the injury on a chair or stool. To remember rest, ice, compression, and elevation, remember that the first letters of the words spell *RICE*.

What You'll Do

■ **Describe** acute and chronic sports injuries.

■ **List** three examples of acute injuries.

■ **List** two examples of chronic injuries.

Terms to Learn

• acute injury

• chronic injury

Start Off

Write

What causes chronic injuries?

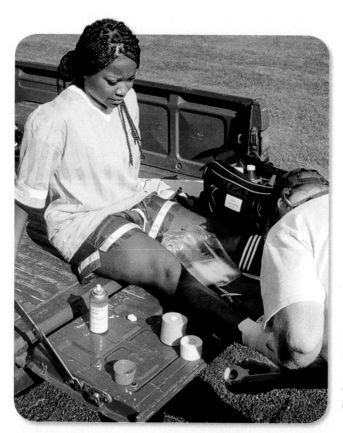

Figure 16 RICE reduces swelling and pain. This girl is using compression and elevation to ease the pain of her injury.

Chronic Injuries

Not all injuries happen suddenly. A **chronic injury** is an injury that develops over a long period of time. Two examples of chronic injuries are stress fractures and tendinitis. A stress fracture is a tiny fracture. Tendinitis is an irritation of a tendon. Increasing physical activity too quickly or exercising too much can cause chronic injuries. They can also happen when you use the wrong equipment or exercise on uneven surfaces.

Your doctor should treat chronic injuries. He or she may ask you to do special exercises. Otherwise, the best treatment for chronic injuries is usually rest. Some chronic injuries can take a few months to heal fully.

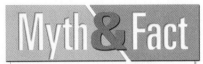

Myth: More exercise is better.

Fact: Too much exercise can lead to chronic injuries. To avoid injury, set reasonable goals and listen to your body when you exercise.

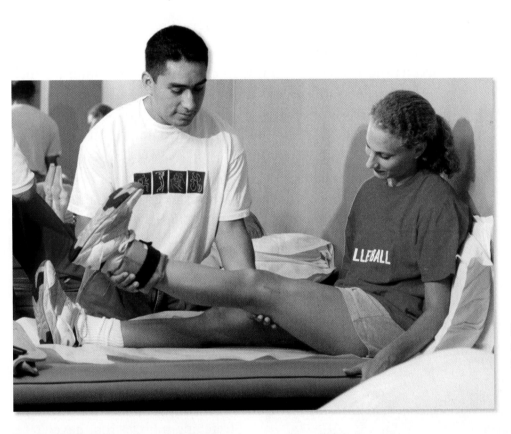

Figure 17 To recover from a chronic injury, you may need to do special exercises.

Lesson Review

Using Vocabulary

1. Compare acute and chronic injuries.

Understanding Concepts

2. What type of injury is a sprain? What type of injury is tendinitis?

Critical Thinking

3. Making Inferences Larissa has been running for three months. Recently, she noticed that her knee hurts. If she has new shoes and has been running on even surfaces, what could have caused her injury?

internet connect
www.scilinks.org/health
Topic: Sports Injury
HealthLinks code: HD4093
HEALTH LINKS Maintained by the National Science Teachers Association

Eight Ways to Avoid Injury

Have you ever seen someone get hurt during a football game or basketball game? If you do physical activities, there is always a chance that you will get hurt.

In this lesson, you will learn eight ways to lower your chances of getting hurt during physical activities.

Warm Up and Cool Down

A *warm-up* is any activity that gets you ready for exercise. Exercising without warming up can lead to acute injuries, such as strains. A warm-up loosens your muscles and increases your heart rate. A warm-up also prepares you mentally for the activity. Walking, jogging, or jumping rope are common warm-ups. You should warm up until you break a light sweat.

A *cool-down* helps the body return to normal after exercise. During a cool-down, the heart returns to its resting rate. A cool-down also keeps muscles from getting tight and sore. Like warm-ups, cool-downs are activities such as jogging or walking.

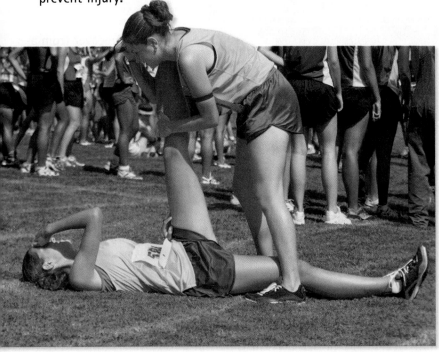

Figure 18 Stretching helps prevent injury.

Stretch

Stretching improves flexibility and may help prevent injury. Stretching relaxes muscles and improves how far your joints can move. You should stretch only after a warm-up or cool-down. Stretching muscles that haven't been warmed up can lead to strains. Many people stretch as part of their cool-downs. Stretch slowly, and do not bounce. Once you feel a mild stretch in a muscle, hold your position. Stretches should be held for about 10 to 30 seconds. Don't hold a stretch if it hurts.

Don't Go Too Fast

To improve your physical fitness, you need to change the frequency, intensity, and time of your workouts. However, increasing these three things too much or too soon can lead to injury. It's also a bad idea to increase all three at once.

If you exercise too frequently, your body doesn't have time to recover between workouts. So you may develop a chronic injury. Increasing intensity too much can make you work too hard or do an exercise wrong. Long workouts cause injury when the body gets too tired to deal with the impact of exercise. You can also lose focus and have an accident. These situations increase your risk of injury.

Improve Your Form

Sometimes, the way you do a physical activity can lead to injury. Poor form can cause injury over time. For example, many runners get stress fractures or tendinitis because they have poor form. Poor form puts more stress on muscles, bones, and joints. Improving your form can keep you from getting hurt.

Weight lifters and dancers use mirrors to watch their form. For other activities, a coach or trainer can make suggestions for improvement. A training partner can watch what you do and tell you how you're doing. It takes a lot of practice to learn how to use the correct form. But improving your form can keep you from getting hurt. It may also help you do better in a sport or activity.

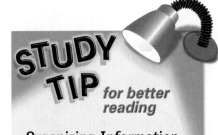

STUDY TIP *for better reading*

Organizing Information
A *mnemonic device* (nee MAHN ik di VIES) is a word or phrase that can help you remember long lists. Sometimes, you can make a word using the first letter of each word or phrase in a list. If you can't make a word, try inventing a silly phrase that uses the first letter of each word in the list. Create a mnemonic device to remember the eight ways to avoid injury!

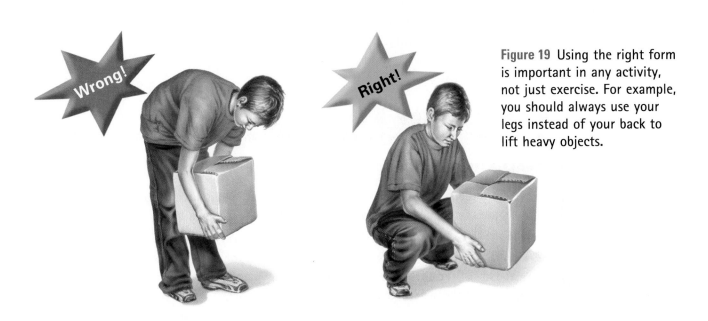

Figure 19 Using the right form is important in any activity, not just exercise. For example, you should always use your legs instead of your back to lift heavy objects.

Take a Break

Rest and recovery are important parts of a fitness program. Getting enough rest gives the body time to repair itself. You should plan rest along with exercise in your fitness program.

You don't have to stop all physical activity to rest. **Active rest** is a way to recover from exercise by reducing the amount of activity you do. Active rest lets your body repair itself. A good fitness program will alternate between hard exercise and active rest. If you plan well, you can avoid overtraining and chronic injuries.

Wear the Right Clothes

Almost every physical activity has special clothing. Most physical activities require clothing that lets you move easily. The right clothing will make you more comfortable as you play. It may also protect you from getting hurt.

Don't forget about the weather when you choose what to wear. Special fabrics keep you warm for cold-weather activities. Other fabrics keep you cool in warm weather. For many warm-weather activities, all you need is shorts and a T-shirt. But, if it's cold, you should dress in layers. Use a hat, sunglasses, and sunscreen to protect yourself from sunburn, even on cloudy days. This tip is very important if you're at the beach or hiking in the mountains.

Shoes are one of the most important pieces of clothing you will use for some activities. Wearing shoes that don't fit correctly or aren't designed for your sport can lead to injury. Most sports shoe stores will have the right shoe for what you do.

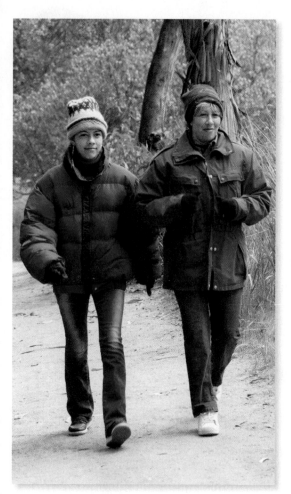

Figure 20 Be sure to wear warm clothes and layers on a cold day!

LIFE SKILLS ACTIVITY

EVALUATING MEDIA MESSAGES

1. Search through popular magazines and Internet sites for an advertisement that uses physical activity to attract customers.

2. How is the physical activity related to this product? If the physical activity is not related, why is the advertiser using it?

3. What age group do you think the advertiser is trying to attract? Why?

4. Is the physical activity being done safely in the ad? If not, what is missing? Why might advertisers leave out safety equipment?

5. Would you buy this product? Why or why not?

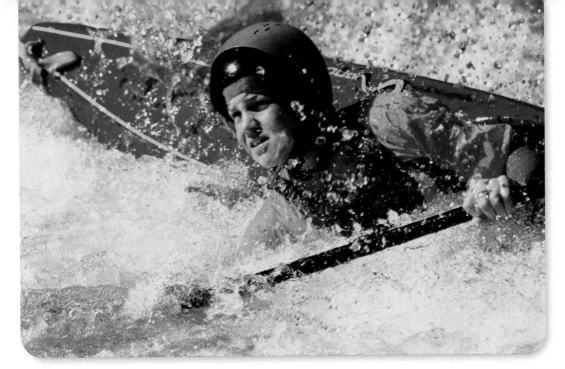

Figure 21 Safety equipment helps protect you from injury during activities.

Use Your Safety Equipment

Many sports have safety equipment. Safety equipment helps protect you from injury. You should always use your safety equipment. For sports such as football and hockey, falls and collisions are common. So, it's dangerous not to use safety equipment. For other activities, accidents happen when you don't expect them. Safety equipment increases enjoyment of physical activities by lowering your chances of injury.

Don't Exercise Alone

Exercising with friends is a good way to protect yourself in case of an accident. If you get hurt and no one is around to help you, an injury can become life threatening. Friends can also make physical activity more exciting. Friends motivate you to continue exercising.

Lesson Review

Using Vocabulary

1. What is active rest?

Understanding Concepts

2. What could happen if you changed the frequency, intensity, and time of your workouts too much? Explain your answer.

3. If someone has poor form, what might happen?

Critical Thinking

4. Making Good Decisions Imagine that it's a cold, sunny day. What do you need to wear to protect yourself if you play soccer with your friends?

Chapter Summary

■ Physical fitness is the ability to do everyday activities without becoming short of breath, sore, or very tired. ■ Four parts of physical fitness are strength, endurance, flexibility, and body composition. ■ Exercise is any physical activity that maintains or improves physical fitness. ■ Frequency, intensity, and time of exercise can be adjusted to help improve fitness. ■ Aerobic exercise uses oxygen to get energy. ■ Anaerobic exercise doesn't use oxygen to get energy. ■ Competition is a contest between two or more people or teams. ■ Weight training is the use of weight to make muscles stronger or bigger. ■ Overtraining happens when someone exercises too much. ■ The two types of injury are acute injuries and chronic injuries.

Using Vocabulary

For each pair of terms, describe how the meanings of the terms differ.

1 aerobic exercise/anaerobic exercise

2 competition/sportsmanship

3 acute injury/chronic injury

For each sentence, fill in the blank with the proper word from the word bank provided below.

body composition	overtraining
active rest	endurance
recovery time	flexibility

4 ___ is a condition that happens when you exercise too much.

5 ___ is the ability to move joints easily.

6 ___ is the ability to do an activity for more than a few minutes.

7 ___ is the amount of time your heart takes to return to its resting heart rate after you exercise.

8 ___ is a fitness technique in which you rest by reducing the intensity of your physical activity.

Understanding Concepts

9 Describe four parts of physical fitness.

10 What five things influence your fitness goals?

11 How do you recognize a good sport?

12 How does weight training for strength development differ from bodybuilding?

13 List seven safety tips for weight training.

14 Describe two weight-training exercises for your upper body.

15 List five warning signs of overtraining.

16 List three examples of acute injuries and two examples of chronic injuries.

17 How does increasing frequency, intensity, and time of exercise affect fitness?

18 How do you avoid injury when changing the parts of FIT?

19 What is the target heart rate zone for a 13-year-old?

20 List eight ways to avoid injury while exercising.

21 How are resting heart rate and recovery time related?

Critical Thinking

Applying Concepts

22 Julio is 14 years old. He can do 6 pull-ups and 40 curl-ups. He can run a mile in a little over 7 minutes. He can also reach past 8 inches on the sit-and-reach test. Based on his results, do you think Julio can try out for the soccer team? Explain your answer.

23 Maria has decided to hike in the mountains by herself. Maria claims that she will be safe because no other people are on the trail. Why is hiking by herself a bad idea?

24 One way to avoid overtraining is to make sure that you get plenty of rest between workouts. What can you do to make sure that you get the rest you need?

Making Good Decisions

25 Your friend has been making excuses for not wanting to play basketball lately. When he does show up to practice, he doesn't play as hard as he used to, and he gets hurt easily. What should your friend do?

26 You played tennis with some friends for the first time last night. This morning, your muscles ached and felt sore. Should you play tennis again tonight? Explain your answer.

27 At the ice-skating rink, your friend shows you a jump that she just learned. But she falls as she lands. She seems to have sprained her ankle. What type of injury does she have? What can you do to help?

Interpreting Graphics

Fitness Test Results for Three 13-Year-Old Boys

Exercise	Boy A	Boy B	Boy C
Pull-ups	3	1	4
Curl-ups	35	20	42
1-mile run (minutes and seconds)	8:46	10:24	7:59
Sit and reach (inches)	6	8	9

Use the table above to answer questions 28–31.

28 Which boy has the best fitness? the worst fitness?

29 Which boy needs to improve his flexibility? his heart and lung endurance?

30 How can the boy who needs to improve his flexibility do so? How can the boy who needs to improve his heart and lung endurance do so?

31 Which boy would be most likely to try out for the soccer team? Explain your answer.

Reading Checkup

Take a minute to review your answers to the Health IQ questions at the beginning of this chapter. How has reading this chapter improved your Health IQ?

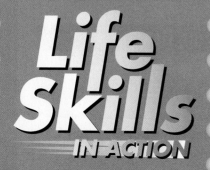

Life Skills IN ACTION

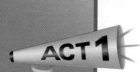

ACT 1

The 4 Steps of Assessing Your Health

1. Choose the part of your health you want to assess.

2. List your strengths and weaknesses.

3. Describe how your behaviors may contribute to your weaknesses.

4. Develop a plan to address your weaknesses.

Assessing Your Health

Assessing your health means evaluating each of the four parts of your health and examining your behaviors. By assessing your health regularly, you will know what your strengths and weaknesses are and will be able to take steps to improve your health. Complete the following activity to improve your ability to assess your health.

Swim Team Tryouts

Setting the Scene

Sonya has gone swimming frequently since she was a little girl. She has always thought of herself as a strong swimmer. So this year, Sonya decides to try out for the school's swim team. Because making the team is so important to her, Sonya wants to make sure she is in good physical condition before the tryouts. She decides to talk to the swim team coach about preparing for the tryouts.

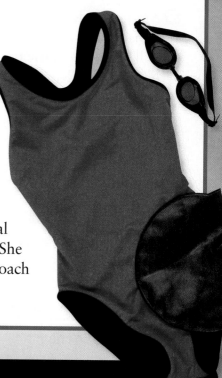

Guided Practice

Practice with a Friend

Form a group of three. Have one person play the role of Sonya and another person play the role of the swim team coach. Have the third person be an observer. Walking through each of the four steps of assessing your health, role-play Sonya assessing her health. The swim team coach can help Sonya by offering advice. The observer will take notes, which will include observations about what the person playing Sonya did well and suggestions of ways to improve. Stop after each step to evaluate the process.

Independent Practice

Check Yourself

After you have completed the guided practice, go through Act 1 again without stopping at each step. Answer the questions below to review what you did.

1. What are some of Sonya's possible strengths and weaknesses?

2. What behaviors may contribute to Sonya's weaknesses?

3. What can Sonya do to overcome her weaknesses?

4. What are some weaknesses in your physical health? How can you address your weaknesses?

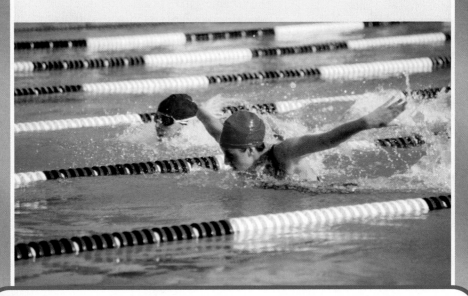

ACT 2 — On Your Own

Sonya's efforts to prepare for the swim team tryouts paid off when she made the team. She was very excited during her first swim meet. However, at the end of her race, Sonya was surprised to learn that she lost and that her finishing time was not very good. Since then, Sonya has been very depressed about her race results. She thinks about her failure all the time and has trouble concentrating on her schoolwork. Make an outline showing how Sonya could use the four steps of assessing your health to assess her health.

CHAPTER 5

Nutrition and Your Health

Lessons

Check out **Current Health** articles related to this chapter by visiting go.hrw.com. Just type in the keyword **HD4CH20**.

92

"I am usually **hungry** by the end of school. I have **soccer practice** after school, so I just grab something from the **vending machine**. The snack that I buy doesn't usually last very long, and I'm starving by the end of practice. What can I do to make sure that I'm not hungry all the time?**"**

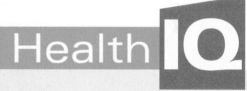

PRE-READING

Answer the multiple-choice questions to find out what you already know about nutrition. When you've finished this chapter, you'll have the opportunity to change your answers based on what you've learned.

1. **Your body needs energy to**
   a. grow.
   b. repair tissues.
   c. fight germs.
   d. All of the above

2. **The process in which your body breaks down food into a form your body can use is called**
   a. hunger.
   b. digestion.
   c. metabolism.
   d. indigestion.

3. **The process in which your body changes nutrients into usable energy is called**
   a. hunger.
   b. digestion.
   c. metabolism.
   d. sleeping.

4. **Tofu and _____ are good sources of protein.**
   a. fruit
   b. vegetables
   c. peanut butter
   d. water

5. **There are _____ different groups in the Food Guide Pyramid.**
   a. five
   b. six
   c. seven
   d. four

6. **The Nutrition Facts label states**
   a. the number of Calories in each serving of food.
   b. the number of servings in a container of food.
   c. the amount of nutrients in each serving of food.
   d. All of the above

ANSWERS: 1. d; 2. b; 3. c; 4. c; 5. b; 6. d

Nutrition and Diet

Josh's grandfather recently survived a heart attack. Now, all of Josh's family members are talking about eating better and improving their diets. Josh wonders how much food can really affect someone's health.

Like Josh, many people may be confused about how food can affect a person's overall health. After all, you need to eat to stay alive, right? The truth is that food contains substances that your body needs to stay healthy. *Nutrition* is the study of how your bodies use the substances in food to maintain our health.

Nutrition and Your Health

Practicing good nutrition means eating foods that are good for you and eating them in the right amounts. Your nutrition affects many of the things you do every day. The substances in food give you the energy you need for learning, studying, staying active, and hanging out with your friends. Your body uses the same substances to grow, repair tissues, and fight germs that cause sickness.

Think about Josh's grandfather. The foods he ate may have played a part in causing his heart attack. Practicing good nutrition will help Josh's grandfather stay healthy from now on.

What You'll Do

- **Explain** how nutrition affects your overall health.
- **Explain** how your body uses food.
- **Identify** six factors that affect your food choices.
- **Explain** how your feelings may affect your food choices.

Terms to Learn

- digestion
- nutrient
- diet

Start Off *Write*

What does it mean to practice good nutrition?

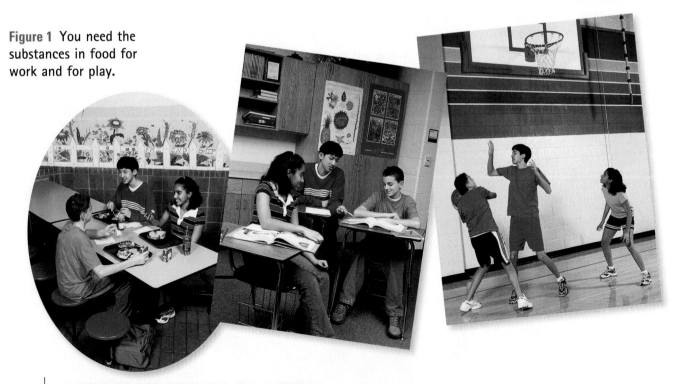

Figure 1 You need the substances in food for work and for play.

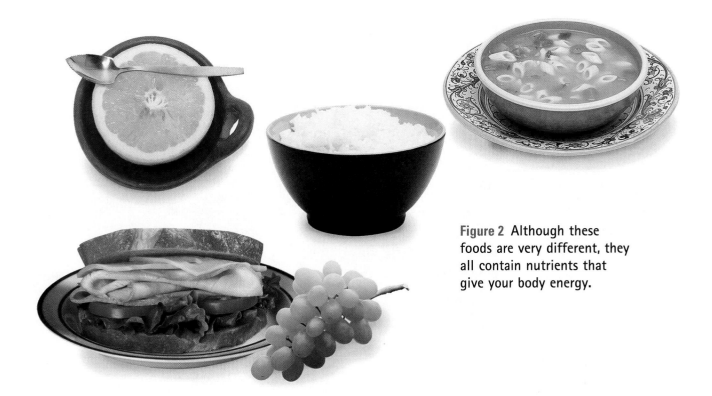

Figure 2 Although these foods are very different, they all contain nutrients that give your body energy.

How Your Body Uses Food

Your body uses food for energy. However, your body can't use food directly for energy. The food must be broken down into a form that your body can use. **Digestion** is the process in which food is broken down into a form your body can use.

Digestion begins when you chew your food. After the food you eat is chewed and swallowed, it passes into the stomach. In the stomach, the food is broken down by a strong acid and other substances. This step turns your food into a thick liquid. The liquid passes into the small intestine, where it is broken down further into nutrients (NOO tree uhnts). **Nutrients** are the substances found in food that your body needs to function properly. The nutrients are absorbed into your blood and delivered to tissues throughout your body. Your body turns the nutrients into usable energy through a process called *metabolism*.

Your body can make some nutrients. But most nutrients come from the foods you eat. For example, your body needs nutrients to fight germs that cause sickness. One way you can get these nutrients is by drinking orange juice. Because not every food has every nutrient, eating a variety of foods is important. This way, you will get all the nutrients you need.

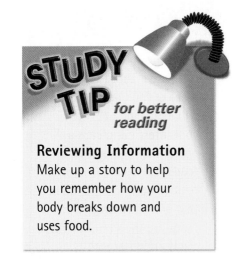

STUDY TIP *for better reading*

Reviewing Information
Make up a story to help you remember how your body breaks down and uses food.

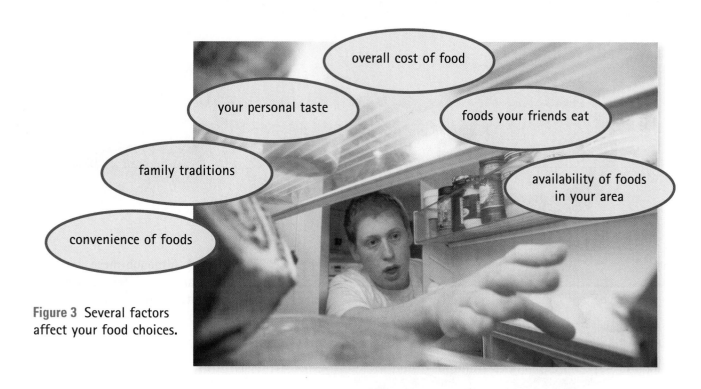

Figure 3 Several factors affect your food choices.

Your Diet and Food Choices

Most people think of a diet as a way of eating to lose weight. Actually, a **diet** is a pattern of eating. Your pattern of eating includes what you eat, how much you eat, and how often you eat. Because your diet includes what kinds of foods you eat, it is affected by your food choices. Many factors influence both your diet and your food choices.

Your personal taste has a lot to do with what you decide to eat. You may eat some foods because they are convenient. For example, you may choose to eat a fast-food burger one night. It is convenient because you can eat it in the car on the way to soccer practice. Often, the cost of food determines the kinds of foods your family buys. Your family traditions or your cultural background may affect the types of foods you decide to eat. You may eat certain foods because your friends like them and because you have come to like these foods, too. Finally, you may eat certain foods because they are available in your local area. The following list shows you six factors that affect your food choices:

- your personal taste
- family traditions
- convenience of foods
- overall cost of food
- foods your friends eat
- availability of foods in your area

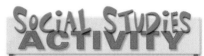

Interview an elderly friend or relative about what types of food he or she ate while growing up. After your interview, create a poster that compares the foods that your friend or relative ate with the foods that you eat today. Which foods are the same? Which foods are different?

Food and Feelings

Most people know when their bodies need nutrients because they get hungry. Feeling hungry is the way your body tells you that it needs more food for energy. Sometimes, people eat even though they are not hungry.

Often, people's feelings can affect how and what they choose to eat. Some people may eat when they are sad or upset. Others may eat when they are happy or want to celebrate. Some people may skip meals if they are nervous. Others may like to eat when they are nervous. Many people like to eat when they are with friends in a social setting. Have you ever gone to a party and eaten snacks even though you had already eaten dinner?

If a person's feelings affect his or her food choices once in a while, it is not a bad thing. However, some people's feelings may affect their food choices all the time. This behavior can be unhealthy because a person may want to eat every time he or she has a particular emotion. Also, the person may choose to eat foods that are unhealthy. By understanding what feelings affect your food choices, you can avoid eating unhealthy foods. You can also avoid eating when you know you are not hungry.

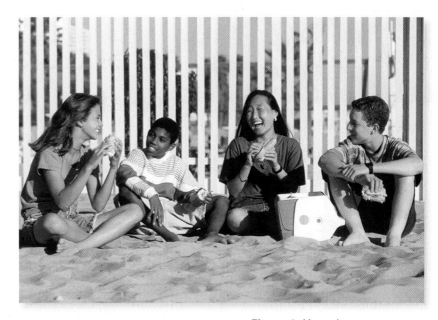

Figure 4 How do your feelings affect what you eat?

Health Journal

Write down everything you eat and drink for one day. Next to each entry, describe how you are feeling when you eat. The next day, take a look at your list. Do you eat only when you are hungry?

Lesson Review

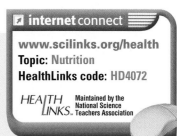

internet connect

www.scilinks.org/health
Topic: Nutrition
HealthLinks code: HD4072

HEALTH LINKS. Maintained by the National Science Teachers Association

Using Vocabulary

1. Use each of the following terms in a separate sentence: *nutrient*, *diet*, and *digestion*.

Understanding Concepts

2. List six factors that influence your food choices.

3. Explain how your nutrition affects your overall health.

4. How does your body use the food you eat?

Critical Thinking

5. Making Good Decisions Your best friend eats large servings of ice cream when she is upset. Lately, she has been eating a big bowl of ice cream every day. You know this behavior may be unhealthy for her. Should you say something to her? If so, what would you tell her?

The Six Classes of Essential Nutrients

The nutrients in food help your body function properly. But what are these nutrients, and where do you get them? Read on to find out!

What You'll Do

- **List** the six classes of essential nutrients.
- **Explain** what each class of essential nutrient does for your body.
- **Identify** foods that are good sources of the essential nutrients.

Terms to Learn

- carbohydrate
- fat
- protein
- vitamin
- mineral

Start Off Write

What is the difference between vitamins and minerals?

The Nutrients You Need

Your body can make some of the nutrients it needs. However most of the nutrients your body needs come from the food you eat. The nutrients that you get from food are called the *essential nutrients.* The six classes of essential nutrients are carbohydrates (KAHR boh HIE drayts), fats, proteins (PROH TEENZ), vitamins (VIET uh minz), minerals (MIN uhr uhlz), and water. Each of these nutrient classes play a special role in your body. Your body uses carbohydrates, fats, and proteins as direct sources of energy. Vitamins and minerals control many body functions. They also help your body use the energy from the other nutrients. Your body uses water to control your body temperature. Water is also used to transport other nutrients throughout your body. The essential nutrients are necessary for your body to function properly. So, eating a variety of foods that contain these nutrients is very important.

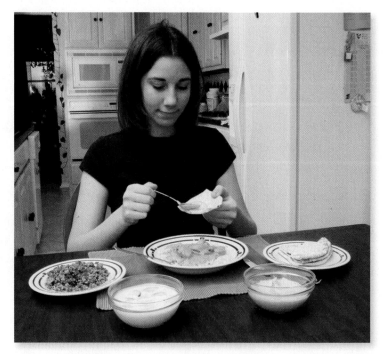

Figure 5 Every food contains different nutrients. It's important to eat a variety of foods so that you get all the nutrients that you need.

Carbohydrates

Carbohydrates provide energy for your body. A **carbohydrate** is a chemical composed of one or more simple sugars. Carbohydrates can be sugars or starches. Sugars are found in foods such as fruit, honey, table sugar, candy, and desserts. Starches are found in foods such as rice, pasta, and bread. Starches are carbohydrates that are made up of many simple sugars. In their natural state, these foods contain fiber, a kind of carbohydrate that cannot be digested in our bodies. Foods that are high in fiber are a part of a healthy diet. Brown rice and whole-wheat bread are good sources of fiber.

Fats

Believe it or not, it's important to have a small amount of fat in your diet. **Fats** are nutrients that store energy and store some vitamins. Fats also help your body produce hormones. Fats can be found in solid or liquid form. Solid fats are found in foods such as butter and margarine. Liquid fats are found in cooking oils and salad dressings. Fats are also found in meats such as steak, pork, or chicken. Fats make some foods taste and smell good. Fried foods and desserts taste good in part because they contain a large amount of fat. Fats contain more Calories than any other nutrient does. If you eat too many foods that are high in fat, you may eat more Calories than you need. In these cases, the unused Calories will be stored as fat in your body. Your body needs only a small amount of fat to function properly. When there is too much fat in your body, it can block the flow of blood to your heart. This blockage may lead to a heart attack when you are older.

Proteins

You can think of proteins as building blocks for your body. **Proteins** are nutrients that are used for building, maintaining, and repairing tissues and cells. Proteins help the body break down and use nutrients for energy. Proteins also help protect the body from germs that cause sickness. Meat, poultry, and fish are good sources of proteins. Milk and cheese are also good sources of protiens. You can also get proteins from beans, nuts, tofu, eggs, whole grains, and vegetables.

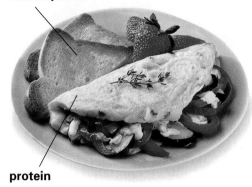

carbohydrate

protein

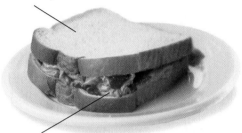

carbohydrate

protein and fat

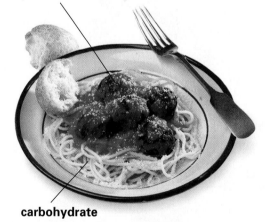

protein and fat

carbohydrate

Figure 6 Most foods contain more than one class of nutrient, but they are often a good source of only one class.

Hands-on ACTIVITY

BROWN BAG TEST

1. Cut a brown paper bag into small squares.

2. Gather a variety of foods, such as cookies, fruit, chips, chocolate, and popcorn. Place a piece of each type of food on a different square.

3. Leave the food on the squares overnight.

Analysis

1. Remove each piece of food from its square. How much oil did each food leave behind?

2. Which foods had the most oil? Which foods had the least?

Vitamins and Minerals

Although you need only small amounts of vitamins and minerals, they are very important to your health. **Vitamins** are organic compounds that control many body functions. **Minerals** are elements that are essential for good health. Vitamins and minerals are found in fresh fruits, vegetables, nuts, and dairy products. The figure below shows you foods that are good sources of some vitamins and minerals.

Without vitamins and minerals, your body would not function properly. For example, a lack of vitamin C can cause scurvy, a disease that affects the gums. Without vitamin A, you may develop night blindness. You also need minerals for healthy growth. Calcium, phosphorus (FAHS fuh ruhs), iron, sodium, potassium, and zinc are just a few of the minerals that your body needs. You need calcium and phosphorus to build strong bones. Sodium and potassium help regulate blood pressure. Iron is necessary for your blood to deliver oxygen to your cells. To avoid health problems, you should eat plenty of fresh fruits, vegetables, and whole grains every day.

Figure 7 Fruits and vegetables are great sources of vitamins and minerals.

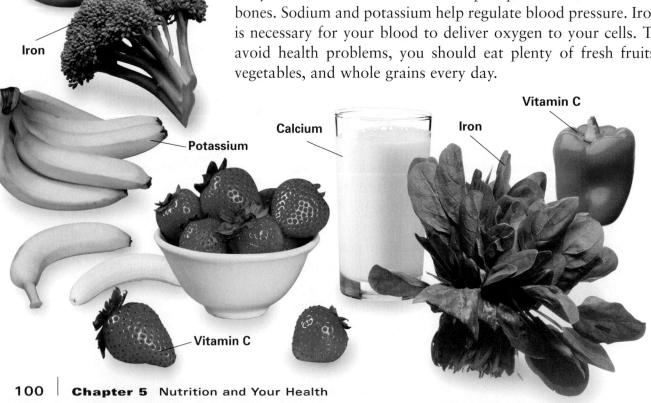

Vitamin C

Iron

Iron

Potassium

Calcium

Iron

Vitamin C

Vitamin C

Water

Water is a very important nutrient. Your body does not get energy from water, but water is needed for most of your body functions. A person can live for several weeks without food. However, without water, the person will die within a few days. The reason is that your body uses water to transport food and nutrients. Water is used to fill the cells and the spaces between the cells in your body. Your body uses water to fill spaces in your joints, and water in your spine is used to absorb shock. Your body uses water to keep your mouth and eyes moist. Your body also uses water to wash away the waste products that your body produces.

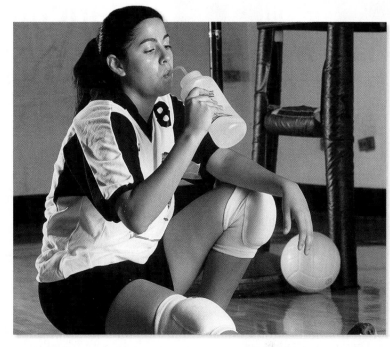

Figure 8 Drinking water is important, especially while you are being physically active.

Water regulates your body temperature. When your body gets too hot, you sweat. As the water evaporates, you feel cooler and your body temperature returns to normal. This keeps you from overheating. If you don't drink enough water each day, you may *dehydrate,* or dry out. If you become dehydrated, your body will not function properly. As a result, you may faint. In extreme cases, you may die. You must drink plenty of water so that you don't dry out.

Drinking water is the best way to replace lost water. But you can get water from other food and drinks. Good sources of water are fruit juices, fruits, vegetables, soups, stews, and milk. A good rule of thumb is to drink 8 to 10 glasses of water every day. If you play sports, you should drink even more.

Lesson Review

Using Vocabulary

1. What are carbohydrates?

2. What are vitamins?

Understanding Concepts

3. List the six classes of essential nutrients. What does each nutrient class do for your body?

4. List three foods that are good sources of protein.

Critical Thinking

5. **Analyzing Processes** Your friend asks you to go ride bikes. It is a very hot day. What will happen if you don't drink enough water?

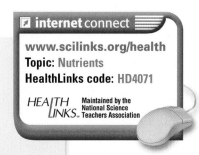

internet connect

www.scilinks.org/health
Topic: Nutrients
HealthLinks code: HD4071

HEALTH LINKS. Maintained by the National Science Teachers Association

Balancing Your Diet

You know that your body needs the nutrients in food to stay healthy. However, you may not know which foods to eat or how much of them to eat to get all the nutrients you need.

Fortunately, there are many tools you can use to help you make healthy food choices. These tools include the Dietary Guidelines for Americans, the Food Guide Pyramid, and the Nutrition Facts label.

The Dietary Guidelines for Americans

A healthy lifestyle involves many steps. These steps include eating a healthful diet and staying physically active every day. The **Dietary Guidelines for Americans** are a set of suggestions to help you develop a healthy lifestyle. These guidelines were developed by the U.S. Department of Agriculture and the U.S. Department of Health and Human Services. Following the dietary guidelines will help you develop healthy eating habits. Having healthy eating habits can help you get enough nutrients every day.

You can think of the dietary guidelines as the ABCs for good health. The ABCs are **a**im for fitness, **b**uild a healthy base, and **c**hoose sensibly. The table below provides more information about these guidelines.

What You'll Do

- **Describe** the Dietary Guidelines for Americans.
- **Describe** how to use the Food Guide Pyramid.
- **Explain** how to read a Nutrition Facts label.
- **Explain** the difference between a serving and a portion.

Terms to Learn

- Dietary Guidelines for Americans
- Food Guide Pyramid
- Nutrition Facts label

Start Off Write

Why is eating a balanced diet important?

TABLE 1 The Dietary Guidelines for Americans	
Aim for fitness	Aim to stay at a healthy weight by being physically active every day.
Build a healthy base	Choose healthy foods by using the Food Guide Pyramid. Eat a variety of whole grains, fresh fruits, and vegetables.
	Keep foods safe to eat by cooking your food fully. Store foods properly by keeping cold foods cold and refrigerating hot foods soon after you are finished with them.
Choose sensibly	Choose foods that are low in salt, sugar, and fat.

The Food Guide Pyramid

To build a healthy diet, you must be able to choose foods that give you the proper nutrients. The **Food Guide Pyramid** is a tool that shows you which foods to eat and how much of each type of food you should eat every day. The pyramid is made up of food groups. A food group is made up of foods that contain similar nutrients. Each food group has its own block, and each block is a different size. A bigger block means you should eat more food from that food group. The number of servings for each group tells you how much food from each food group you should eat daily.

The bread group has the largest block. So, you need more foods from the bread group in your daily diet than you need from any other group. The exact amount you should eat depends on your age and weight. But the Food Guide Pyramid suggests you should eat 6 to 11 servings of bread each day.

Figure 9 The Food Guide Pyramid

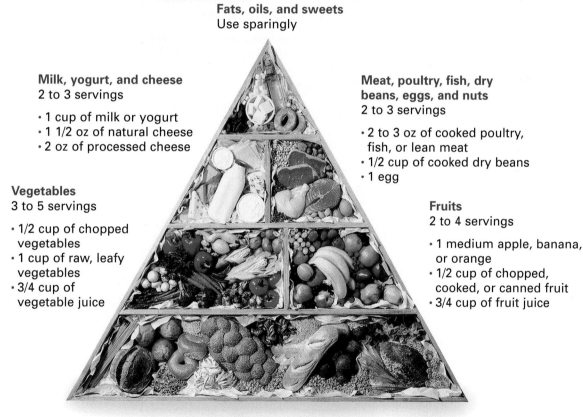

Fats, oils, and sweets
Use sparingly

Milk, yogurt, and cheese
2 to 3 servings

• 1 cup of milk or yogurt
• 1 1/2 oz of natural cheese
• 2 oz of processed cheese

Meat, poultry, fish, dry beans, eggs, and nuts
2 to 3 servings

• 2 to 3 oz of cooked poultry, fish, or lean meat
• 1/2 cup of cooked dry beans
• 1 egg

Vegetables
3 to 5 servings

• 1/2 cup of chopped vegetables
• 1 cup of raw, leafy vegetables
• 3/4 cup of vegetable juice

Fruits
2 to 4 servings

• 1 medium apple, banana, or orange
• 1/2 cup of chopped, cooked, or canned fruit
• 3/4 cup of fruit juice

Bread, cereal, rice, and pasta
6 to 11 servings

• 1 slice of bread
• 1 oz of ready-to-eat cereal
• 1/2 cup of rice or pasta
• 1/2 cup of cooked cereal

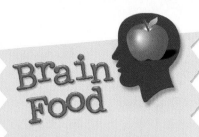

Many teens in the United States do not get enough calcium or iron in their daily diet. They also do not get enough of vitamins A and C. Drinking milk and eating leafy green vegetables and fresh fruit will help you get these nutrients.

The Nutrition Facts Label

A useful tool for finding out what nutrients are in a food is the Nutrition Facts label. The **Nutrition Facts label** is a label found on the outside packages of food and states the number of servings in the container, the number of Calories in each serving, and the amount of nutrients in each serving. The Daily Values section states what amount of your daily nutrient need is in one serving of the food. For example, the chicken soup below has 15 percent of your daily need of vitamin A. You can tell whether a food is high or low in a nutrient by looking at its percent daily value. A percent daily value of 5 percent or less means that the food is low in that nutrient. A percent daily value of 20 percent or more means that the food is high in that nutrient.

Figure 10 The Nutrition Facts Label

Serving information

Number of Calories per serving

Percentage of daily value of nutrients per serving

Nutrition Facts

Serving Size 1/2 cup (120 ml)
Servings per Container 2.5

Amount per Serving	Prepared
Calories	70
Calories from Fat	25

	% Daily Value
Total Fat 2.5 g	4%
Saturated Fat 1 g	5%
Cholesterol 15 mg	5%
Sodium 960 mg	40%
Total Carbohydrate 8 g	3%
Dietary Fiber less than 1 g	4%
Sugars 1 g	
Protein 3 g	
Vitamin A	15%
Vitamin C	0%
Calcium	0%
Iron	4%

*Percent Daily Values are based on a 2,000 calorie diet. your daily values may be higher or lower depending on your calorie needs:

	Calories	2,000	2,500
Total Fat	Less than	65g	80g
Sat Fat	Less than	20g	25g
Cholesterol	Less than	300mg	300mg
Sodium	Less than	2,400mg	2,400mg
Total Carbohydrate		300g	375g
Dietary Fiber		25g	30g
Protien		50g	60g

What Is a Serving Size?

A serving size is a standard amount of food that allows foods to be compared with one another. The Nutrition Facts label shows you information about the nutrients in one serving of a packaged food. The Food Guide Pyramid also uses serving sizes. For example, 1 cup of milk is one serving of the milk group. One medium apple is one serving of the fruit group. Keep in mind that serving sizes for a food are not always the same, especially on packaged foods. Also, remember that how much you actually eat is very important; the number of servings that you eat depends on you.

What Is a Portion?

A *portion* of food is the amount of food you want to eat. Often, a portion is not the same as a serving. For example, imagine you are going to eat a can of soup. The Nutrition Facts label states that the can of soup contains two servings. If you eat the whole can of soup, you would be eating two servings. Our portion sizes depend on how much we want to eat. It is important to note that most restaurants provide portions that are larger than one serving. For instance, in some restaurants, one hamburger (or one portion) could equal three servings in the meat group. Be sure to use the Food Guide Pyramid and the Nutrition Facts label to know how many servings of foods from each food group you need. Then, you can choose your portions wisely.

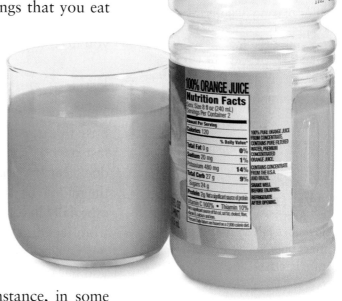

Figure 11 The glass you see here contains a serving of juice. How does that amount compare with the amount in the bottle?

Lesson Review

Using Vocabulary

1. What are the Dietary Guidelines for Americans?

2. What is the Food Guide Pyramid?

Understanding Concepts

3. Use the Food Guide Pyramid to create a menu for 1 day. Be creative by choosing foods that are not shown on the pyramid.

Critical Thinking

4. Analyzing Ideas Describe how you would use the Nutrition Facts label to eat foods that are low in fat.

5. Making Inferences Suppose you are keeping track of how many Calories you eat. Why is it important to pay attention to the serving size of each food you eat?

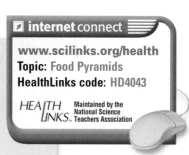

internet connect

www.scilinks.org/health
Topic: Food Pyramids
HealthLinks code: HD4043

HEALTH LINKS. Maintained by the National Science Teachers Association

Building Healthful Eating Habits

What You'll Do

■ **Explain** why eating a healthy breakfast is important.

■ **Describe** three strategies for making healthy snack choices.

■ **List** seven ways to eat healthily at a fast-food restaurant.

■ **List** six ways to eat healthily at home.

Start Off
Write

How does eating breakfast affect your ability to concentrate in class?

Every morning, Jimmy's dad makes Jimmy eat breakfast. But Jimmy isn't always hungry in the morning. Why do you think his dad wants him to eat breakfast?

Breakfast is a very important meal because it gives you the energy you need to start the day.

Eating a Healthy Breakfast

Many teens skip breakfast in the morning. Often, they are too busy to eat, or they do not feel hungry. However, skipping breakfast may affect a person in many ways. First, most people who don't eat breakfast become hungry, irritated, or light-headed by the middle of the morning. They may have trouble concentrating, especially in class. Eating a healthy breakfast usually prevents you from feeling this way. In the morning, your body has been without food all night and needs nutrients from food. The nutrients you get from breakfast will be used for energy at different times. So, if you eat breakfast, you will continue to have energy over a length of time. If you can't eat breakfast in the morning, be sure to bring a healthy, mid-morning snack to school. The figure below shows some ideas for a healthy breakfast.

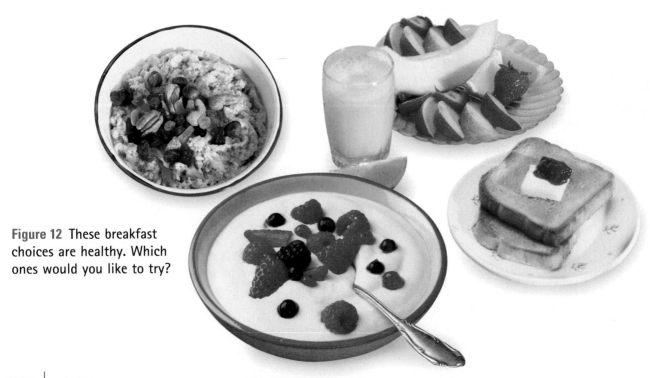

Figure 12 These breakfast choices are healthy. Which ones would you like to try?

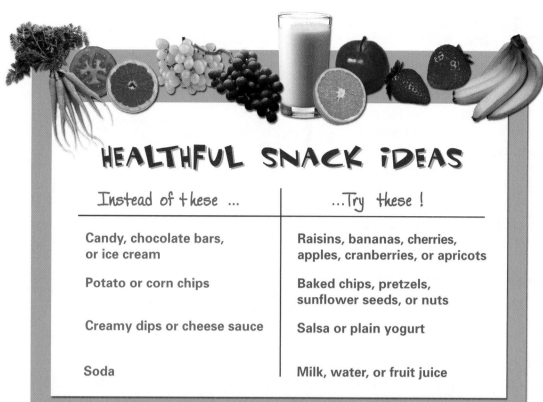

HEALTHFUL SNACK IDEAS

Instead of these ...	...Try these !
Candy, chocolate bars, or ice cream	Raisins, bananas, cherries, apples, cranberries, or apricots
Potato or corn chips	Baked chips, pretzels, sunflower seeds, or nuts
Creamy dips or cheese sauce	Salsa or plain yogurt
Soda	Milk, water, or fruit juice

Figure 13 Many snack foods are high in fat, sugar, or salt. Try these snack ideas for a healthy treat.

Snacking Well

Snacks are the foods you eat between meals. Believe it or not, eating snacks is not a bad thing! In fact, eating a snack is a good idea because doing so keeps you from being too hungry at mealtimes. If you are too hungry, you may eat more food than you need. However, the type of snack you choose is important. Unfortunately, many snack foods, such as cookies and chips, are high in fat, sugar, and salt. Also, eating too many snacks may cause you to be full at mealtimes. If you feel full, you may not feel like eating lunch or dinner.

Choosing snacks that are good for you is easy. First, choose to eat sugary or salty snacks only once in a while. These snacks include candy bars, chocolate, hard candies, and chips. Second, choose foods that are low in fat. For example, choose to eat fresh fruit, crackers, yogurt, or vegetables. Bring a snack with you if you know you will be away from home. Bringing a snack from home will keep you from buying a snack from the vending machine. Third, choose healthful snack foods that you will enjoy. You will be more likely to eat healthfully if you are eating something you like! Take a look at the figure above for some healthy snack ideas.

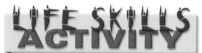

LIFE SKILLS ACTIVITY

PRACTICING WELLNESS

Try making this great trail mix for a healthy snack!

The ingredients include 1 cup unsalted, shelled nuts, 1 cup sunflower seeds, 1 cup raisins, 1/2 cup dried apricots. Mix all the ingredients together in a large bowl. Store the trail mix in an airtight container, and enjoy!

MAKING GOOD DECISIONS

You and your friends decide to eat dinner at Charlie's Take-Out in the mall. The menu at this restaurant is shown at right. Next to each item, you will find how many grams of carbohydrates (C), protein (P), and fat (F) are found in each food. Based on what you have learned, choose a healthy meal from the menu.

Charlie's Take Out

Main Meals	C	F	P
Hamburger	45	21	36
Grilled Chicken Sandwich	38	13	27
Bean Taco	25	16	1
Hot Dog	0	13	5
Tuna Sandwich	29	4	27

Sides & Drinks	C	F	P
French Fries	30	13	2
Side Salad	4	0.3	1
Baked Potato	82	0.3	7
Soda	51	0	0
Iced Tea	1	0	0

Eating Out

Eating out is a normal part of most people's lives. Many teens choose to eat at fast-food restaurants. It is OK to eat fast-food meals once in a while. But if you eat fast-food meals more than once a week, you may be eating more fat and salt than you need.

If you must eat at fast-food restaurants, choose healthful meals. Many restaurants offer salads or grilled meals. Grilling is a method of cooking that is usually low in fat. If low-fat choices are not available, you can choose not to eat the entire portion.

There are several ways to make your fast-food meal healthier. For example, when you use dressing, ask for one that is low in fat. You can use mustard or ketchup instead of mayonnaise. You should try to avoid using mayonnaise because it is high in fat. Also, you can avoid the extra foods that come with your meal, such as bacon or extra cheese on a hamburger. Try eating salsa instead of cheese sauce. Finally, you can order water with your meal instead of ordering a soda.

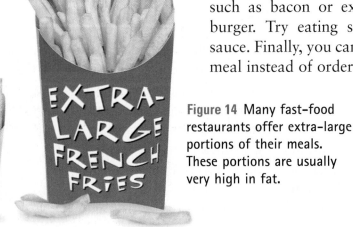

Figure 14 Many fast-food restaurants offer extra-large portions of their meals. These portions are usually very high in fat.

10 g of fat   29 g of fat

Eating at Home

Eating healthy meals at home can be fun and easy. Encourage whoever prepares meals at home to make healthy choices by using the Food Guide Pyramid and the Dietary Guidelines for Americans. If you prepare a meal for yourself, you can follow these suggestions, too. Choose whole-wheat bread for a sandwich. Use a tomato sauce on pasta rather than a creamy sauce. Be sure to have plenty of vegetables with your meals. You can easily prepare a salad with lettuce, tomatoes, carrots, and other fresh vegetables that you like. If you like eggs, choose to eat an omelet or scrambled eggs instead of fried eggs. You can also try jam on breads and bagels instead of butter. Finally, try drinking water, milk, or juice instead of soda.

Health Journal

For 1 day, write down everything that you eat. Then, on a second day, plan what you are going to eat on that day. Follow your plan. Compare what you ate when you didn't plan and what you ate when you did plan. Which day did you eat more healthful foods?

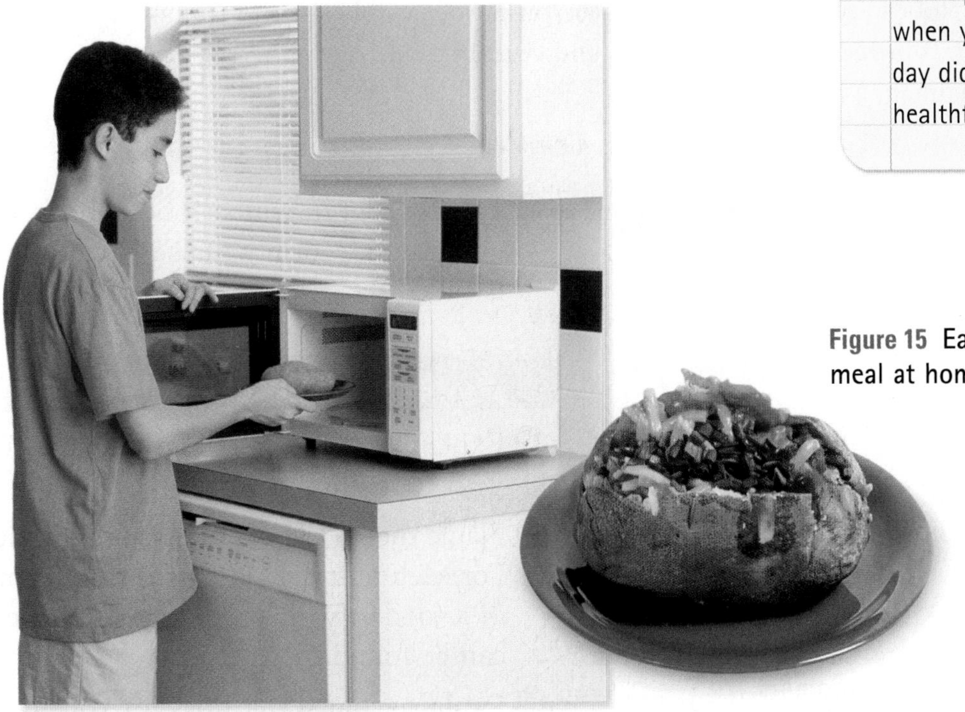

Figure 15 Eating a healthy meal at home can be easy!

Lesson Review

Understanding Concepts

1. Explain why eating a healthful breakfast is important.

2. List three ways to make healthy snack choices.

3. Describe seven ways to make healthy choices at a fast-food restaurant.

4. List six strategies for eating healthily at home.

Critical Thinking

5. Imagine that you have to stay after school for soccer practice. What can you do to make sure that you have a healthy snack before practice?

Chapter Summary

■ Nutrition is the study of how your body uses the food you eat to maintain your health. ■ Your diet is a pattern of eating that includes what you eat, how often you eat, and how much you eat. ■ The six classes of essential nutrients are carbohydrates, fats, proteins, minerals, vitamins, and water. ■ The Dietary Guidelines for Americans, the Food Guide Pyramid, and the Nutrition Facts label are tools you can use to make healthy food choices. ■ Eating a healthy breakfast prevents you from feeling hungry, irritated, or lightheaded during the first half of the school day. ■ Eating a healthy snack between meals prevents you from eating too much at mealtimes. ■ Choosing foods low in fat and salt when you eat out will help you maintain a healthy diet. ■ Including plenty of fruits and vegetables in your meals at home will help you maintain a healthy diet.

Using Vocabulary

For each pair of terms, describe how the meanings of the terms differ.

❶ Food Guide Pyramid/Nutrition Facts label

❷ carbohydrate/protein

For each sentence, fill in the blank with the proper word from the word bank provided below.

nutrients	digestion
diet	carbohydrate
fats	proteins
vitamin	mineral
Dietary Guidelines for Americans	Nutrition Facts label Food Guide Pyramid

❸ A ___ is a pattern of eating.

❹ Nutrients that supply the body with energy for building and repairing tissues are ___.

❺ Nutrients that store energy and some vitamins are ___.

❻ A tool that shows you which foods to eat and how much of each type of food you should eat every day is the ___.

❼ The process in which food is broken down into a form your body can use is called ___.

Understanding Concepts

❽ Explain how your feelings may affect your food choices.

❾ Name the six classes of essential nutrients. For each nutrient class, give one example of a food in which that type of nutrient can be found.

❿ Explain what water does for your body.

⓫ Which nutrients provide your body with energy?

⓬ What is the difference between a serving and a portion?

⓭ Why can eating a snack between meals be good for you?

⓮ What are some healthy breakfast choices?

⓯ How many glasses of water should you drink every day?

Critical Thinking

Applying Concepts

16 Imagine that you are using the Food Guide Pyramid to plan a meal to eat before your volleyball game. From which food groups will you choose most of your foods?

17 Explain how you can use the Nutrition Facts label to choose a food that is high in calcium.

18 Given what you now know about eating healthfully, list two habits that you would like to change. Then, list two ways you could change your eating habits.

19 If 1 cup of milk is considered a serving, and you buy a gallon of milk, how many servings of milk do you have? According to the Food Guide Pyramid, how many days will the gallon of milk last you?

20 The cheeseburger you ate for lunch today contained 14 grams of fat, 35 grams of carbohydrate, and 12 grams of protein. If 1 gram of carbohydrate contains 4 Calories, 1 gram of fat contains 9 Calories, and 1 gram of protein contains 4 Calories, how many Calories did the cheeseburger contain?

Making Good Decisions

21 You are trying to decide what to eat for a snack. After looking around the kitchen, you find a bag of potato chips, a bagel, some strawberries, and a banana. Suppose that you have basketball practice in 1 hour. Which foods will you choose for your snack? Which foods will give you the most energy for basketball practice?

Interpreting Graphics

Nutrition Facts	
Serving Size 1 cup (228 g)	
Servings per Container 2	
Amount per Serving	
Calories 250	
	% Daily Value
Total Fat 12 g	18%
Cholesterol 30 mg	15%
Sodium 470 mg	20%
Carbohydrates 31 g	10%
Protein 5 g	
Vitamin A	4%
Vitamin C	2%
Calcium	20%
Iron	4%

Use the Nutrition Facts label for Macaroni and Cheese above to answer questions 22–27.

22 How many Calories are in the entire box of macaroni and cheese?

23 Which vitamins and minerals are found in this box of macaroni and cheese?

24 Would a serving of macaroni and cheese from this package of be considered high in sodium or low in sodium?

25 Is this food high in calcium? Explain your answer.

26 How many total grams are in this box of macaroni and cheese?

27 Is this food high in iron? Explain your answer.

Reading Checkup

Take a minute to review your answers to the Health IQ questions at the beginning of this chapter. How has reading this chapter improved your Health IQ?

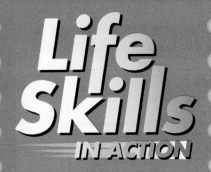

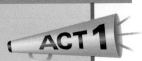

Making Good Decisions

You make decisions every day. But how do you know if you are making good decisions? Making good decisions is making choices that are healthy and responsible. Following the six steps of making good decisions will help you make the best possible choice whenever you make a decision. Complete the following activity to practice the six steps of making good decisions.

What's for Lunch?

Setting the Scene

Simon and his friend Tabitha need to eat a quick lunch before returning to their volunteer jobs at the hospital. The line in the hospital cafeteria is very long, so they decide to go to the fast-food restaurant next door. As they look over the menu, Tabitha says that she wants to eat something healthy. Simon agrees but is unsure of what to pick.

Frank's Take Out

Main Meals		Sides & Drinks	
Hamburger	1.00	French Fries	1.00
Cheeseburger	1.50	Side Salad	1.50
Grilled Chicken Sandwich	1.50	Baked Potato	1.00
		Soda	1.00
Hot Dog	1.00	Iced Tea	1.25
Tuna Sandwich	1.00	Chocolate Brownie	.75
		Frozen Yogurt	.75

The **6** Steps of Making Good Decisions

1. Identify the problem.
2. Consider your values.
3. List the options.
4. Weigh the consequences.
5. Decide, and act.
6. Evaluate your choice.

Guided Practice

Practice with a Friend

Form a group of three. Have one person play the role of Simon and another person play the role of Tabitha. Have the third person be an observer. Walking through each of the six steps of making good decisions, role-play Simon and Tabitha deciding what to eat for lunch. Use the menu shown above when you reach step 3. The observer will take notes, which will include observations about what the people playing Simon and Tabitha did well and suggestions of ways to improve. Stop after each step to evaluate the process.

Independent Practice

Check Yourself

After you have completed the guided practice, go through Act 1 again without stopping at each step. Answer the questions below to review what you did.

1. What values should Simon and Tabitha consider before choosing what to eat?

2. What are the healthy food options that Simon and Tabitha can choose from?

3. What are some possible consequences of selecting an unhealthy food option?

4. How can you evaluate the food choices at a restaurant?

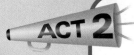

On Your Own

After eating lunch, Tabitha tells Simon that she is tired and doesn't want to go back to work at the hospital. She asks Simon to tell their supervisor that she got sick at lunch and had to go home. Simon doesn't want to do it, but Tabitha offers to buy him dessert if he does. Write a short story describing how Simon could use the six steps of making good decisions in this situation.

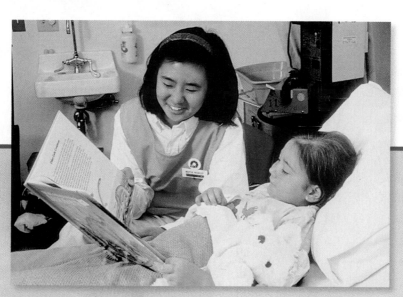

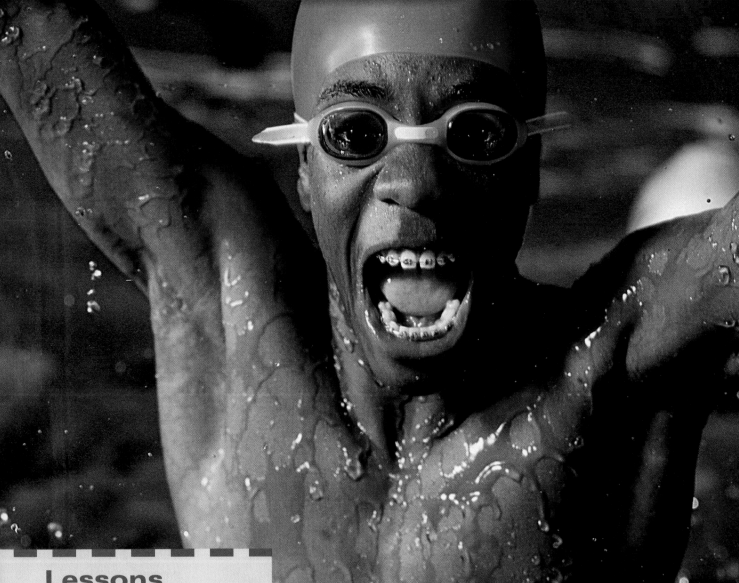

CHAPTER 6

A Healthy Body, a Healthy Weight

Lessons

Check out **Current Health** articles related to this chapter by visiting **go.hrw.com**. Just type in the keyword **HD4CH21**.

" I used to think I was **too skinny.**

So, I decided to join the **swim team** to build more **muscle.**

Now, I feel much better about my body, and I am keeping a healthy weight. **"**

Health IQ

PRE-READING

Answer the following true/false questions to find out what you already know about body image and eating disorders. When you've finished this chapter, you'll have the opportunity to change your answers based on what you've learned.

1. Eating disorders affect only girls and women.

2. Too much exercise can be bad for you.

3. You can maintain your weight by eating well and staying physically active.

4. Your body image is important only when you are going out with your friends.

5. A person with a healthy body image wants to change his or her body in some way.

6. Following fad diets is not harmful to your health.

7. Your body image affects how you face new challenges.

8. The photographs you see on TV and in magazines can influence your body image.

9. If you eat more food than your body needs to get energy for your daily activities, you will gain weight.

10. Eating disorders are only a phase, and most people don't suffer from them for a long time.

11. Having a healthy body image can boost your confidence.

12. Your body image does not affect your self-esteem.

13. Unhealthy eating behaviors can lead to eating disorders.

14. Obesity may result in health problems such as diabetes or stroke.

ANSWERS: 1. false; 2. true; 3. true; 4. false; 5. false; 6. false; 7. true; 8. true; 9. true; 10. false; 11. true; 12. false; 13. true; 14. true

What Is Body Image?

Sudeep is shorter and thinner than most of the boys at school. The day of the big race in gym class, some of his classmates laughed at him because he's so small. Sudeep ignored them and focused on running as fast as he could.

Instead of letting the comments about his small size bother him, Sudeep focused on his goal. He is comfortable with his body. Sudeep has a healthy body image.

Your Body Image

Your **body image** is the way you see and imagine your body. Your body image is important because it affects many aspects of your life.

How you feel about your body can affect the way you handle many situations. If you feel comfortable with yourself and your body, you will be more likely to have confidence when you are faced with new challenges. For example, you may have more confidence when trying a new activity, or you may feel more confident in class. If you are uncomfortable with your body, you may want to change how your body looks. The desire to change can lead to unhealthy behaviors.

Your body image is especially important at your age because your body is changing a lot. You will most likely grow taller and develop more muscle mass. Most teens gain weight as they grow and as their body changes. Feeling good about your body will help you deal with these changes in a positive way.

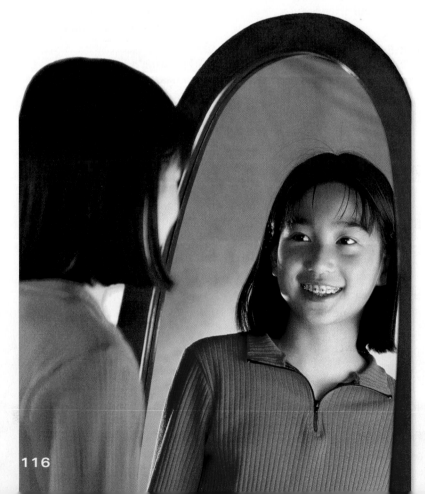

Figure 1 Your body image is the way you see and imagine your body. This teen is comfortable with her body and has a healthy body image.

What Is a Healthy Body Image?

To have a healthy body image is to accept and feel good about your body. People who have a healthy body image are comfortable with their appearance. They like and accept their bodies. They do not constantly compare themselves to other people in their lives. Nor do they always compare themselves to the people they see on TV or in magazines. People who have a healthy body image do not usually want to change their bodies. And their healthy body image gives them more confidence to handle new challenges.

What Is an Unhealthy Body Image?

To have an unhealthy body image is to feel uncomfortable with your body. People who have an unhealthy body image often compare their body with others. And people who have an unhealthy body image are very unhappy with their appearance. In fact, they may not see themselves accurately.

Many people feel somewhat unhappy with their body. They may feel unhappy with their weight, their hair, their legs—any part of their body. This is normal. However, some people are extremely unhappy about their body. Their body image keeps them from spending time with other people or from trying new things. Their body image may also keep them from being active in class, which can hurt their grades. Often, these people want very much to change their bodies. They may drastically change their eating habits, which can be dangerous.

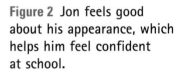

Health Journal

Each day for the next three days, write down two things that you like about your appearance. Think about the items on your list when you feel down about your appearance.

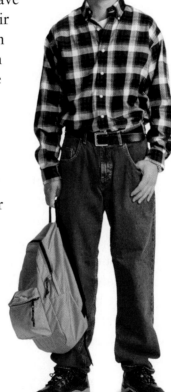

Figure 2 Jon feels good about his appearance, which helps him feel confident at school.

Lesson Review

Using Vocabulary

1. What is body image?

Understanding Concepts

2. Describe the characteristics of a person who has an unhealthy body image.

Critical Thinking

3. Making Inferences How can your body image affect how you feel on your first day at a new school?

internet connect

www.scilinks.org/health

Topic: Body Image

HealthLinks code: HD4019

HEALTH LINKS. Maintained by the National Science Teachers Association

Building a Healthy Body Image

What You'll Do

- **Identify** three influences on your body image.

- **Describe** how I statements can help you build a healthy body image.

Start Off
Write

How can your friends affect your body image?

Lexi loves teen magazines. She enjoys reading about celebrities and looking at the latest fashion trends. Sometimes, though, Lexi thinks that she'll never be thin enough to look good in the clothes that the models wear.

Lexi tends to compare herself to the models she sees in magazines. She thinks that if she doesn't look like the models, she doesn't look good.

The Media and Your Body Image

Did you know that the media can influence your body image? The media includes TV, movies, magazines, and music videos. TV shows and magazines usually show unrealistic images of men and women. Many magazines and TV programs show girls and women who are unusually thin. They also show boys and men who are unusually muscular.

Some people think that they should look like the models in magazines or the actors on TV. They may even feel ugly or fat compared with the models and actors. But the people shown on TV and in magazines are not typical. In fact, if you look around your classroom, you will probably find that most of your classmates do not look like models or actors. Most of your classmates are not that thin or that muscular. The unrealistic images of people that magazines and TV tend to show can lead a teen to develop an unhealthy body image.

Figure 3 Often, the images in magazines and on TV give us the wrong impression of what is "normal."

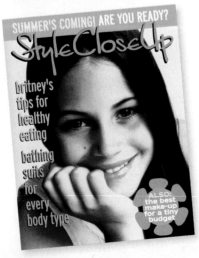

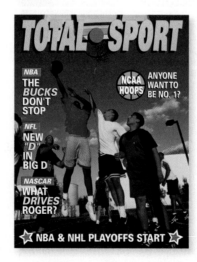

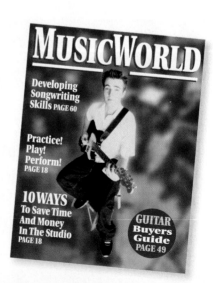

Family, Friends, and Body Image

You will face many physical and emotional changes as a teen. When you go through periods of change, you may be sensitive to the comments of others. Your family, friends, and even your teachers and coaches may make comments about your appearance. Most likely, these people do not want to hurt you. But sometimes these comments can hurt your feelings. If you already feel bad about your body, hearing negative comments may lead you to develop an unhealthy body image. If you feel good about your body, you can deal with these comments in a positive way. Also, remember that your family, friends, teachers, and coaches are usually very supportive when you are feeling uncomfortable about your body.

"I" Statements

So, what do you do when someone teases you about your appearance? One of the best things to do is to share your feelings by using "I" statements. An "I" statement tells someone how you feel by using a statement that begins with the word *I* instead of the word *you*. The table below shows some examples of "I" statements.

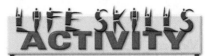

TABLE 1 Staying Positive with "I" Statements

Situation	Example
Your friend tells you that you need to fix your hair, but you already spent half an hour trying to make your hair look nice.	Tell your friend, "I appreciate your opinion, but I think that my hair looks fine."
A classmate suggests that you need to lose weight in order to be more popular.	You can tell your classmate, "I am comfortable with how I look. I don't feel that I should change anything about my body."

Lesson Review

Understanding Concepts

1. Explain how magazines and TV can influence your body image.

2. Write an "I" statement you would use if your brother told you that your nose was big.

Critical Thinking

3. **Analyzing Ideas** Explain how having a healthy body image can help you handle negative comments in a positive way.

Eating Disorders

What You'll Do

- **Identify** two characteristics of a fad diet.
- **Describe** three possible causes of eating disorders.
- **Describe** three types of eating disorders.

Terms to Learn

- fad diet
- eating disorder
- anorexia nervosa
- bulimia nervosa
- binge eating disorder

Start Off *Write*

How do eating disorders develop?

> Johanna went on a fasting diet to lose 10 pounds. She wanted to look thinner for the school dance. Johanna did not think about how unhealthy she was being by not eating.

Johanna did not realize that she was developing an *unhealthy eating behavior*. Fasting to lose weight is one example of an unhealthy eating behavior.

Unhealthy Eating Behavior

Many people feel the need to have a perfect body to be accepted or popular among their peers. Some people may change their eating habits to become thinner or more muscular. For example, people may skip meals, eat only certain foods, or eat large amounts of food at one time. They may also use diet pills or follow unhealthy diets. These types of eating habits are called *unhealthy eating behaviors* and can be very harmful.

The most common unhealthy eating behavior is following a fad diet. **Fad diets** are eating plans that promise quick weight loss with little effort. Most fad diets require you to buy special products, such as pills or shakes. Fad diets often require you to avoid many foods that are good sources of essential nutrients.

Unhealthy eating behaviors can affect a teen's growth, development, and ability to learn. Unhealthy eating behaviors may develop into an eating disorder. Eating disorders are illnesses that severely affect a person's body image and eating habits.

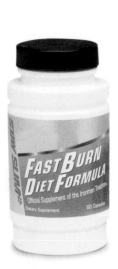
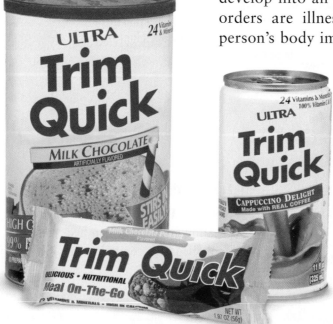

Figure 4 Fad diets usually require you to buy special products, which can be expensive.

Overexercising

In addition to changing their eating habits, some people increase their physical activity to lose weight. Regular exercise is healthy, but some people exercise too much. When a person exercises harder and for a longer period of time than is healthy, that person is *overexercising*. People may overexercise because they are concerned about their weight or because they feel the need to be better at athletics. These people risk getting injured and usually feel tired all the time. They may also feel depressed. Unfortunately, most people don't realize that too much exercise can be dangerous.

What Is an Eating Disorder?

Both unhealthy eating behaviors and overexercising can be dangerous. They can harm a person's growth and development. Or they can develop into an eating disorder. An **eating disorder** is a disease in which a person has an unhealthy concern with his or her body weight and shape. Eating disorders are very complex. They can be caused by many factors. Three factors are low self-esteem, emotional problems, and poor body image. Other factors are pressure from peers to be thin and a history of physical or emotional abuse.

Eating disorders are dangerous to a person's physical and emotional health. Some physical effects of eating disorders include dangerous digestive problems and heart failure. Some emotional effects are depression and anxiety. Eating disorders can affect anyone—boys, girls, men, and women of all cultures and ethnicities. Examples of eating disorders are anorexia nervosa (AN uh REKS ee uh nuhr VOH suh), bulimia nervosa (boo LEE mee uh nuhr VOH suh), and binge eating disorder. People who develop anorexia nervosa or bulimia nervosa often suffer from poor body image and low self-esteem. People who develop binge eating disorder often suffer from emotional problems and low self-esteem.

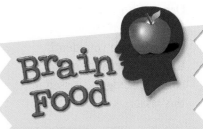

Brain Food

In the United States, 5 million to 10 million girls and women and 1 million boys and men struggle with eating disorders.

TABLE 2 Some Causes of Eating Disorders
Depression
Feelings of lack of control in one's life
History of physical or sexual abuse
Troubled family and personal relationships
Low self-esteem
Unhealthy body image

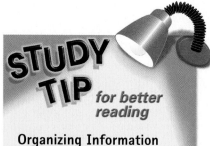

Anorexia Nervosa

Anorexia nervosa is a disease in which a person has a great fear of gaining weight. **Anorexia nervosa** is an eating disorder that includes self-starvation, an unhealthy body image, and extreme weight loss. People who develop anorexia nervosa also suffer from low self-esteem. They are very scared of becoming fat even though they are very thin. They usually starve themselves or eat only foods that are low in Calories and fat. They may spend more time playing with food than eating it. They may also wear many layers of clothing to hide their weight loss. If left untreated, a person with this disease may develop kidney and heart problems. In severe cases, a person suffering from anorexia nervosa may starve to death.

Bulimia Nervosa

Bulimia nervosa is a disease in which a person has difficulty controlling how much he or she eats. **Bulimia nervosa** is an eating disorder in which a person eats a large amount of food and then tries to rid their body of the food. A person who has this disease usually eats large amounts of food at one time, which is called *bingeing* (BINJ ing). After bingeing, the person may make himself or herself vomit. Or he or she may take laxatives or diuretics to eliminate some of the food. The act of ridding the body of food is called *purging* (PUHRJ ing). This "binge and purge" cycle damages a person's health. The person will suffer from a lack of nutrients. And the acid that comes up from the stomach when a person vomits eats away at the gums and teeth. A person with bulimia may also have swollen jaws and cheeks and stained teeth.

TABLE 3 Some Symptoms of Anorexia Nervosa and Bulimia Nervosa	
A person with anorexia nervosa may...	**A person with bulimia nervosa may...**
eat only low-fat or low-Calorie foods	spend a lot of time thinking about food
play with his or her food but not eat it	steal food or hide food in strange places
wear baggy clothes to hide his or her thinness	take trips to the bathroom immediately after eating
overexercise	make himself or herself throw up after eating
	overexercise

Binge Eating Disorder

People who have binge eating disorder often feel as though they cannot stop themselves from eating. **Binge eating disorder** is a disease in which a person has difficulty controlling how much he or she eats but does not purge. In many cases, a person who has this disease suffers from depression as well. People who suffer from this disease usually become very overweight. In many cases, a person may become obese. *Obesity* is a condition in which a person has a large percentage of body fat. Obesity results in many health problems such as increased cholesterol levels, high blood pressure, diabetes, and increased risk for heart disease, stroke, and cancer.

Giving and Getting Help

If you think you or a friend may have an eating disorder, it is very important that you tell a trusted adult about your feelings. This adult may be a parent or teacher. You can also talk to the school nurse, school counselor, or even a doctor. An adult can help you or a friend get professional help as soon as possible. Eating disorders are serious diseases that can damage your health. Even though getting help may be very hard, it is the best decision for your health.

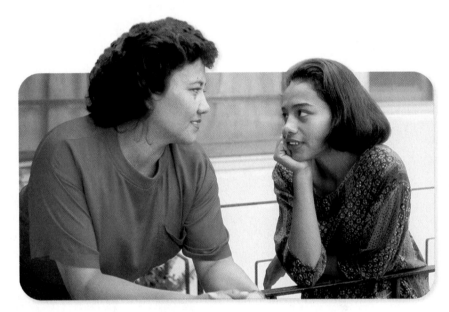

Figure 5 The first step in getting help for an eating disorder is to talk to a parent or other trusted adult.

Lesson Review

Using Vocabulary

1. What are two characteristics of a fad diet?

2. What is an eating disorder?

Understanding Concepts

3. Describe three types of eating disorders.

4. Why are eating disorders dangerous to a person's health?

5. What are three possible causes of eating disorders?

Critical Thinking

6. Making Good Decisions You notice that your friend has been exercising a lot lately. He is also very concerned about how his body looks. You think that he is developing unhealthy eating behaviors. Would you talk to your friend? If so, what would you say?

Lesson 4 Managing Your Weight

What You'll Do

- **Describe** how to find your healthy weight range.
- **Describe** five factors that affect your weight.
- **Describe** how to keep a healthy weight.
- **Explain** how your feelings can affect your eating habits.
- **List** five ways to make healthy food choices.

Terms to Learn

- healthy weight range

Start Off Write

How can you maintain your weight healthfully?

Lauren wants to maintain her weight. She is often confused about which foods to eat and which foods to avoid. Lauren wishes that she didn't have to worry about food so much.

Many teens wonder how to maintain, gain, or lose weight. However, most of these teens do not consider how to manage their weight healthfully.

Your Healthy Weight Range

The first step in managing your weight healthfully is to determine your healthy weight range. Your **healthy weight range** is an estimate of how much you should weigh depending on your height and your body frame. Every person has a unique body shape and size. So, determining exactly how much a person should weigh is impossible. There is no ideal weight for a person.

So, how do you determine your healthy weight range? The body mass index, or BMI, is a calculation that can help you find your healthy weight range. You can find a BMI table in the appendix of this book. You can also ask your family doctor to help you determine what weight range is healthy for you.

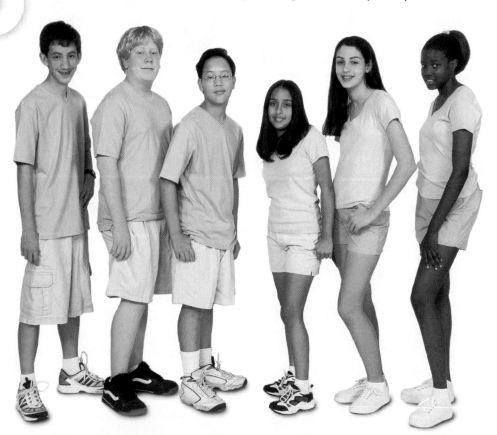

Figure 6 There is no such thing as a normal body shape or size.

What Affects Your Weight?

Many factors affect your weight. You inherit traits for body size and shape from your parents. These traits play a role in your height and weight as you become an adult. Here are some other factors that may affect your weight:

- Teens go through a period of rapid growth, which can cause a natural, healthy weight gain.
- Hormonal changes, especially in girls, can cause changes in a teen's weight.
- The types of food you eat can affect your weight.
- Your level of physical activity can affect your weight.

Keeping a Healthy Weight

Eating a healthy diet and balancing the food you eat with physical activity will help you keep a healthy weight. Your body uses the food you eat for energy. You use some of this energy to keep your body systems working. You use some of it for exercise, such as riding your bike or playing sports.

If you eat more food than your body can use for your daily activities, you will gain weight. If you eat the same amount of food that your body needs daily, you will maintain your weight. Similarly, if your body uses more energy than the energy you get from the food you eat, you will lose weight.

After you find your healthy weight range, you should balance the amount of food you eat with enough physical activity to stay in your healthy weight range.

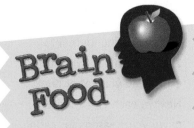

Figure 7 Balancing the food you eat with physical activity helps you stay in your healthy weight range.

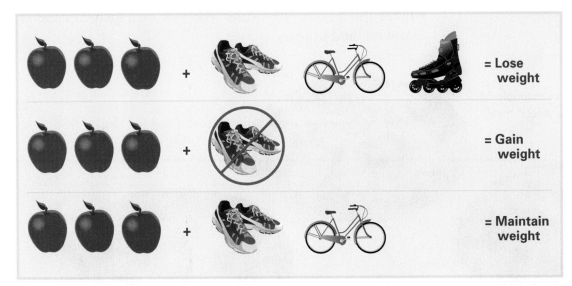

= Lose weight

= Gain weight

= Maintain weight

Why Do You Eat?

Do you know why you eat when you eat? You may think that the answer is because you are hungry. Most people eat when they are hungry. However, other reasons may affect your decision to eat. Sometimes, your emotions may make you feel like eating even if you are not hungry. Or they may make you feel like not eating at all. Here are some situations that may affect your decision to eat:

- nervousness
- anger
- sadness
- happiness
- a family gathering or a friend's party
- a holiday, such as Thanksgiving

Sometimes, when your feelings affect the way you eat, your food choices may be unhealthy. If you know how your feelings affect your eating habits, you can make healthful food choices.

Eating Healthfully

Eating a well-balanced diet is a good way to keep a healthy weight. Here are some tips for making good nutritional choices:

- Eat plenty of fresh fruits and vegetables every day.
- Drink water or juice rather than soda with each meal.
- Eat lean meat, chicken, or fish.
- Limit the amount of fried foods that you eat, such as french fries and potato chips.
- Limit the amount of sweets that you eat, such as candies, cookies, and cakes.

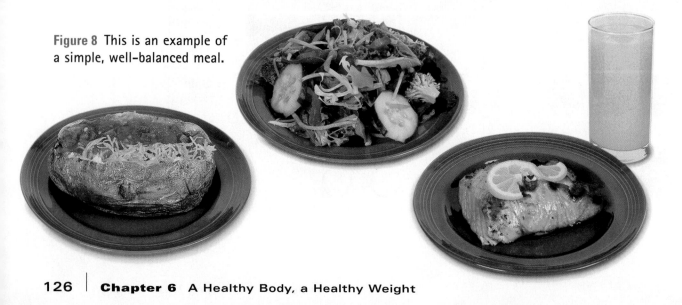

Figure 8 This is an example of a simple, well-balanced meal.

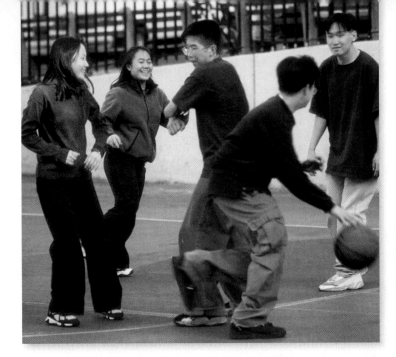

Figure 9 Going outside and having fun with your friends is a great way to stay physically active.

Staying Physically Active

Being physically active is a great way to keep a healthy weight. Being physically active does not mean you have to play sports. You don't even have to follow an exercise routine to be physically active. Activities such as in-line skating and riding bikes are great ways to stay physically active. You can also stay physically active by helping out around the house, gardening, or walking around the neighborhood. It is great if you enjoy playing sports or exercising. However, you don't have to be an athlete to enjoy being physically active. Regular physical activity can help you feel good about your body. These feelings will help you build a healthy body image. Being regularly active will also help you keep a healthy weight.

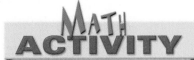

The energy you get from food is measured in units called Calories. Suppose you ate a cheeseburger for lunch. The cheeseburger contained 300 Calories. If running around the track uses 480 Calories an hour, how long would you have to run to use all the energy you got from the cheeseburger?

Lesson Review

Vocabulary

1. How do you find your healthy weight range?

Understanding Concepts

2. Explain how to stay within your healthy weight range.

3. Explain how your feelings may affect your eating habits.

4. Describe five factors that influence your weight.

Critical Thinking

5. **Applying Concepts** Imagine your family doctor told you that you are below your healthy weight range. Make a plan that will help you get to a healthy weight. Suppose your doctor said that you are over your healthy weight range. How would your plan change?

Chapter Summary

■ Your body image is the way you see and imagine your body. Your body image can affect many aspects of your life. ■ If you have a healthy body image, you will be less likely to want to change your body for unhealthy reasons. ■ Your body image is influenced by the media, your family, and friends, and your teachers and coaches. ■ You can maintain your healthy body image by using "I" statements to deal with unkind remarks from other people. ■ Unhealthy eating behaviors, such as dieting, can develop into an eating disorder. ■ Eating disorders are very dangerous and may result in death. ■ Each person has a different healthy weight range. You can keep a healthy weight by eating well and staying active.

Using Vocabulary

For each pair of terms, describe how the meanings of the terms differ.

1 anorexia nervosa/bulimia nervosa

2 fad diet/eating disorder

For each sentence, fill in the blank with the proper word from the word bank provided below.

> healthy weight range
> fad diet
> bulimia nervosa
> binge eating disorder
> eating disorder
> body image

3 The way you see, imagine, and feel about your body is called your ___.

4 ___ is an illness in which a person eats a large amount of food and then purges.

5 An illness in which a person is overly concerned about his or her body weight and shape is a(n) ___.

6 An eating plan that promises quick weight loss is called a(n) ___.

Understanding Concepts

7 Explain how to keep a healthy weight by eating well and staying physically active.

8 Describe the importance of telling an adult if you suspect your friend has an eating disorder.

9 How can your level of physical activity affect your weight?

10 Why is having a healthy body image important?

11 Describe three factors that influence your body image. How do these factors influence you?

12 What is a healthy weight range? Does every person have the same healthy weight range? Explain your answer.

13 What are some feelings that may affect your eating habits?

14 List five ways to make healthy food choices.

15 Explain the difference between healthy body image and unhealthy body image.

16 Explain how using "I" statements can help you build a healthy body image.

Critical Thinking

Making Inferences

17 Megan compares herself to the teens she sees in magazines. She thinks that she needs to look like the teen models in order to be popular at school. She decides to go on a diet. Does Megan have a healthy body image? What could happen to Megan if she continues to diet?

18 Michael admits to you that he has a problem controlling how much he eats. He tells you that sometimes he just can't stop eating, and afterwards he feels ashamed of himself. Michael asks you to not tell anyone about his problem. What kind of problem does Michael have? What will happen to him if he does not get help from an adult? What can you do to help him?

Using Refusal Skills

19 Tracy tells you that she purges after she eats lunch. She tells you that if you purge every day after lunch for the next week, you will be thinner for the school dance. Tracy tells you that purging is okay because you are going to do it for only a short period of time. What will you say to Tracy?

20 Rebecca brings diet pills to school. You overhear Rebecca telling your best friend that one pill will help your friend burn more Calories than if she exercised for 1 hour. Your friend is tempted to try the pills. How can you help your friend refuse Rebecca's diet pills?

Interpreting Graphics

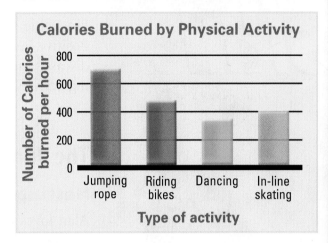

Calories Burned by Physical Activity

Use the figure above to answer questions 21–23.

21 Imagine that you are trying to maintain your healthy weight. Your food intake for the day was 2,500 Calories. How many hours would you have to jump rope to burn half of these Calories?

22 Your friend Rachel dances for 1 hour every day after school. She does not dance on the weekends. How many Calories does Rachel use for dancing in 1 week?

23 Tom in-line skates for 2 hours each week. He also rides his bike for 3 hours each week. How many Calories does Tom use for these two physical activities each week?

Reading Checkup

Take a minute to review your answers to the Health IQ questions at the beginning of this chapter. How has reading this chapter improved your Health IQ?

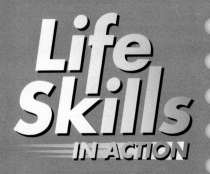

Life Skills IN ACTION

The 4 Steps of Practicing Wellness

1. Choose a health behavior you want to improve or change.
2. Gather information on how you can improve that health behavior.
3. Start using the improved health behavior.
4. Evaluate the effects of the health behavior.

Practicing Wellness

Practicing wellness means practicing good health habits. Positive health behaviors can help prevent injury, illness, disease, and even premature death. Complete the following activity to learn how you can practice wellness.

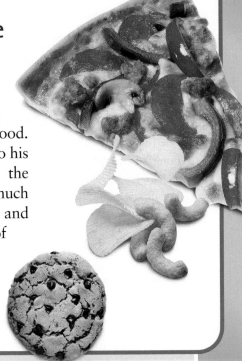

The Junk Food Junkie

ACT 1

Setting the Scene

Alan loves eating junk food. He uses all of his allowance to buy pizza, chips, and other junk food. One day, a dietitian gives a talk to his health class. During her talk, the dietitian shows the class how much fat is in a serving of french fries and how much sugar is in a can of soda. Alan is surprised to learn how unhealthy junk food is and begins to think about changing his eating habits.

Guided Practice

Practice with a Friend

Form a group of three. Have one person play the role of Alan and another person play the role of the dietitian. Have the third person be an observer. Walking through each of the four steps of practicing wellness, role-play Alan learning to improve his eating habits. Alan can talk to the dietitian to gather information about nutrition. The observer will take notes, which will include observations about what the person playing Alan did well and suggestions of ways to improve. Stop after each step to evaluate the process.

Independent Practice

Check Yourself

After you have completed the guided practice, go through Act 1 again without stopping at each step. Answer the questions below to review what you did.

1. In addition to talking with the dietitian, how can Alan find information about good eating habits?

2. What are some specific examples of what Alan could do to improve his health behavior?

3. How could Alan evaluate the effects of changing his eating habits?

4. What are some ways that you can improve your eating habits?

ACT 2

On Your Own

Alan has been eating better for a month, and he is feeling great. Improving his eating habits has caused him to think about his overall health. Alan wonders if he is getting enough exercise. He spends most of his afternoons watching TV or playing video games. Make a poster showing how Alan could use the four steps of practicing wellness to begin an exercise program.

Mental and Emotional Health

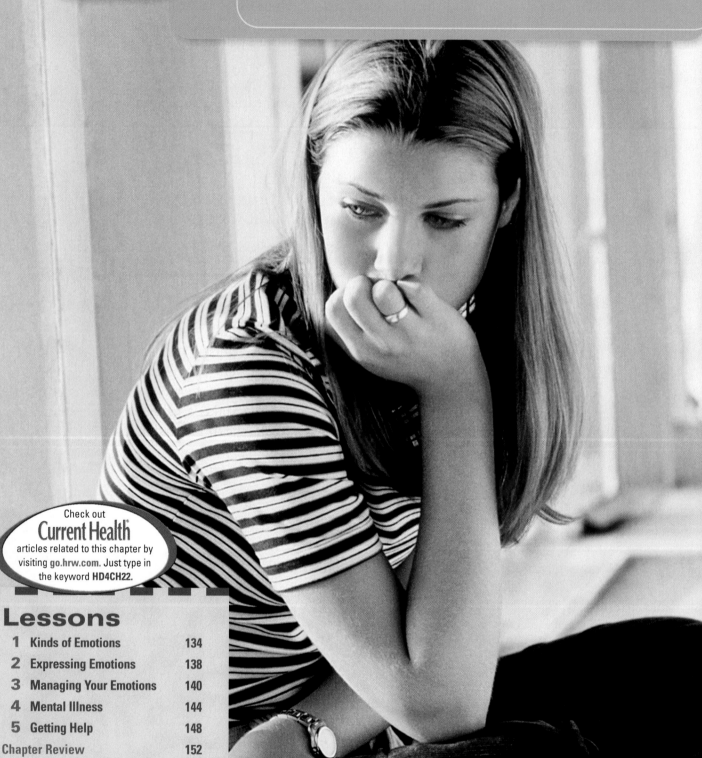

Check out
Current Health
articles related to this chapter by
visiting **go.hrw.com**. Just type in
the keyword **HD4CH22**.

Lessons

" I never knew that **depression** could be so **serious** until my dad was **diagnosed** with it. He said that it was different from just feeling **sad.** He goes to therapy and takes medicine, and he is becoming much more like himself again. "

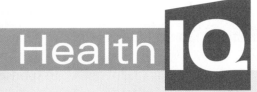

Health **IQ**

PRE-READING

Answer the following multiple-choice questions to find out what you already know about mental and emotional health. When you've finished this chapter, you'll have the opportunity to change your answers based on what you've learned.

1. Mental illness
a. is very rare.
b. happens only to people who have a weak mind.
c. cannot be treated.
d. affects thoughts, emotions, and behavior.

2. Which of the following statements is true?
a. Teens can't manage their emotions.
b. Hormones have nothing to do with emotions.
c. Most teens are happy and well adjusted.
d. It is normal to be depressed when you are a teenager.

3. Which of the following statements is true?
a. Depression means being sad.
b. Depression will go away if something good happens.
c. Depression is a disorder that can lead to suicidal thinking.
d. People who have depression are lazy.

4. A trigger is
a. a person, thing, or event that causes an emotional response.
b. a way of using body language to communicate.
c. a way of thinking about emotional problems.
d. a behavior used to cope with emotional stress.

5. Bipolar mood disorder
a. is an illness that affects moods.
b. includes a happy period called mania.
c. is bad only during periods of depression.
d. is an anxiety disorder.

ANSWERS: 1. d; 2. c; 3. c; 4. a; 5. a

Kinds of Emotions

Hatim is confused about his emotions. Lately, he has been feeling really sensitive about everything. He finds himself arguing with his parents more often. He also gets upset at his friends a lot.

Being confused about new feelings is normal. Dealing with confusing feelings is part of good mental health. **Mental health** is the way people think about and respond to events in their lives.

Teen Emotions

People respond to the world around them with thoughts, actions, and emotions. An **emotion** is a feeling produced in response to a life event. Emotions are caused by chemical changes in the brain that affect how the body feels. Emotional reactions help people understand relationships, danger, success, and loss.

Both personality and experience influence a person's emotional responses. People are born with tendencies to respond to life in a certain way. But as they grow and experience more situations, people learn and change their emotional responses. Much of this learning happens during the teen years. Teens take on many new roles and responsibilities as they grow and mature. Reacting to these changes can produce unfamiliar feelings. Teens can learn and mature from these experiences and the emotions the experiences produce.

Teen emotions are also affected by the changes happening in their bodies. During the early teen years, the body produces new hormones. A **hormone** is a chemical that helps control how the body grows and functions. These chemicals can affect the brain and sometimes cause mood swings. Most teens find healthy ways to deal with the emotional changes they experience.

What You'll Do

- **Explain** how teens' changing lives and bodies affect their emotions.
- **Describe** how emotions can be pleasant or unpleasant.
- **Explain** how emotions can have physical effects.

Terms to Learn

- mental health
- emotion
- hormone
- emotional health

Start Off Write

How could unpleasant emotions be helpful to a person?

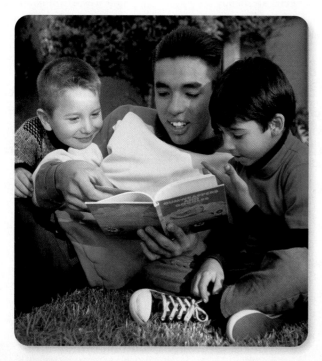

Figure 1 New responsibilities, such as babysitting, can cause teens to feel new emotions.

From Sadness to Happiness

Moods can range from very sad to very happy. Having such a wide range of moods is normal. Feeling a range of emotions is part of good emotional health. **Emotional health** is the way a person experiences and deals with feelings. Experiencing one emotion all the time—even happiness—would be unhealthy.

Unpleasant emotions, such as sadness, can be valuable. Sadness can help us remember and appreciate a loss. If a pet dies, sadness can help you understand how important the pet was to you. Sadness can also help you realize when you need to make changes in your life. Sadness about not doing well in school can help you decide to study more often or ask for help.

Emotions become unhealthy when they get in the way of relationships and responsibilities. For example, sadness is healthy. But skipping class because you are sad is unhealthy. Dealing with emotions in healthy ways keeps them from becoming unhealthy. Talking with someone when you are sad is a healthy way to deal with sadness.

Recognizing your emotions can help you deal with them in healthy ways. Your emotions can be easier to recognize when you know where they lie on an emotional spectrum. An *emotional spectrum* is a range of emotions organized by how pleasant they are. The figure below shows an emotional spectrum.

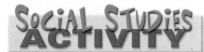

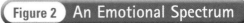

Figure 2 An Emotional Spectrum

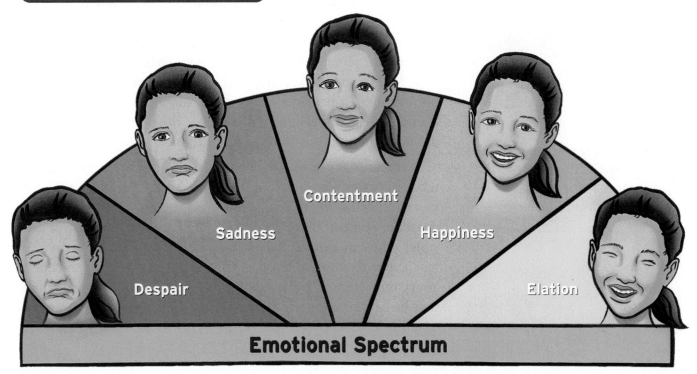

Contentment

Sadness

Happiness

Despair

Elation

Emotional Spectrum

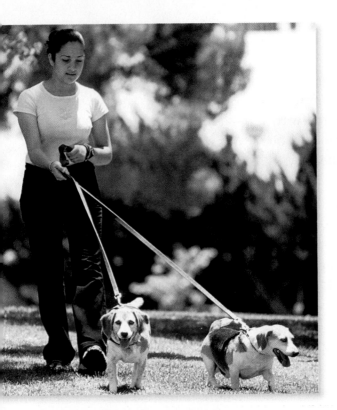

Figure 3 If you like dogs, you might have a good first impression of a person who also likes dogs.

Love and Hate

The emotions that range from love to hate help us know how we feel about parts of life. Love and like help us understand how much we value objects, events, or relationships. Hate and dislike let us know when we do not value these things.

There are many ways to value something. You might like the taste of chocolate. You might love playing basketball. Or, love can be a reaction to a family member, a friend, or a romantic interest. People can also experience hate in different strengths. You might dislike peas but hate snakes.

Sometimes, feelings of dislike or hate are based on prejudice (PREJ oo dis). *Prejudice* is an unfair judgment made before a person knows anything about someone or something. For example, if a person you don't know reminds you of something that you dislike, you may be tempted to dislike that person. But after you get to know the person, you may find out that you really like him or her. Avoiding prejudice can help you clearly understand your values. You can avoid prejudice by learning more about the differences between people that make them unique.

What's Useful About Anger?

Anger is an emotion of strong disappointment and displeasure that forms when hopes are not met. Anger can be helpful if it is dealt with in healthy ways. But anger can be unhealthy if it is misdirected at people who are not at fault. *Misdirection* is aiming your feelings at a person who did nothing to cause those feelings. For example, a baseball player might get angry if he strikes out. He could react by yelling at a coach or the umpire. These people did not cause him to strike out, so his anger is misdirected.

Managing anger in a healthy way begins with figuring out what hopes or desires were not met. After you figure this out, you can decide whether meeting these desires is possible. If it is possible, you can try to meet them another way. If it is not possible, you can think about a new set of hopes that is within reach. For example, the baseball player could realize that he is angry with himself for not being a better player. He may realize that he cannot expect a home run every time. He may decide to practice harder so that he can do better in the future.

Myth & Fact

Myth: A person can tell if he or she is going to like or dislike another person the first time they meet.

Fact: Many times your impression of a person changes after you get to know the person better.

Physical Effects of Emotions

During an emotional response, chemical changes in the brain cause changes in the body. For example, when a person is scared, chemicals are released into the blood. These chemicals prepare the body to escape or defend itself. They increase heart and breathing rates, and they prepare the muscles to react quickly. These physical changes can help you recognize that you are afraid.

Many of the physical effects that occur in an emotional response vary from person to person. However, pleasant emotions, such as happiness, usually have comfortable physical effects. These emotions sometimes even improve physical health by lowering blood pressure and heart rate. But sadness and worry can bring headaches or feelings of tiredness. And stressful emotions can increase heart rate, blood pressure, and muscle tension. Anger may even cause hot flashes and shaking. Tension in your body can sometimes be a sign that you should deal with your emotions.

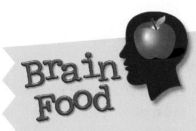

Brain Food

When animals are in stressful or dangerous situations, they show many of the same physical signs of fear as humans do. These signs have led some researchers to wonder if animals have emotions, too.

TABLE 1 Physical Responses to Fear

Increased heart rate, blood pressure, and breathing rate
Hair stands on end
Lightheadedness
Trembling, shaking, and chills or hot flashes
Sweating

Lesson Review

Using Vocabulary

1. What are emotions?

2. How is mental health related to emotional health?

Understanding Concepts

3. What life changes affect teen emotions?

4. How can emotions be pleasant or unpleasant?

Critical Thinking

5. **Analyzing Ideas** What physical signs could tell you that someone is angry?

6. **Making Predictions** Which emotions are more likely to be fair—those based on facts or those based on prejudice? Explain your answer and give an example.

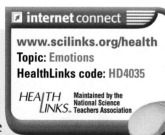

internet connect

www.scilinks.org/health
Topic: Emotions
HealthLinks code: HD4035

HEALTH LINKS Maintained by the National Science Teachers Association

What You'll Do

■ **Explain** why people express and communicate emotions.

■ **List** four effective ways to communicate.

■ **Describe** how a person can use creative expression.

Terms to Learn

• verbal communication
• active listening
• body language
• creative expression

Start Off

Write

How can body language express emotions?

Expressing Emotions

Amy could tell that Deena was not being honest. Deena insisted she was fine. But her body was slouched, and she was frowning.

Amy knew from Deena's behavior that she was sad. Understanding other people is one part of communication. Being able to express your own emotions is the other part.

Communicating Emotions

Communication allows people to understand each other. When other people understand your emotions, they can share your joy or help you solve problems. People use both verbal and nonverbal communication.

Verbal communication is expressing and understanding thoughts and emotions by talking. Words can be used to express emotions clearly so problems can be resolved. For verbal communication to be effective, someone must hear and understand a speaker. An active listener does this. **Active listening** is not only hearing but also showing that you understand what a person is saying. Asking questions and listening to answers encourages the other person to keep talking. Making eye contact is another signal that you are paying attention.

Body language is a way to express thoughts and emotions with the face, hands, and posture. Body language is nonverbal communication. Eye contact can express your interest in another person. Facial movements, such as smiles and frowns, can express happiness or sadness. And a slouched body posture shows a lack of energy or confidence. By being aware of body language, people can avoid sending others the wrong messages. Someone pacing and clenching his or her fists in anger can be very scary. However, that person may not realize how scary these behaviors look.

Figure 4 Noticing body language can help you understand another person.

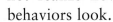

Expression as Release

Why is expressing emotions important? Communication can solve problems and clear up misunderstandings between people. But expressing emotions can feel good even when it does not solve a person's problems. People often feel better after crying or telling someone about feeling sad. Expressing emotions allows people to release physical and emotional tension.

Sometimes, discussing emotions with other people is hard. When communicating with others is difficult, you can express emotions through creative expression. **Creative expression** is using an art to express emotion. This type of expression includes painting, sculpting, acting in a play, dancing, writing a poem, keeping a journal, and playing music. Creative expression is a healthy way to release emotional tensions.

Not all ways of expressing emotions are healthy. Fighting, vandalism, or hurting oneself are unhealthy ways of expressing emotions. Healthy emotional expression never damages oneself, other people, or property.

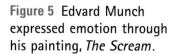

COMMUNICATING EFFECTIVELY

Choose an emotion, and express it through a creative project. The project could be a drawing, a sculpture, or a story.

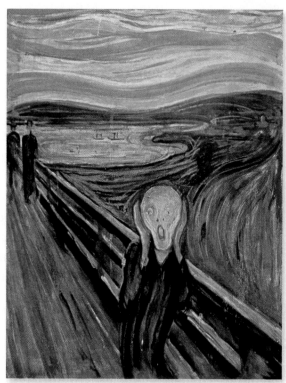

Figure 5 Edvard Munch expressed emotion through his painting, *The Scream*.

Lesson Review

Using Vocabulary

1. What is active listening?

Understanding Concepts

2. What are four effective ways to communicate?

3. Why do people express emotions and communicate?

Critical Thinking

4. Making Inferences What emotions do you think Edvard Munch was expressing when he painted *The Scream*? Do you notice any body language in the painting? Consider both facial expression and body posture.

Managing Your Emotions

Shayla was worried about her friend Ellie. Ellie's parents were getting divorced. Shayla couldn't believe that Ellie wasn't affected, but Ellie didn't act sad.

People deal with stress in many ways. Sometimes, not thinking about unpleasant emotions is easier. But being able to deal honestly with emotions is part of good emotional health.

Dealing with Unpleasant Emotions

It is normal to have unpleasant emotions sometimes. These emotions may help you learn from a situation or motivate you to solve problems. But unpleasant emotions can become unhealthy if they are not dealt with properly.

Sometimes, you can deal with unpleasant emotions by simply thinking about them in a new way. Focusing on only the bad parts of a situation is called **negative thinking.** Trying to think about the good parts of a situation may help you feel differently. **Positive self-talk** is the process of thinking about the good parts of a bad situation. Positive self-talk about a bad situation may include ideas such as these: "This situation won't last forever," "I will have other chances," and "It doesn't always happen like this." Being able to think of a bad situation in a positive way can help you cope until the situation improves. Positive thinking can help you feel better.

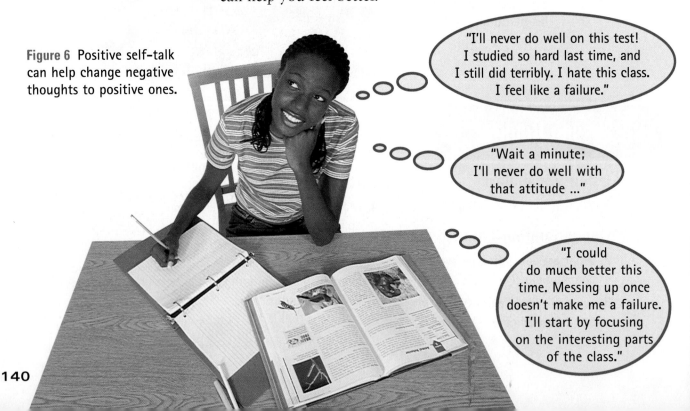

Figure 6 Positive self-talk can help change negative thoughts to positive ones.

"I'll never do well on this test! I studied so hard last time, and I still did terribly. I hate this class. I feel like a failure."

"Wait a minute; I'll never do well with that attitude ..."

"I could do much better this time. Messing up once doesn't make me a failure. I'll start by focusing on the interesting parts of the class."

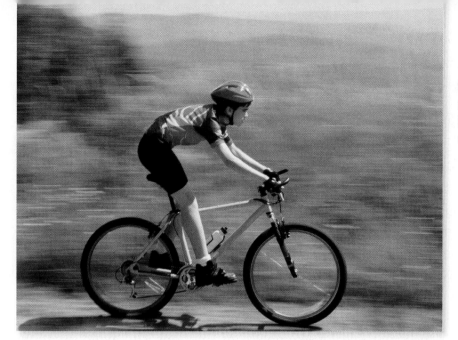

Figure 7 Fun activities, such as riding a bike, can be a good way to cope with stress.

Coping with Stress

Stress is the body's response to new or unpleasant situations. Sometimes, we ignore problems to delay dealing with stress. Other times, we deal with problems immediately. A famous doctor named Sigmund Freud (SIG muhnd FROYD) called our responses to stress defense mechanisms. **Defense mechanisms** are behaviors we use to deal with stress.

Healthy defense mechanisms help you deal with emotions in a useful way. For example, humor can help relieve stress by focusing on the amusing parts of a tough situation. Defense mechanisms are unhealthy if they cause you to ignore your emotions or the issues that cause them. *Devaluation* is a defense mechanism in which someone transfers unpleasant feelings about a situation to specific people. Thinking negatively about others allows that person to ignore the negative situation. If you are aware of defense mechanisms, you can avoid the behaviors that keep you from dealing honestly with emotions.

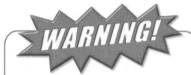

Avoiding Emotions

While it may be easier to ignore unpleasant emotions, avoiding your emotions can prevent you from solving the problems that cause them. In fact, the problems could even get worse.

LIFE SKILLS ACTIVITY

COPING

Imagine that you just moved to a new school, started a new babysitting job, had a fight with your parents, and sprained your wrist. These things have caused you to feel a lot of stress. Write and illustrate a short story showing at least five different ways that you could cope with stress in this situation. Point out which strategies are healthy and which are unhealthy. Explain how the unhealthy strategies could affect you in negative ways.

Finding Your Triggers

One way to deal with unpleasant emotions is to avoid situations that cause them. You can do this by figuring out what triggers your different emotions. A **trigger** is a person, situation, or event that influences emotions. If you recognize that certain situations always make you feel badly, you can try to avoid those situations.

Once you know what triggers your emotions, you can also seek out situations that trigger pleasant emotions. For example, if you know that music makes you happy, you could join a music group or listen to music more often. Spending time doing healthy things that you enjoy can improve your emotional health.

Knowing your triggers can also help you to be more aware of your emotions. If you know that a particular situation triggers certain emotions, you can recognize those feelings more easily when they happen. Once you recognize emotions, you can deal with them more effectively. Dealing with emotions quickly can keep them from becoming problems.

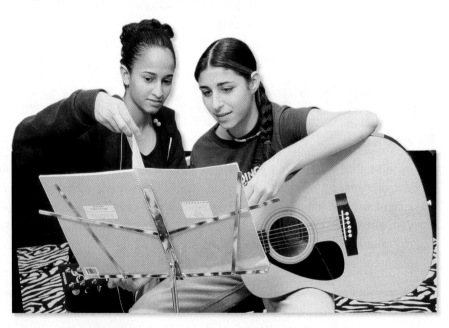

Figure 8 An activity such as playing music may trigger pleasant emotions.

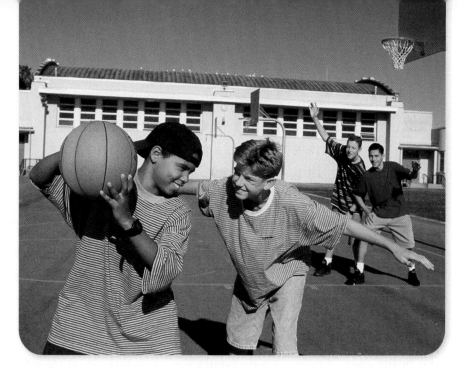

Figure 9 Activites that improve physical health can also improve emotional health.

Influences You Can Control

Everyone has unpleasant emotions from time to time. These emotions can be healthy, but sometimes they are stressful. One way to reduce the impact of stressful emotions is to improve your social and physical health.

Filling your life with people, activities, and healthy habits can improve social and physical health. Building close relationships is valuable. Friends and family members can help you cope with emotional problems. Finding activities that you enjoy can help you express yourself and feel good about yourself. Exercising and eating right can also improve your self-esteem. Improving these aspects of your life will make rough times easier to handle.

Lesson Review

Using Vocabulary

1. What is a defense mechanism?

2. Use the term *trigger* in a sentence.

Understanding Concepts

3. How can defense mechanisms be healthy or unhealthy?

4. Name two habits that can influence emotional health.

Critical Thinking

5. Making Inferences Suppose you are disappointed about not doing well on a test. What are three ways to handle the disappointment?

6. Analyzing Ideas Your friend just moved away, and you feel terrible. Write a paragraph in which you use positive self-talk to feel better.

Mental Illness

Lana thought something was wrong with her mother. Lana's whole family was going to a party for her brother's graduating class. But Lana's mother refused to go because she was afraid of crowds.

Lana's mother has an intense fear of crowds. Controlling her fear is very difficult because she has a mental illness. Illness can affect mental and emotional health just as it can affect physical health.

What Is Mental Illness?

The brain usually responds to events with normal thoughts and emotions. But sometimes brain chemistry is disrupted, which causes thoughts and emotions to get out of control. This disruption may result in a mental illness. A **mental illness** is a disorder that affects a person's thoughts, emotions, and behaviors.

Nobody knows what causes the changes in brain chemistry that lead to mental illness. Some people may be born with a tendency to have these disorders. Some people develop mental illness when stressful life events cause changes in the brain.

Medicines can help treat mental illness by balancing the brain's chemistry. *Therapy*, or talking about thoughts and changing behaviors, can also help people. With continuing medicine and therapy, many people who have mental illness can live regular lives.

What You'll Do

- **List** two factors that can cause mental illness.
- **Explain** how depression is different from sadness.
- **Describe** bipolar mood disorder and schizophrenia.
- **Describe** three anxiety disorders.

Terms to Learn

- mental illness
- depression
- phobia

Start Off
Write

How can you tell if someone is depressed?

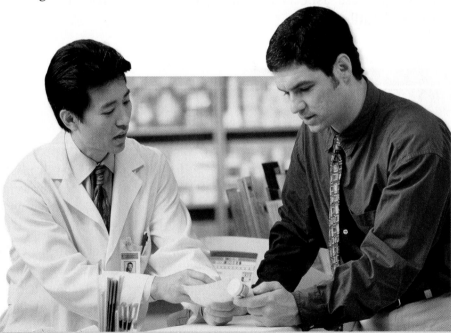

Figure 10 Medicine can be used to help treat mental illness.

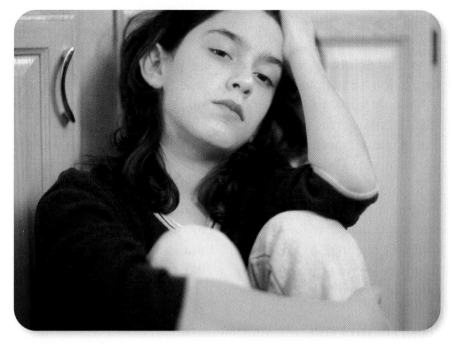

Figure 11 Depression may sometimes lead to suicide. Luckily, there are ways to treat depression.

Depression

A mental illness that affects a person's moods is called a *mood disorder*. Depression is a mood disorder in which a person is extremely sad and hopeless for a long time.

Depression differs from healthy sadness. People with depression can become sad or hopeless for no reason. And these feelings last two weeks or longer in a depressed person.

The following behaviors can be signs of depression:

- being unable to enjoy daily activities
- sleeping either more or less than normal
- overeating or not having an appetite
- feeling tired or lacking energy
- moving slowly or being unable to sit still
- having difficulty concentrating or making decisions
- using alcohol or other drugs
- feeling guilty, irritable, or hopeless without cause
- thinking about death or hurting oneself

If you think you or someone you know is depressed, you should find help immediately. The most dangerous part of depression is the possibility of suicide. *Suicide* is the act of killing oneself. Depression can feel so painful and hopeless that a person would rather be dead. However, depression can be treated successfully. With treatment, people who were depressed can feel happy to be alive.

Myth & Fact

Myth: Depressed people are just lazy.

Fact: People that are depressed must cope with unbalanced brain chemistry that keeps their minds and bodies from working properly.

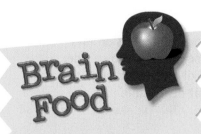

Bipolar Mood Disorder

Bipolar mood disorder is a mood disorder in which a person has depression sometimes and mania other times. This disorder is commonly known as manic depression. *Mania* is an excited mood that is associated with excessive energy or irritation. During mania, people need very little sleep. Their thoughts may become disorganized. They may talk fast and be difficult to interrupt.

In some cases, people who have bipolar mood disorder break from reality. They may *hallucinate* (huh LOO si NAYT), or hear and see things that do not exist. They may also have *delusions* (di LOO zhuhnz), or false beliefs. For example, they may believe that they know a famous person well. Bipolar mood disorder can often be controlled with medicine and therapy.

Schizophrenia

Schizophrenia (SKIT suh FREE nee uh) is a mental illness that affects thoughts and behaviors more than it affects moods. In fact, people who have schizophrenia may show very little emotion despite the difficulties they face. Schizophrenia causes people to hallucinate and have delusions. It can cause a person's thoughts to become so disorganized that other people cannot understand that person's speech. In some cases, people who have schizophrenia remain "frozen" in one position for a long time.

This disorder can take over a person's life. However, with proper treatment, people who have schizophrenia can often live as regular members of a community.

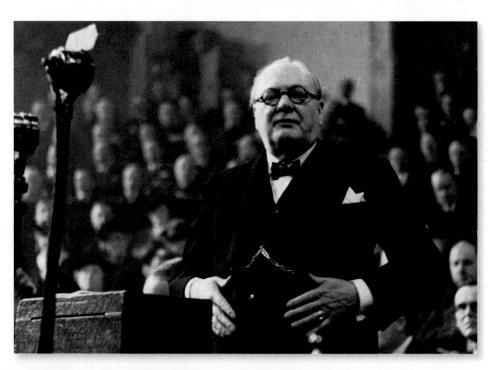

Figure 12 Winston Churchill, who was the prime minister of Great Britain during WWII, had bipolar mood disorder and yet he led an extraordinary life.

Anxiety Disorders

Anxiety (ang ZIE uh tee) *disorders* are mental illnesses that cause extreme nervousness, worry, or panic. There are several types of anxiety disorders. They can be classified by how long the nervous feelings last and by what triggers the feelings.

Feelings of anxiety that happen in brief spurts without a trigger or warning can be signs of *panic disorder*. These brief periods of extreme anxiety are called *panic attacks*. During panic attacks, people get very scared and may think they are having a heart attack. They may shake, feel light-headed, and have a hard time breathing.

If panic attacks are triggered by certain situations, the attacks can be signs of a phobia (FOH bee uh). A **phobia** is a strong, abnormal fear of something. Many people have phobias of animals, such as snakes, or situations, such as flying in airplanes. Some people even have phobias of other people.

Some people feel anxiety about thoughts that they have over and over again. These repeating thoughts are called *obsessions*. When people develop repeating behaviors in response to these thoughts, those people have *obsessive-compulsive disorder (OCD)*. For example, a person with OCD might try washing repeatedly to avoid the anxiety of thinking about dirt. OCD and most other anxiety disorders can be treated with medicines and therapy.

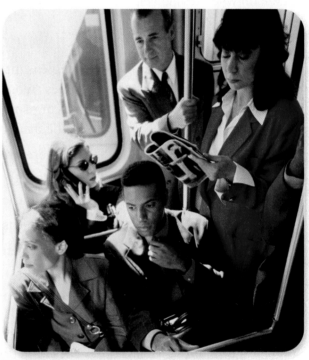

Figure 13 Fear of people or crowded places can cause people to avoid crowds.

Lesson Review

Using Vocabulary

1. What is a phobia?

2. How is depression different from sadness?

Understanding Concepts

3. What are two factors that might cause the brain changes that lead to mental illness?

4. Describe three anxiety disorders.

5. Describe bipolar mood disorder and schizophrenia.

Critical Thinking

6. **Identifying Relationships** What are the similarities and differences between depression and a medical problem that does not affect the brain, such as high blood pressure?

internet connect

www.scilinks.org/health

Topic: Schizophrenia
HealthLinks code: HD4085

Topic: Bipolar Disorder
HealthLinks code: HD4014

Topic: Anxiety Disorders
HealthLinks code: HD4010

HEALTH LINKS. Maintained by the National Science Teachers Association

Getting Help

Martin had not slept well for three nights, and he couldn't concentrate at school. He was very sad that his best friend moved across the country. Would he need help getting through this?

Unpleasant emotions that last for a long time can be scary. Asking for help dealing with emotions can only make things better. And sometimes it can keep problems from getting worse.

Knowing When to Get Help

Unpleasant emotions are very uncomfortable. You may sometimes wonder if you need help dealing with these feelings. Asking someone for help is always OK. Finding help is nothing to be ashamed of or embarrassed about.

There are several signs that can help you know when finding help is especially important. You should tell someone if:

- unpleasant emotions last for a long time or happen often
- unpleasant emotions frequently happen for no reason
- your emotions interfere with relationships or responsibilities

It is best to try solving these problems quickly, before they become even more serious.

Emotions and thoughts that cause you to want to hurt yourself or others are serious warning signs. If you have thoughts about hurting yourself or others, you should get help immediately.

What You'll Do

- **Describe** how to know when you need help for an emotional problem.

- **List** three sources of help for emotional problems.

- **Explain** when to find help for others who have emotional problems.

Terms to Learn

- therapist
- psychiatrist

Start Off
Write

What should you do to help a friend who is depressed?

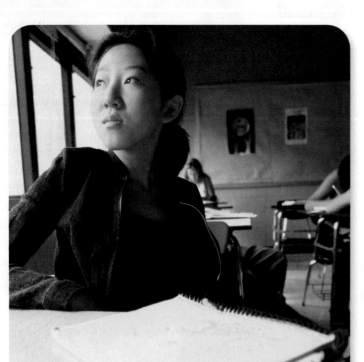

Figure 14 When emotions interfere with duties or relationships, it is time to get help.

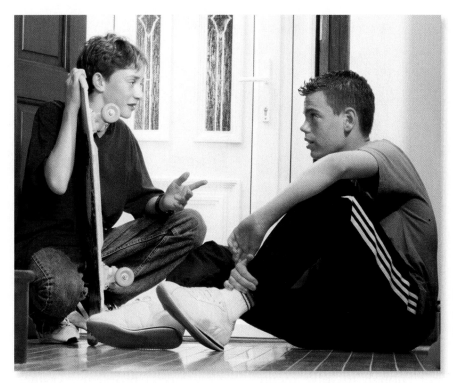

Figure 15 Talking to friends about problems can help you stay emotionally healthy.

Friends and Family

When people have emotional problems, they often turn to people they know for help. Friends, family, and trusted adults can be an important resource for working out emotional problems. These people can help you see your problem from another point of view. They may be able to share stories of similar situations they have experienced. Knowing that others have had similar problems can be comforting.

Sometimes, people are uncomfortable talking to friends or family about personal problems. This can happen when a problem is private or embarrassing. It can also happen when family or friends are part of the problem. In these cases, a friend or family member's involvement could prevent that person from understanding the problem. When family and friends are not a comfortable source of help, people in the community can help. Community resources include teachers, principals, school counselors, doctors, clergy, anonymous hotlines, and peer counseling groups. Because these people are not involved in the situation, their help will be *impartial,* or without prejudice.

Talking about emotional problems can be difficult. It is helpful to prepare a plan of action before you have problems. This preparation includes identifying people that could help you if you had a problem. It can also be helpful to talk with friends and family about emotions when things are going well. This can make you more comfortable discussing emotions with them when problems come up later.

Health Journal

Make a table in your Health Journal. For a week, keep track of all the triggers that make you angry, happy, or sad. Note whether you exercise each day and how much sleep you get each night. Does exercise or sleep affect your emotions? How do you feel after talking to a friend about your emotions?

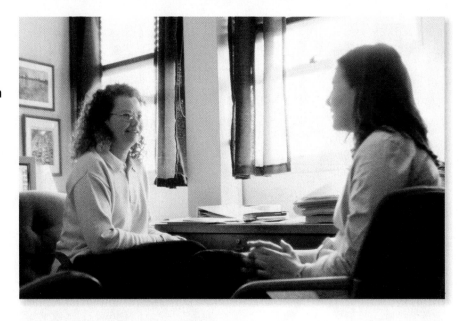

Figure 16 Professionals can give you a fresh point of view on your problems.

Professionals

Sometimes, talking to friends, family, or community members is not enough to solve mental and emotional problems. Trained mental health professionals can help treat serious problems and mental illness.

A **therapist** is a professional who is trained to treat emotional problems by talking about them. Therapists, such as counselors and social workers, try to change the way people think, feel, and act. Through talking, people can learn the cause of their thoughts and feelings or learn new ways to manage their emotions.

Psychiatrists (sie KIE uh trists) are medical doctors that understand how the brain and body affect emotions and behavior. Psychiatrists may use medicine and therapy to treat people who have a mental illness. Often, people who have a mental illness need this treatment to help them recover.

Successful Response to Treatment for Depression

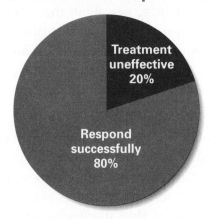

Treatment uneffective 20%

Respond successfully 80%

Figure 17 Most people who get professional treatment for depression recover, but many do not get help.

Source: American Psychiatric Association.

Finding Help for Others

People do not always seek help for their emotional problems. This could be because they are embarrassed. Or they could think that they are able to handle the problem on their own. If someone you know suffers from an emotional problem and is not asking for help, you can encourage that person to find help.

When a person has a mental illness, he or she may be unable to get help alone. Letting a serious emotional problem or mental illness go untreated is very dangerous. People with these problems can suffer greatly. They may even end up hurting themselves or others. If you believe that someone might hurt himself or herself or someone else, it is important that you get help for that person. You may save a life.

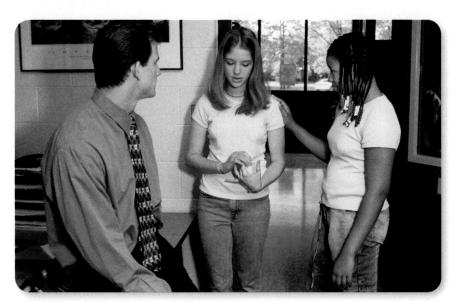

Figure 18 Getting help for a friend with an emotional problem or mental illness can save that friend's life.

Lesson Review

Using Vocabulary

1. What is the difference between a therapist and a psychiatrist?

Understanding Concepts

2. When should you get help for an emotional problem?

3. What are three sources of help for emotional health problems?

4. When should you help a friend who has emotional problems?

Critical Thinking

5. Applying Concepts Carlos has had an emotional problem for 1 month. He thought it would go away on its own, but now he feels worse. He talked to his family, but that didn't help either. What should he do now?

6. Making Predictions What are possible negative outcomes of not asking for help if a friend is having emotional problems?

Chapter Summary

■ Emotions are feelings that are produced in response to life events. ■ Hormones and changing responsibilities affect teens' emotions. ■ Having a full range of emotions is healthy. ■ Expressing emotions helps people solve problems, understand others, and release tension. ■ Positive self-talk can overcome negative thinking. ■ Defense mechanisms are ways to cope with stress. ■ Knowing your triggers can help you avoid unpleasant emotions. ■ A mental illness is a disorder that affects emotions, thoughts, and behavior. ■ Family members, friends, community members, and professionals can help people who have emotional problems. ■ Encouraging someone to get help for an emotional problem can save that person's life.

Using Vocabulary

For each pair of terms, describe how the meanings of the terms differ.

1 mental health/emotional health

2 verbal communication/body language

For each sentence, fill in the blank with the proper word from the word bank provided below.

active listening	mental illness
triggers	hormones
defense mechanism	positive self-talk
creative expression	therapist
negative thinking	depression

3 ___ are chemicals that help control how the body grows and functions.

4 ___ is one way to encourage someone to talk and communicate.

5 ___ is a way to think about the good parts of a bad situation.

6 ___ is a mental illness that includes extreme sadness.

7 Knowing your ___ helps you avoid situations that cause unpleasant emotions.

8 Using a(n) ___ is a way to cope with stress.

Understanding Concepts

9 How do changes in teens' bodies and in their lives affect their emotions?

10 Are pleasant emotions healthier than unpleasant emotions? Explain.

11 How can emotions affect a person physically?

12 Why is it helpful to express emotions?

13 What are some effective ways to communicate emotions?

14 When might a person want to use creative expression?

15 How do social and physical health affect mental and emotional health?

16 What are two things that can affect brain chemistry and lead to a mental illness?

17 How is depression different from sadness?

18 What is bipolar mood disorder?

19 What is schizophrenia?

20 How would you know if you needed help for an emotional problem?

Critical Thinking

Applying Concepts

21 Julia just turned thirteen. She moved to a new school and had to make new friends. She started babysitting after school, and her parents put her in charge of taking care of the family dog. Lately, Julia has felt emotionally confused and overwhelmed. Why do you think she might feel confused about her emotions?

22 Imagine that you are helping your family get ready for a big reunion. You have been working hard all day, and your sister yelled at you because she thought you weren't helping enough. As you walk home from the grocery store with party supplies, the bag of groceries breaks and milk spills all over the street. How could you use positive self-talk to overcome negative thinking in this situation?

23 Erik really hates it when his friend Robert teases him about his big feet. Robert is just joking and doesn't know that Erik is upset. What might happen if Erik doesn't express his emotions to Robert?

Making Good Decisions

24 Alex went to the park every day after school to play basketball. There were two courts there, and the bigger one was always full of older kids. When Alex tried playing with the older kids, he got really nervous. When he got home after playing with them, he felt sad and exhausted. What could Alex do to avoid this trigger for sadness?

25 Rita's friend Leigh has been sad for several weeks. Rita notices that Leigh doesn't eat much at lunch and that she looks really tired. Rita tries to talk to Leigh about her emotions, but Leigh will not discuss her problem. What can Rita do to help Leigh?

26 Use what you have learned in this chapter to set a personal goal. Write your goal, and make an action plan by using the Health Behavior Contract for mental and emotional health. You can find the Health Behavior Contract at go.hrw.com. Just type in the keyword HD4HBC06.

Name _____ Class _____ Date _____

Health Behavior Contract

Mental and Emotional Health

My Goals: I, _____, will accomplish one or more of the following goals:
I will practice good communication skills.
I will use positive self-talk to overcome negative thinking.
I will find an activity that triggers pleasant emotions.
Other: _____

My Reasons: By improving my ability to communicate, to think through emotional problems, and to trigger pleasant emotions, I will improve my mental and emotional health.
Other: _____

My Values: Personal values that will help me meet my goals are
_____
_____

My Plan: The actions I will take to meet my goals are
_____
_____

Evaluation: I will use my Health Journal to keep a log of actions I took to fulfill this contract. After 1 month, I will evaluate my goals. I will adjust my plan if my goals are not being met. If my goals are being met, I will consider setting additional goals.

Signed _____
Date _____

Reading Checkup

Take a minute to review your answers to the Health IQ questions at the beginning of this chapter. How has reading this chapter improved your Health IQ?

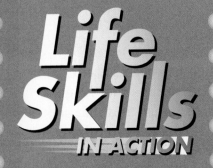

Communicating Effectively

Have you ever been in a bad situation that was made worse because of poor communication? Or maybe you have difficulty understanding others or being understood. You can avoid misunderstandings by expressing your feelings in a healthy way, which is communicating effectively. Complete the following activity to develop effective communication skills.

ACT 1

Sean's Sadness

Setting the Scene

Sean's parents have been fighting a lot. It seems like they fight every night. Sean hates listening to their fights but doesn't know how to make them stop. All of the anger in the house is upsetting him, and he wonders if he somehow caused his parents' unhappiness. He feels sad all the time, and he is having trouble sleeping and concentrating on his schoolwork. Sean decides to talk to his father about his problems.

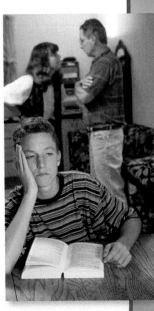

The 4 Steps of Communicating Effectively

1. Express yourself calmly and clearly.
2. Choose your words carefully.
3. Use open body language.
4. Use active listening.

Guided Practice

Practice with a Friend

Form a group of three. Have one person play the role of Sean and another person play the role of Sean's father. Have the third person be an observer. Walking through each of the four steps of communicating effectively, role-play Sean talking with his father about his problems. Sean should tell his father how the fights between him and his mother are affecting his mental and emotional health. The observer will take notes, which will include observations about what the person playing Sean did well and suggestions of ways to improve. Stop after each step to evaluate the process.

Independent Practice

Check Yourself

After you have completed the guided practice, go through Act 1 again without stopping at each step. Answer the questions below to review what you did.

1. Why is it important for Sean to express himself calmly and clearly?

2. What specific body language could Sean use when he is talking with his father?

3. What should Sean's father do to show that he is actively listening to what Sean is saying?

4. Why is it important to use good communication skills when explaining your feelings to someone?

ACT 2 On Your Own

After several talks with his parents, Sean now understands that their fighting is not his fault. He is starting to feel better mentally and emotionally. One day, Sean's parents tell him that they are getting a divorce and that he will live with his mother. Sean doesn't like the arrangement because he wants to be able to spend time with his father. Make a flowchart showing how Sean could use the four steps of communicating effectively to tell his parents how he feels.

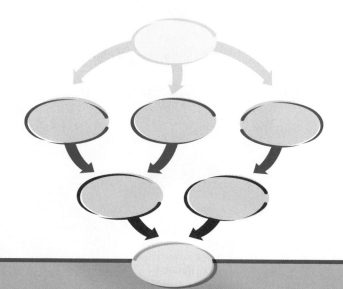

Managing Stress

Check out
Current Health®
articles related to this chapter by
visiting go.hrw.com. Just type in
the keyword **HD4CH23**.

> **When my grandmother got sick, she came to live with us.** That was two years ago.
> I had to give up **my bedroom**, but that was OK.
>
> Now, my grandmother needs help all the time. My mom can't do everything, so my sister and I help her. I love my grandmother, and I want to help my mom. But sometimes I just want to get away.

Health IQ

PRE-READING

Answer the following multiple-choice questions to find out what you already know about managing stress. When you've finished this chapter, you'll have the opportunity to change your answers based on what you've learned.

1. **Which of the following statements is true?**
   a. You can manage much of the stress in your life.
   b. You should avoid all stress.
   c. Good stress does not exist.
   d. Asking other people to help you manage your stress is a bad idea.

2. **Ignoring stress**
   a. will make the stress go away.
   b. can make the stress worse.
   c. helps a person manage stress.
   d. None of the above

3. **Stress can be caused by**
   a. schoolwork.
   b. family problems.
   c. running in a race.
   d. All of the above

4. **The physical effects of stress include**
   a. quick energy boost.
   b. slowed digestion.
   c. an increased heart rate.
   d. All of the above

5. **A defense mechanism is**
   a. a type of medical procedure that prevents malaria.
   b. a short-term way to handle stress.
   c. used by doctors to stop disease.
   d. a type of play in football.

6. **The stress response is**
   a. a reaction that occurs only before a big test.
   b. a physical change in your body as a result of puberty.
   c. a natural response to something new or threatening.
   d. always caused by mental problems.

ANSWERS: 1. a; 2. b; 3. d; 4. d; 5. b; 6. c

Stress Is Only Natural

What You'll Do

- **Discuss** stress as a natural part of life.
- **Distinguish** between positive stress and distress.
- **Identify** three sources of stress in your life.

Terms to Learn:

- stress
- stressor
- distress
- positive stress

Start Off
Write

What does the word *stress* mean to you?

> Kris plays basketball for her school team. Kris is usually very relaxed, but her stomach gets upset right before each game. Sometimes she even throws up.

Waiting for the game to start is stressful for Kris. Her body responds to the tension with an upset stomach. Kris's response is not unusual—everyone experiences stress at one time or another.

Stress Is Part of Life

Stress is the combination of a new or possibly threatening situation and your body's natural response to it. Stress can be physical, mental, emotional, or social. Some situations are stronger stressors than others are. A **stressor** is anything that triggers a stress response. A stressor may be something small, such as not being able to find your favorite shirt. Or a stressor may be something big, such as a serious illness or the death of a parent. You have control over some stressors. For example, you can study more for an upcoming test. But other stressors, such as moving to a new school, cannot be controlled.

How you react to a stressor is important. Different people have different reactions to the same stressor. Something that is not stressful to you may be stressful to one of your friends. Knowing that stressors come in all sizes will help you deal with stress when it comes. And knowing that you can control some stressors but not others may help you react to a stressor in a positive way.

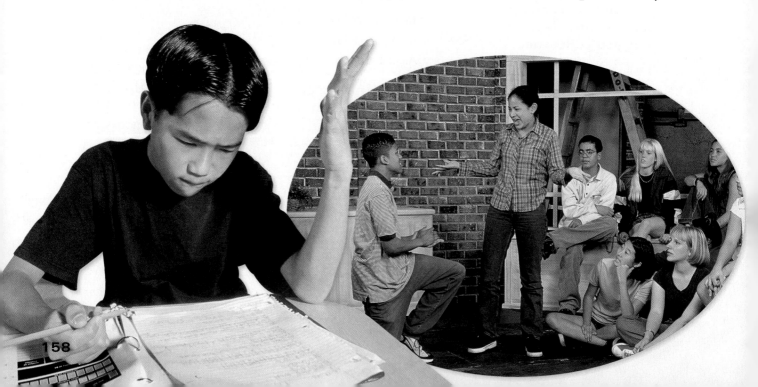

Distress and Positive Stress

When you hear the word *stress*, you may think of something negative or harmful. **Distress** is any stress that keeps you from reaching your goals or that makes you sick. Distress can leave you feeling tired and depressed or may make you lose sleep. It can keep you from studying properly. Distress may affect your relationships and damage your health. Sometimes, distress is caused by a major stressor, such as fighting with your best friend. But distress is often caused by a collection of minor problems that pile up. If you are rushing to get dressed and are worried because you are late, breaking your shoelace just adds to the stress you already feel.

Some kinds of stress are good for you. **Positive stress** is stress that makes you feel good. It is triggered by something that makes you excited or happy, such as having a special birthday party, winning a speech tournament, or making a basketball team. Positive stress can help you reach your goals. And positive stress usually leaves you feeling relaxed and calm.

A new or changing situation may produce either distress or positive stress. Some changes are more stressful than others. Something that wasn't a stressor in the past can be stressful now if you aren't prepared for it. Or you may find that something that once caused you distress, such as speaking in front of your class, now makes you excited. How you react to a stressor often determines whether you feel distress or positive stress.

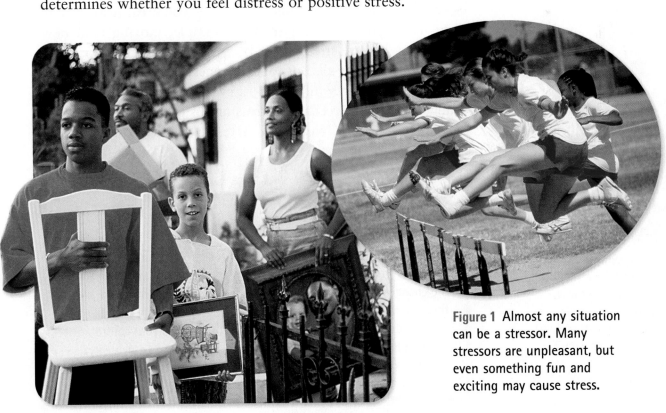

Figure 1 Almost any situation can be a stressor. Many stressors are unpleasant, but even something fun and exciting may cause stress.

Stress Inventory

- Arguing less with friends - 26
- Arguing less with parents - 29
- Having a brother or sister leave home - 33
- Having another adult, such as a grandparent, move in - 34

- Experiencing the serious illness of a brother or sister - 44
- Achieving an outstanding personal goal - 45
- Beginning middle school - 45
- Arguing with parents more - 46

- Changing physical appearance (braces or glasses) - 47
- Seeing more arguments between parents - 48
- Being rejected for an extracurricular activity - 48
- Moving to a new school district - 52

less stress

Figure 2 Each of the life changes in this stress inventory has been given a point value. When your life changes add up, you may begin to feel the effects of stress.

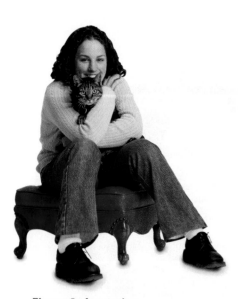

Figure 3 Accepting responsibility for a new pet may be a stressor to some people. Does this change cause positive stress or distress? Why?

Stress In Your Life

Teens face a variety of stressors. Common stressors are breaking up with a boyfriend or girlfriend, arguing more with your parents, or having trouble with a brother or sister. More-serious stressors include seeing your parents argue more or finding out that your parents are divorcing. If you make a list of stressors in your own life, some will be more serious than others.

The effect that a particular stressor will have on someone may be hard to measure. A change that causes you great distress may seem minor to someone else. For example, moving to a new school may be very stressful to you. Someone else may not mind changing schools at all. But some changes, such as the death of a parent, are very stressful to almost everyone. Some common life changes that cause teenagers stress are listed in Figure 2. These stressors are listed from the least stressful to the most stressful.

LIFE SKILLS ACTIVITY

ASSESSING YOUR HEALTH

Use the list of life changes in Figure 2 to total the points for the changes you have gone through in the last year. Analyze your results. Do your stressors come from a particular part of your life, such as family, school, or friends? Are your stressors things over which you have some control, such as schoolwork or relationships? Or are they things that are beyond your control, such as moving to a new city? Can you eliminate any stressors?

- **Getting into trouble at school - 54**
- **Beginning to go out on dates - 55**
- **Failing a grade at school - 62**
- **Death of a close friend - 65**
- **Involved with drugs or alcohol - 70**
- **Death of a brother or sister - 71**
- **Divorce of parents - 84**
- **DEATH OF A PARENT - 94**

more stress

Personal Stress Inventory

People suffering from stress sometimes take a personal stress inventory. They list all the life changes they have faced in the last year. Each change, such as those listed in Figure 2, is given a point value. Life changes that are less stressful or are somewhat stressful have lower point values. Stressors that are more stressful or extremely stressful have higher point values.

Doctors know that high levels of stress or stress over a long period of time can increase a person's chances of getting sick. For instance, a score of 300 points or more for a year shows that the person has gone through major life changes. Someone with a score that high has almost certainly experienced stress. He or she must be careful to protect his or her physical and emotional health. Protect your own health. Do a stress inventory occasionally and watch for the warning signs of stress.

Health Journal

Review your list of life changes and the total points for the list. Now think back over the last year. Try to remember if you have had any health problems, such as headaches, colds, or other illnesses. Do you think the health problems may be related to stressful events?

Lesson Review

Using Vocabulary

1. What is stress?

2. Define *stressor*, and identify three stressors in your life.

Understanding Concepts

3. Which is more harmful to your health: positive stress or distress? Explain your answer, and give examples.

Critical Thinking

4. **Identifying Relationships** You and a friend are talking about his personal stress inventory. Most of his stressors are things that he can control or change. Explain how adding stressors beyond his control might affect his health.

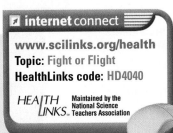

internet connect

www.scilinks.org/health
Topic: Fight or Flight
HealthLinks code: HD4040

HEALTH LINKS. Maintained by the National Science Teachers Association

The Effects of Stress

Adriana moved to a new city far from her old home and all of her old friends. Now Adriana always seems tired. Her mother thinks Adriana is suffering from stress.

What You'll Do

■ **Describe** the body's response to stress.

■ **Distinguish** between physical effects and mental or emotional effects of stress.

Terms to Learn:

● stress response

● fatigue

Start Off
Write

Describe how your body responds when something scares you.

Adriana's mother may be right. Stressors can cause physical and mental reactions, including tiredness. And reactions caused by stressors can be either short-term or long-term.

Physical Effects of Stress

When you face a stressor, your brain analyzes the situation quickly. For example, imagine that you are walking along and suddenly a strange dog runs up to you and starts barking and growling. Your brain must decide if this stressor is important or not. Is the dog dangerous or just looking you over? If your brain decides the dog is a threat, it orders the release of *epinephrine* (EP uh NEF rin). Epinephrine is a hormone that triggers your body's stress response. The **stress response** is a set of physical changes that prepare your body to act in response to a stressor. The stress response is also called the "fight-or-flight" response because the release of epinephrine gives you a quick burst of energy. This energy boost prepares your body either to fight the stressor physically or to run from it. Figure 4 shows the major physical changes that make up the stress response.

Most of the stress response changes go away when the stressor is gone. But if you do not relieve your stress or eliminate the stressor, you may suffer long-term physical effects.

One common effect of long-term stress is fatigue. **Fatigue** is physical or mental exhaustion. Physical fatigue can cause aches and pains all over your body. It also makes you feel extremely tired. Other long-term effects of stress include stomachaches, headaches, and changes in appetite. Stress can weaken your immune system. It may cause high blood pressure or make asthma worse.

More blood goes to brain

Hearing and vision sharpen

Heart beats faster and harder

Breathing speeds up

Epinephrine release gives energy boost

More blood goes to legs and arms

Figure 4 The stress response produces specific physical reactions.

Other Effects of Stress

Repeated or long-term stress can also cause mental, emotional, and social effects. Mental effects include confusion and memory problems. Emotional effects include sleeplessness, anxiety, and sadness. One of the most serious long-term effects of stress is psychological (SIE kuh LAHG i kuhl) fatigue. Psychological fatigue is much like physical fatigue. They both make you feel extremely tired or exhausted. Psychological fatigue can be very hard to relieve. It can even lead to depression. More emotional and mental effects of stress are shown in Table 1.

Social effects of stress may be as harmful as other effects. If you are always angry, relationships with your family may be harmed. If you are sad all the time, your friends may not understand why. If you are depressed, you may not want to be around anyone else. Severe stress can be dangerous.

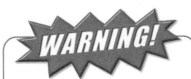

WARNING!

Stress has been shown to lower a person's IQ by 10 to 15 points. You are likely to make more mistakes during a stressful time.

Table 1 Emotional and Mental Effects of Stress	
Emotional effects	**Mental effects**
depression	boredom
anger	confusion
distrust	memory problems
frustration	lack of concentration
guilt	psychological fatigue
sadness and crying	anxiety
sleeplessness, insomnia	poor decision making
irritability, irrational behavior	become accident prone
jealousy	

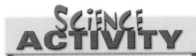

SCIENCE ACTIVITY

Research the relationship between long-term stress and disease. Make a poster that shows how long-term stress affects the body.

Lesson Review

Using Vocabulary

1. What do you call the set of physical changes that prepare your body to act in response to a stressor?

Understanding Concepts

2. Describe the difference between physical effects of stress and mental or emotional effects of stress.

3. Why is the stress response called the "fight-or-flight" response?

Critical Thinking

4. Analyzing Ideas Discuss fatigue and the reasons why it can be so hard to deal with. Include a discussion of how fatigue interacts with other effects of stress.

Lesson 3

Defense Mechanisms

Doug and Wes were best friends. Now, Wes has a new friend and doesn't spend time with Doug anymore. To cope, Doug acts as if nothing has changed. Wes just ignores Doug.

What You'll Do:

- **Describe** two defense mechanisms.

- **Explain** how defense mechanisms can be helpful or harmful.

Terms to Learn:

- defense mechanism

Start Off
Write

Describe a time when you were angry at yourself but blamed someone else.

Losing a friend can be a strong stressor. The loss may affect you emotionally and physically, depending on how you handle it. Some ways of dealing with stress are better than others.

Short-Term Ways to Handle Stress

The best way to end the stress response is to deal with the stressor. If you act to solve the problem, the effects of stress will not pile up. For example, Doug may just need to talk to Wes. The two of them may be able to fix their friendship. In the long term, Doug may have to make new friends. But talking to Wes may relieve Doug's stress right away.

When the release of epinephrine triggers the stress response, the body wants to take action. It wants to do something physical. So, one way to relieve physical effects of stress is to exercise to burn off energy. Exercise helps your body return to normal. That is why exercise also helps relieve mental or emotional effects of stress.

To relieve mental or emotional effects of stress quickly, people sometimes rely on defense mechanisms. A **defense mechanism** is a short-term, automatic way to protect yourself from being hurt emotionally. It is a way of managing distress or coping with distress. Defense mechanisms are ways you have learned to deal quickly with distress. Your defense mechanisms help you maintain your self-esteem. And you may not even realize you are using a defense mechanism.

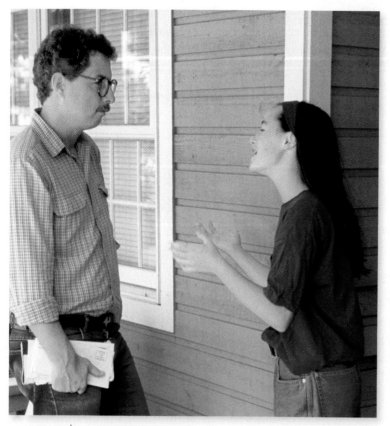

Figure 5 Defense mechanisms, such as rationalization, are short-term ways to handle emotional stress.

TABLE 2 Common Defense Mechanisms

Mechanism	Description
Daydreaming	using your imagination to escape an unpleasant situation
Denial	refusing to accept reality
Projection	putting negative feelings on someone else
Rationalization	making excuses for or justifying behavior to avoid a problem or to gain acceptance
Regression	expressing emotions like anger or disappointment in very childlike ways
Repression	blocking out unpleasant thoughts or memories

Defense Mechanisms—Good or Bad?

Defense mechanisms are unconscious and automatic. Doug and Wes are a good example. Doug uses *denial,* a common defense mechanism, to deal with the changed friendship. Doug, in his mind, denies that anything has changed. He acts as he always has. That way, Doug avoids the hurt feelings and distress from losing a friend. Wes doesn't know that he is hurting Doug's feelings. He doesn't think about Doug at all. Wes blocks out all thoughts about Doug. This is called *repression.*

In the short term, Doug and Wes use defense mechanisms to feel good about themselves. But neither one has faced the real problem—they may end up having no friendship at all. Defense mechanisms can manage your distress. They do not fix the problem. It is important to recognize stress and to know when you are using a defense mechanism. Then you can usually find a way to solve the problem.

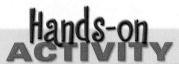

Hands-on ACTIVITY

STRESSORS

1. Select one stressor in your life. Identify one or more defense mechanisms you use to cope with the stressor.
2. List the benefits and problems of using the defense mechanisms.
3. Working as a class, do a survey to see how many different defense mechanisms you and your classmates use.

Analysis

1. Make a bar graph that shows all of the defense mechanisms you and your classmates use and the frequency of each one.
2. Discuss why some defense mechanisms are more common than others.

Lesson Review

Using Vocabulary

1. Define *defense mechanism.*
2. Explain the difference between denial and repression.

Understanding Concepts

3. Explain how defense mechanisms can be used in a healthy way.

Critical Thinking

4. **Making Good Decisions** Explain how you can avoid always relying on defense mechanisms to handle distress.
5. **Analyzing Ideas** How can daydreaming be harmful?

Managing Distress

What You'll Do

- **Identify** physical, mental, or emotional signs of distress.

- **Discuss** ways to manage distress.

- **Identify** ways to avoid or prevent distress.

Terms to Learn

- stress management
- relaxation
- redirection
- reframing

Start Off
Write

How can planning ahead help you manage stressors?

Moesha is very shy. In one of her classes, she has to give a speech. Moesha is so worried about the assignment that she cannot sleep and has an upset stomach.

There are many ways to react to stress. Moesha's not being able to sleep is one reaction. But knowing when you are distressed and doing something to relieve the distress is a better reaction.

Signs of Distress

Your stress response usually follows certain steps:

1. A stressor appears, and you interpret it as unpleasant or threatening.

2. You respond physically, mentally, and emotionally to the stressor—this is when you may begin to show signs of distress.

3. If you don't stop distress, the signs of distress may become long-lasting effects.

When you know what causes you distress, you can take steps to solve the problem. Some common warning signs of distress are listed in Table 3. These warning signs can help you learn whether something is a stressor for you. If you have one or more of these signs, you may be distressed. Recognizing your distress will help you deal with it as soon as you can. If you don't deal with it, you may become ill or depressed. Fortunately, there are ways to manage, stop, and even avoid distress. But all good stress management plans start with recognizing the sources of distress in your life.

TABLE 3 Warning Signs of Distress	
Physical signs	**Emotional and mental signs**
headaches	nightmares
teeth grinding	frustration
fatigue	mood swings
heart pounding	depression
	forgetfulness

Managing Your Stress

You can't stop all the stress in your life, but you can manage much of it. **Stress management** is the ability to handle stress in healthy ways. Stress management is part of mental, emotional, and physical health.

Two common ways to manage stress are relaxation and redirection. **Relaxation** is doing something to take your mind off the problem and to focus on something else that is not stressful. Relaxing activities include listening to music, reading a book, and going for a walk. **Redirection** is taking energy from your stress response and directing it into an activity that is not stressful. For example, jogging or riding your bike burn off energy caused by stress.

Another way to manage stress is to reframe the stressor. **Reframing** is looking at the situation from another point of view and changing your emotional response to the situation. Reframing often lets you find something positive about the situation. When you reframe a stressor, you may reduce distress caused by seeing the situation only in a negative way. For example, failing a quiz can be distressful. But if you look at the questions you got wrong, you can study that material and do better on the final test.

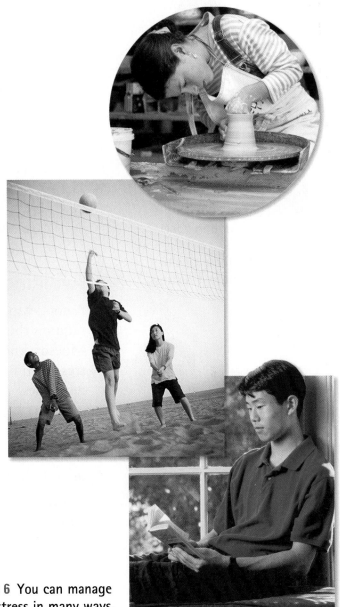

Figure 6 You can manage your stress in many ways.

Hands-on ACTIVITY

STRESS MANAGEMENT

1. Conduct an anonymous class survey in which each student lists three ways that he or she usually manages stress.

2. Compile the class results in a table that shows how often each stress management technique is used.

Analysis

1. Create a bar graph that shows the results of your survey and the information in the table.

2. In a group, select one of the ways of managing stress from the class list. Create a skit that shows a stressful situation and demonstrates the use of the stress management technique that your group selected. Have the class guess which way to manage stress your skit portrays.

3. What other ways to manage stress could you have used in the same situation?

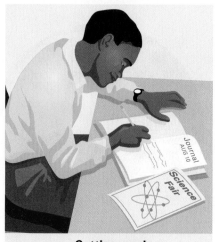

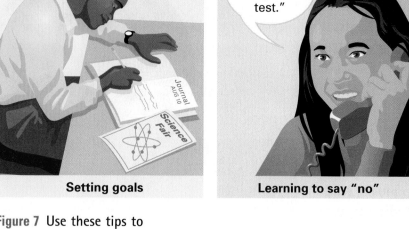

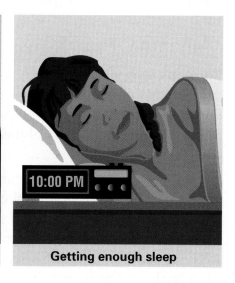

Setting goals

Learning to say "no"

"No, I have to study for a test."

Getting enough sleep

10:00 PM

Figure 7 Use these tips to avoid or to prevent distress.

Brain Food

Laughter is a natural way to avoid or relieve stress temporarily. When you are stressed, watching a funny movie or being with people who are laughing and having a good time helps.

Avoiding Distress

A good way to deal with distress is to avoid it. Avoiding distress requires thinking ahead and doing some planning. For example, Moesha knows that she is shy. She can avoid some of her distress by finishing her speech ahead of time and then practicing a few times.

Another way to avoid distress is to build up your confidence. You cannot be an expert at everything, but you can be good at some things. When you develop a skill, such as taking good notes, use it to help you avoid distress whenever you can. Be confident!

Stressors that you face repeatedly—in school, at home, or in another place—are stressors you can plan to avoid. Avoiding stressors takes practice. You have to learn what situations cause you distress. With experience, you can identify potentially stressful situations. Then, you can plan to avoid them. For example, by marking the dates of major tests on a calendar, you can avoid the distress of having to study for the test at the last minute. Other ways to avoid the effects of distress include getting plenty of exercise and sleep, setting goals, and taking some time just for yourself.

LIFE SKILLS ACTIVITY

COPING

Imagine that you have to move to a new city. List 5 to 10 things about moving that may cause you distress. Now list at least one way to manage or to avoid each of the stressors you have listed.

For example, imagine that you are moving to a city you have never heard of. What are some ways you could learn more about the city?

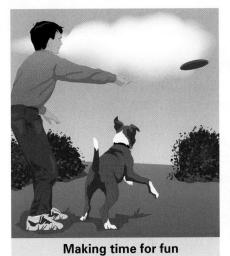

Making time for fun

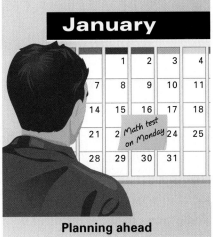

Planning ahead

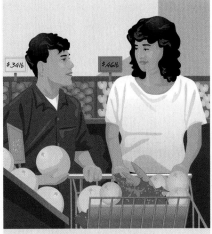

Staying healthy

Preventing Distress

The best way to prevent distress is to be prepared. Think of a situation that causes you distress. What about the situation is so stressful? When you know what the stressor is, make plans to cope with it. For example, you may worry about the first day of school each year. It may be difficult for you to meet new people and start new classes. How can you prevent some of that distress? One way may be to visit the school to learn where your classrooms are. Another way would be to meet a good friend at school and help each other through the first day.

There will always be stress, good and bad, in your life. You cannot live totally stress free. But you can set goals and make choices that keep stress under control. If stress ever becomes more than you can handle by yourself, get help quickly! Stress won't just go away. When stress is bad, find a friend, especially an adult you can trust, to help you. Don't be afraid to ask—everyone needs help sometimes.

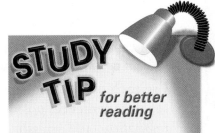

STUDY TIP *for better reading*

Reviewing Information
Use the highlighted vocabulary words and the red headings to create a concept map that summarizes the chapter. Be sure to use connecting words or phrases to link the vocabulary words and important concepts.

Lesson Review

Using Vocabulary

1. Define *stress management.*

Understanding Concepts

2. List six warning signs of distress. Include physical and mental or emotional signs of stress.

3. Explain two ways to manage stress.

4. Explain how planning ahead can help you avoid distress.

Critical Thinking

5. Making Inferences Why is learning how to manage distress in our lives a good idea?

Chapter Summary

■ Stress is a natural part of your life. Stress can come from a wide variety of sources. ■ Stress can be positive or negative. Negative stress is called *distress*. ■ Something that causes stress is called a *stressor*. ■ Stress can cause physical, mental, emotional, and social effects. Some of the effects of stress may be very serious. ■ People often handle stress in the short term by using defense mechanisms. Common defense mechanisms include daydreaming, denial, rationalization, and repression. ■ You can manage most of your distress. Some distress can be avoided, and some distress can even be prevented entirely. ■ An effective way to manage distress is to know what causes your distress and to plan ahead.

Using Vocabulary

1 Use each of the following terms in a separate sentence: *positive stress, fatigue, relaxation,* and *stressor.*

For each sentence, fill in the blank with the proper word from the word bank provided below.

stress	defense mechanism
distress	stress management
positive stress	relaxation
stress response	redirection
denial	repression

2 The way your body reacts to a stressor is called the ___.

3 ___ is taking your mind off your stress and focusing on something that is not stressful.

4 Taking energy produced by the stress response and using it in a nonstressful activity is called ___.

5 The combination of an unpleasant situation and your body's natural response to it is called ___.

6 ___ is blocking out unpleasant thoughts or memories.

7 When you make plans to handle something stressful, you are doing ___.

8 A ___ is a way to handle stress in the short term.

9 ___ is stress that helps you reach a goal and makes you feel good.

10 ___ is refusing to accept reality.

Understanding Concepts

11 Describe three major stressors in your life.

12 Explain how major life changes may affect different people differently.

13 Why is the stress response called the "fight-or-flight" response?

14 Explain why managing and preventing distress are important.

15 Explain why relieving stress is important.

16 Describe three long-term mental and emotional effects of stress.

17 Can defense mechanisms be helpful? harmful? Explain your answers.

18 Is all stress bad? Explain your answer.

Critical Thinking

Identifying Relationships

19 Teresa plays on a softball team. Sometimes she feels that she has extra energy, that she can run faster than usual, and that she can see the ball better when the pitcher pitches it. Explain why Teresa may be experiencing stress.

20 Efrain made a list of stressors in his life. He realized that some of the stressors were beyond his control. Describe ways that Efrain can manage those stressors even though he cannot control them.

21 Jada always seems excited by changes and challenges. Her twin brother, James, gets nervous and can't sleep when he faces the same events. Explain how the way in which Jada and James each view a stressor can affect the way they respond to it.

Making Good Decisions

22 You and your friend have a major test coming up. Both of you are worried about it. Your friend tells you that he is losing sleep and can't concentrate because he is so worried. What can you do to help him?

23 Jimmy is a good student. He and his friend Carlos want to start a band. Jimmy's parents are worried that Jimmy won't have time to do his schoolwork and to play in a band. Jimmy is distressed because his parents may not let him start the band. What can Jimmy do to reassure his parents that his schoolwork won't suffer?

Interpreting Graphics

Brandon's Personal Stress Inventory for the Last 12 Months

Having fewer arguments with his friends	26
Having another adult move into his home	34
Achieving an outstanding personal goal	45
Moving to a new school district	52
Divorce of parents	84

Use the table above to answer questions 24–27.

24 What does this table tell you about Brandon?

25 Based on the information in this table, would you be looking for signs of distress in Brandon? Explain your answer.

26 Which items in the table might help reduce Brandon's distress level?

27 Imagine that another year has gone by. Brandon has made some good friends at his new school, and he has made the basketball team. Brandon still has a good relationship with both his parents. Predict how these factors may affect Brandon's stress level. Explain your prediction.

Reading Checkup

Take a minute to review your answers to the Health IQ questions at the beginning of this chapter. How has reading this chapter improved your Health IQ?

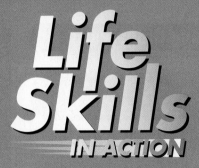

Life Skills IN ACTION

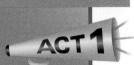
ACT 1

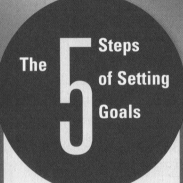

The 5 Steps of Setting Goals

1. Consider your interests and values.
2. Choose goals that include your interests and values.
3. If necessary, break down long-term goals into several short-term goals.
4. Measure your progress.
5. Reward your success.

Setting Goals

A goal is something that you work toward and hope to achieve. Setting goals is important because goals give you a sense of purpose and achieving goals improves your self-esteem. Complete the following activity to learn how to set and achieve goals.

The Procrastinator

Setting the Scene

Zach is a procrastinator—he usually waits until the last minute to do things. He doesn't do his homework until the night before it is due, and he does his chores only after his parents are mad that he hasn't already finished them. It is now 2 weeks until the end of school, and Zach has many projects due in the next week. Zach hasn't started any of them, and he is feeling stressed because he doesn't know if he will be able to finish them all.

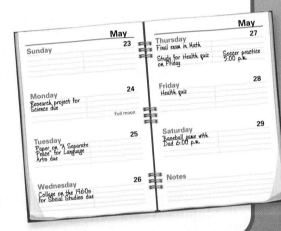

Guided Practice

Practice with a Friend

Form a group of two. Have one person play the role of Zach, and have the second person be an observer. Walking through each of the five steps of setting goals, role-play Zach setting goals to help him finish his projects and manage his stress. The observer will take notes, which will include observations on what the person playing Zach did well and suggestions of ways to improve. Stop after each step to evaluate the process.

Independent Practice

Check Yourself

After you have completed the guided practice, go through Act 1 again without stopping at each step. Answer the questions below to review what you did.

1. Suppose one of Zach's projects is a research project for Science. How could Zach divide this project into short-term goals?

2. How could setting short-term goals help Zach reduce his stress?

3. How could Zach measure his progress on his school projects?

4. Think about one of your school projects. What long-term and short-term goals can you set to finish this project?

ACT 2 On Your Own

Zach managed to finish all of his school projects in time to turn them in. He had to work very hard to finish everything, and he decided never to procrastinate again. At the start of the next school year, Zach's Language Arts teacher gives the class a month-long group project. The other members of Zach's group are worried about the size of the project. Imagine you are Zach, and make a pamphlet for the group members explaining how to use the five steps of setting goals to finish the project without getting stressed.

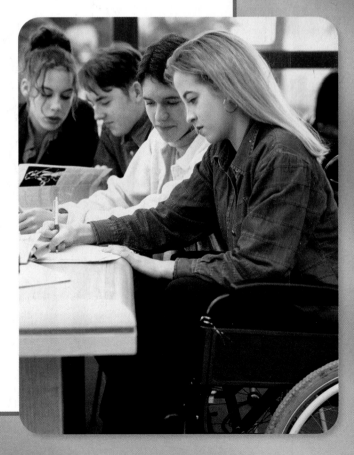

CHAPTER 9

Encouraging Healthy Relationships

Lessons

Check out **Current Health** articles related to this chapter by visiting **go.hrw.com**. Just type in the keyword **HD4CH24**.

> **My little brother, Ray, was born deaf.** I'd be **careful** when watching any kid, but I have to be **really careful** when I watch him. He can't hear things like cars and dogs. When we play in the yard, I listen for both of us.

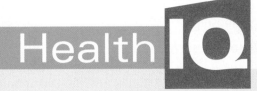

PRE-READING

Answer the following multiple-choice questions to find out what you already know about relationships. When you've finished this chapter, you'll have the opportunity to change your answers based on what you've learned.

1. Body language
a. is a way of talking to your body.
b. communicates information and feelings without words.
c. is rarely helpful in communication.
d. All of the above

2. Personal responsibility is
a. doing your part.
b. keeping promises.
c. accepting the consequences of your actions.
d. All of the above

3. Abuse is
a. sometimes the victim's fault.
b. always the victim's fault.
c. never the victim's fault.
d. All of the above

4. The best way to cope with neglect is to
a. tell a trusted adult as soon as possible.
b. ask your peers for advice.
c. wait until someone asks about it.
d. keep it a secret.

5. A community is made stronger through
a. tolerance.
b. neglect.
c. aggressive behavior.
d. None of the above

6. Sexual abstinence
a. shows that you care about yourself and others.
b. prevents many complications in your life.
c. prevents pregnancy.
d. All of the above

ANSWERS: 1. b; 2. d; 3. c; 4. a; 5. a; 6. d

Building Relationships

You have relationships with many people. Relationships take work to keep them healthy. When you work on your relationships, you improve your social health.

What You'll Do

- **Explain** how relationships can help you stay healthy.
- **Explain** how healthy relationships are like teams.
- **Explain** how people communicate by using words and body language.
- **Identify** how assertive behavior can help you learn and grow.

Terms to Learn

- relationship
- personal responsibility
- body language
- behavior

Start Off
Write

How do you let people know how you feel?

A **relationship** is an emotional or social connection between two or more people. You have relationships with your family, your friends, and your neighbors. All of these connections affect you. Many of these relationships are different, but similar skills are used to keep all relationships healthy.

Keeping You Healthy

When people in relationships are good to each other, they can help keep each other safe and healthy. People in healthy relationships look out for each other and help each other make good choices. They don't put each other in danger. You can have healthy relationships with your family and friends. Listen carefully, cooperate, and let people know what you need. Keeping your relationships healthy takes work, skill, and responsibility.

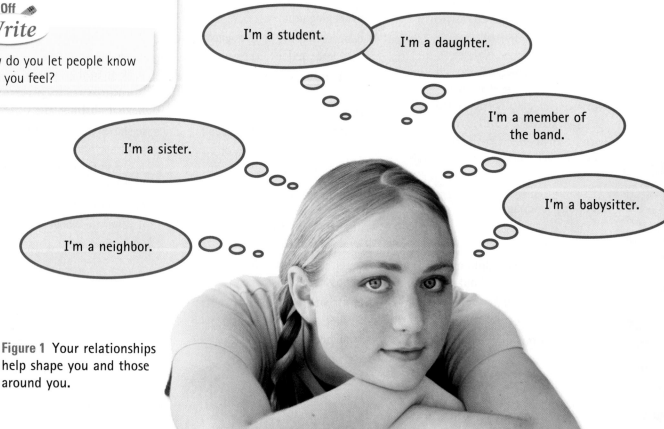

Figure 1 Your relationships help shape you and those around you.

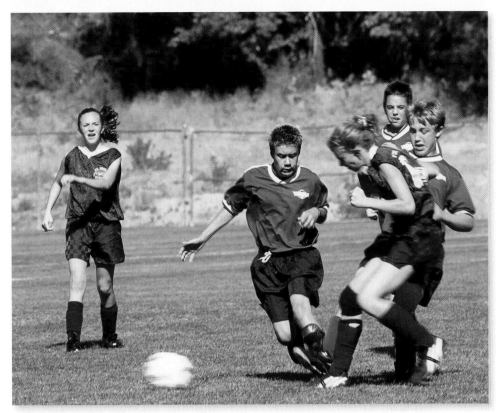

Figure 2 For a team to be effective, each player has to be responsible for his or her actions. For a relationship to thrive, each person has to take responsibility for himself or herself.

Teamwork

For relationships to be healthy, everybody in the relationship has to take personal responsibility. **Personal responsibility** is doing your part, keeping promises, and accepting the consequences of your actions. Taking personal responsibility shows that you are reliable and caring. You know what is expected of you. You let people know what you need, and you do your best to help others. When you are responsible, you correct your mistakes and learn from them. Everybody makes mistakes. When responsible people make a mistake, they don't blame anyone else. They apologize, fix the problem as well as they can, and learn how to keep from making the same mistake again.

Being responsible in a relationship is like being on a team. On a sports team, every player's position matters. For the team to be successful, all of the players have to work hard at their individual positions. And if one player struggles in his or her position, the other players help out.

You can show responsibility and teamwork every day at home by doing chores, being on time, and helping your brothers and sisters. Taking care of small problems that you see around you shows that you care about your role in your family. If you see trash in the yard, pick it up. If you are having an argument with a brother or sister, settle it calmly. Taking responsibility at home helps you learn to be responsible in all of your relationships.

Communicating Clearly

Healthy relationships are impossible if people do not understand each other. So, another important skill in healthy relationships is the ability to communicate clearly. Using good communication skills helps people share thoughts and feelings.

Good communication begins with speaking clearly. Think about what you are going to say before you speak. Face your listeners. Ask questions to make sure you are being understood.

You should also use good listening skills. Look at the person who is speaking. Make eye contact. Nod to let him or her know that you understand. If you are not sure what someone is saying, politely ask the person to clarify the message.

Using Body Language

Communication is more than expressing ideas and feelings with words. It is also understanding body language. **Body language** is a way of communicating by using the look on your face, the way you hold your hands, and the way you stand. The figure below identifies some common body language messages. Sending the same message clearly through both your words and your body language helps get your message across.

LANGUAGE ARTS ACTIVITY

Good speaking and listening skills do more than help us get along. They can save lives. Write a story about someone who uses good communication skills to help someone else who is in danger.

Figure 3 Reading body language is a skill. Body language uses the face, hands, and body position.

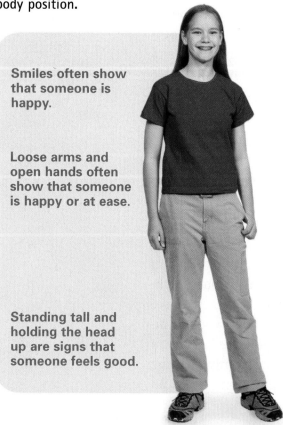

Smiles often show that someone is happy.

Loose arms and open hands often show that someone is happy or at ease.

Standing tall and holding the head up are signs that someone feels good.

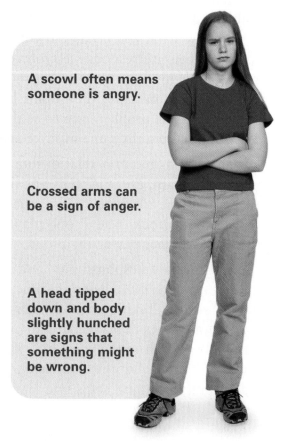

A scowl often means someone is angry.

Crossed arms can be a sign of anger.

A head tipped down and body slightly hunched are signs that something might be wrong.

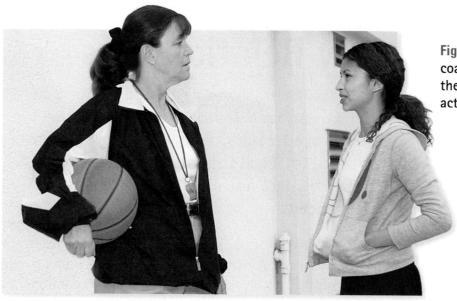

Figure 4 Politely asking a coach why you did not make the team is one example of acting assertively.

Choosing Behavior

You communicate by using words and body language, but you also communicate through your behavior. **Behavior** is the way you choose to act or respond. Acting on your thoughts and feelings in a way that respects the thoughts and feelings of others is being *assertive*.

What does acting assertively look like? Here's an example: If you tried out for a team and were not chosen, you may feel sad and angry. But how would you choose to behave? You could do nothing. You could blame others. Or you could be assertive. You could respectfully speak to the coach. You could ask why you didn't make the team. You could ask for tips on how to improve so that you could make the team next time. When you choose to be assertive, you take responsibility for what happened and help yourself succeed.

Myth & Fact

Myth: It is rude to be assertive.

Fact: Real assertiveness is respectful and sincere. It is not rude.

Lesson Review

Using Vocabulary

1. Define *relationship*, and explain how relationships help you stay healthy.

Understanding Concepts

2. Explain how understanding body language and using good speaking and listening skills help communication.

3. Explain how taking personal responsibility in a relationship is like being on a team.

Critical Thinking

4. Applying Concepts Ken wants to try out for a role in a play, but he has never acted before. How can Ken behave assertively to help him get a part?

Family Relationships

Family relationships are important. You learn your first lessons about language, values, traditions, and cooperation in your family. Families are alike in their importance. But not all families have the same structure.

Families have different forms. You may live with two parents, or you may live with only your mom or your dad. You may live in a *blended family,* which is made when two families combine, or with an extended family. Your *extended family* can include grandparents, aunts, uncles, and cousins. Sometimes, extended families, such as the family in the figure below, get together for reunions. Yet no matter what your family looks like, everyone plays an important role.

Roles for Everybody

Being a family is a lot of work. Food must be cooked, dishes must be cleaned, and laundry must be washed. If you have a yard or pet, those things will also need care. There is enough work for everyone to have a role. Your role depends on what your family needs. Different families have different roles to fill. Your parents have probably told you what they expect of you. You may have chores to do and a room to keep clean. For your family to function smoothly, everyone must do his or her part.

What You'll Do

- **Explain** why there are a lot of family roles.
- **Describe** four ways that families nurture.
- **Describe** five ways to show respect.
- **Describe** two ways you can work through small family problems.
- **Identify** four serious problems and a way to deal with them.

Terms to Learn

- nurturing
- neglect
- abuse

Write

Why is respect important in all family relationships?

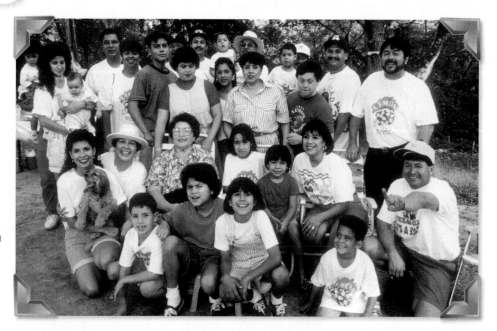

Figure 5 The Limon family gets together for a reunion every year.

Nurturing

All of the roles in a family have the same basic purpose: to nurture. **Nurturing** (NUR chuhr ing) is providing the things that people need in order to live and grow. People in families nurture by providing

- love and acceptance
- the things needed for survival, such as food, clothing, and housing
- protection from danger and rules to keep everyone safe
- instruction in skills and values

Adults are usually responsible for most of the nurturing in a family. But you can help nurture, too. Help your brothers and sisters by being a good role model and by showing them love and acceptance.

Respect

Healthy relationships are based on respect. To respect people is to be considerate of them and to let them know they are important. When you show respect to the members of your family, you send the message that you care about their thoughts and feelings. Showing respect helps you trust each other and strengthens your relationships. Here are some ways to show respect for your family:

- Follow family rules.
- Keep your word.
- Discuss disagreements respectfully.
- Treat family members' property and rooms as you would like yours to be treated.
- Listen carefully when people speak to you, and respond politely.

Respecting your family members helps you trust and rely on each other. Being able to trust and rely on each other makes living together more pleasant. And getting through hard times is easier if you have the help of people who care about you.

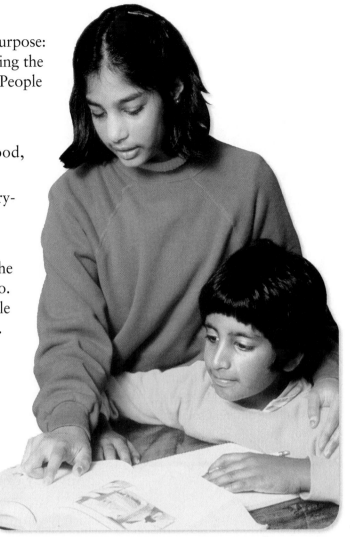

Figure 6 You can help provide nurturing by taking care of your brothers and sisters.

Minor Problems

Learning to work through everyday problems is a skill everybody needs to learn. When you have a minor problem, you can often resolve it yourself. Problems such as arguments between brothers and sisters can usually be solved if the people involved listen to each other, work together, and look for a solution that works for everyone.

One way to work on problems as a family is to hold regular family meetings. At a family meeting, the whole household meets to talk openly about everyone's thoughts and feelings. Everyone gets a chance to speak, and everyone listens carefully. By treating everyone's concerns respectfully, people can take care of minor problems before they grow into major problems.

Serious Problems

Not all problems are easy to handle. Some problems are more serious. Serious problems include neglect (ni GLECKT) and abuse (uh BYOOS). **Neglect** is the failure of a parent or responsible adult to provide for a child's basic needs, such as food, clothing, and shelter. **Abuse** is treating someone in a harmful or offensive way. Some forms of abuse are described in the table below. All forms of abuse and neglect are wrong.

Anybody can become a victim of abuse or neglect. Abuse and neglect can hurt a person physically and emotionally. Victims can have injuries to their bodies. They can feel worthless and powerless. But victims are valuable people who deserve to live safe, healthy lives. Help is available, and all victims should get help. If you know of anyone being abused or neglected, help that person by reporting the problem as soon as you can.

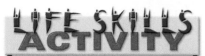

LIFE SKILLS ACTIVITY

COPING

In small groups, role-play the following scenario:

Beth and her brother argue every night about which TV shows to watch.

How can Beth and her brother settle this problem? Try to find three solutions. When you are finished, have each group share solutions. Make a list of all the different solutions you find.

TABLE 1 Identifying Forms of Abuse	
Problem	**Description**
Physical abuse	harmful treatment that causes injury to the body; sometimes results in cuts, burns, and broken bones
Emotional abuse	the repeated use of harsh words or threatening actions to control another person; treating a person as though he or she is worthless
Sexual abuse	any forced sexual contact or any sexual contact with a child

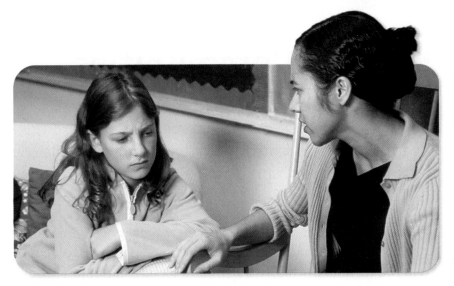

Figure 7 Talking to a counselor can help you solve many problems.

Help

Talking about serious problems is difficult. Many people who have been abused are afraid or ashamed. But there is nothing shameful about being abused or neglected. Abuse or neglect can happen to anyone and is never the victim's fault. Where can people who have been abused or neglected get help? The first step is to talk to a trusted adult, such as

- an adult family member (a parent, a grandparent, an aunt, or an uncle)
- someone at school (a teacher, a school nurse, a coach, or a counselor)
- a police officer or a firefighter

Any of these people will know how to help and should help. But if the first adult told about the abuse does not help, the victim should keep telling adults until the abuse stops.

Health Journal

If you had a friend with a serious problem, whom could you tell? In your Health Journal, make a list of trusted adults in your life. What do these people have in common?

Lesson Review

Using Vocabulary

1. What does *nurturing* mean?

Understanding Concepts

2. What are four ways that families nurture?

3. Define four serious family problems, and describe what should be done about them.

4. Explain why there are a lot of family roles.

5. Describe five ways of showing respect to your family.

Critical Thinking

6. Making Good Decisions Rosa and her brother both think that the other does not help enough around the house. Describe two ways they could work on their problem.

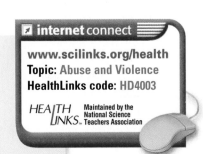

internet connect

www.scilinks.org/health
Topic: Abuse and Violence
HealthLinks code: HD4003

HEALTH LINKS Maintained by the National Science Teachers Association

Lesson 3

Healthy Communities

What You'll Do

- **Explain** why tolerance is needed in communities.

- **List** five ways to keep a community healthy.

Terms to Learn

- community
- tolerance

Start Off
Write

What do you have in common with your neighbors?

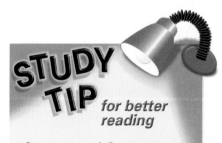

STUDY TIP *for better reading*

Compare and Contrast
How are healthy communities like healthy families? How are they different? Make a chart that compares and contrasts families and communities.

Scott and his friends walk by a vacant lot every day on their way to school. The lot is filling with trash. Scott and his friends want to make the lot cleaner and safer. They'd like to plant a community garden.

Scott and his friends are part of a neighborhood community. A **community** is made up of people of who have a common background or location or who share similar interests, beliefs, or goals. Neighborhoods, schools, and teams are examples of communities.

Practicing Tolerance

Members of a community share some common interests. But in every community, people have differences. Because of differences, tolerance (TAHL urh uhns) is needed to keep communities healthy. **Tolerance** is the ability to respect differences in people and to accept people for who they are. By respecting differences in each other, people in a community can learn from each other. Tolerance also strengthens a community. People with different backgrounds and talents help the community solve problems in different ways. When you have more ways to solve problems, you are more likely to find good solutions.

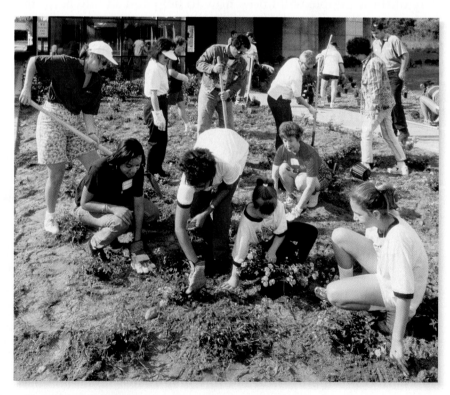

Figure 8 Healthy communities work together and use everybody's strengths. People of all ages can help make a community garden.

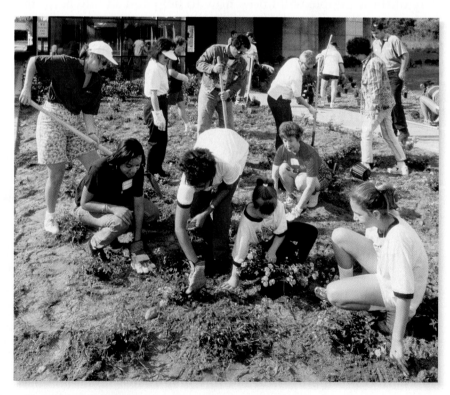

Figure 8 Healthy communities work together and use everybody's strengths. People of all ages can help make a community garden.

Living in Communities

You are a member of many communities, including your neighborhood and your school. Doing your part helps keep these communities healthy. You help when you

- obey rules and laws
- practice tolerance
- take part in community activities
- respectfully point out problems
- work with others to find solutions to community problems

Being part of a community can also be fun. For example, being a member of a band and having a role in a play are ways to spend time with people who like to do the things you like to do.

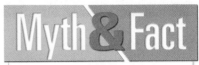

Myth: Members of healthy communities always agree with each other.

Fact: Members of healthy communities often disagree. Learning to accept each other in spite of differences helps strengthen communities.

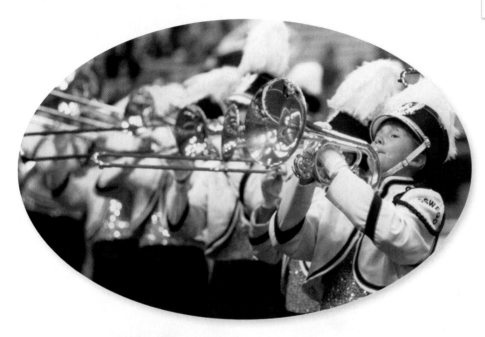

Figure 9 A marching band is a community made of individuals who like to play music. The band plays music best when all members of this community work together.

Lesson Review

Using Vocabulary

1. What is tolerance?

2. Define *community*, and give three examples of communities.

Understanding Concepts

3. How do communities benefit from tolerance?

4. List five ways you can be a responsible member of a community.

Critical Thinking

5. Identifying Relationships Larone is in the school band, which plays at school concerts, at football games, and in town parades. How does Larone's role in one community help the other communities he is a part of?

Building Friendships

What You'll Do

- **Explain** why healthy friendships are important.
- **Describe** how supporting your friends can help them stay healthy.
- **Describe** three messages sent by healthy forms of affection.
- **Describe** how to identify and resolve an unhealthy relationship.

Terms to Learn

- friendship

Start Off
Write

Why should you support your friends?

Miriam has been thinking about helping dogs at the animal shelter. She called the shelter and found out that the shelter needs volunteers to walk dogs. She mentioned her idea to her friend Leah, who said she would help, too. Miriam was glad to start her new project with a friend.

Doing projects together can build a friendship. A **friendship** is a relationship between people who enjoy being together, who care about each other, and who have similar interests. Good friends help each other by demonstrating and encouraging good character. Good character helps you maintain healthy friendships.

Identifying Healthy Friendships

Your friends do more than hang around with you and make you laugh. They help you make decisions that are good for you. They support your goals and help you do your best work in school.

Friends also respect your beliefs and values. Good friends would never ask you to do anything that would go against your values or the values of your family. The number of friends you have does not matter. What does matter is making sure that the friends you do have are caring and respectful.

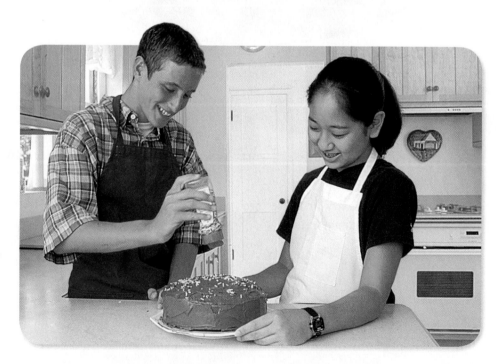

Figure 10 Friends enjoy being together, care about each other, and have similar interests.

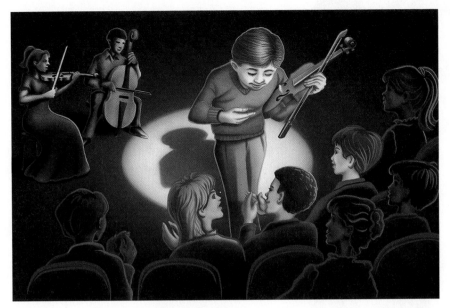

Figure 11 You can support your friends by cheering for them at a performance.

Supporting Each Other

One of the most important benefits of friendship is the support you give each other. Supporting your friends in healthy ways shows your commitment to helping them succeed. You can support your friends by

- helping them reach healthy goals
- cheering for them at a game or performance
- helping them with a project or chores
- studying or exercising together
- standing by them when they say no to unhealthy choices

You are always responsible for choosing your own behavior. Your friends are responsible for theirs, too. But you can help each other by supporting healthy choices.

Speaking Up

Supporting your friends does not mean agreeing with every choice they make. If you think a friend is making an unhealthy choice, say so. Sometimes changing someone's mind takes only one person's voice or actions. Stating your honest opinion about a friend's decision can be hard to do. But being honest with each other is an important part of friendship.

When friends support each other, they influence each other. Influencing friends to make good decisions is *positive peer pressure*. It can be hard to make a healthy choice by yourself. People who see friends making good decisions will often have the courage to make good decisions themselves.

Myth & Fact

Myth: You are responsible for your friends' decisions.

Fact: Supporting your friends is important, but each person is responsible for his or her own decisions.

LIFE SKILLS ACTIVITY

MAKING GOOD DECISIONS

In pairs or groups, discuss how you could use positive peer pressure to help in the following scenario: Two peers are asking your friend to help them cheat on a quiz.

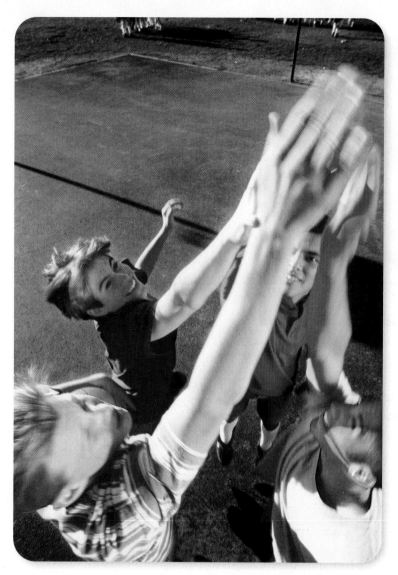

Figure 12 Friends can show affection by giving a high-five.

Showing Affection

Healthy relationships are strengthened when people show affection. Showing affection lets people know that you like them. Your affection shows your friends you think they are valuable. Knowing that someone thinks that they are valuable helps your friends feel good about themselves. This may help your friends make decisions that are good for them. Giving affection also shows your friends that they are not alone, even during difficult times.

Some forms of affection are simpler than others. A smile is usually easy and says a lot. Writing a letter or card can be more difficult. Sometimes expressing affection in words is easier if you first plan what you want to say.

Not everybody likes or appreciates the same forms of affection. Never show affection in a way that is unwelcome. For example, some people don't like to be touched. Don't touch them. And be sure to tell people if they are showing you affection in a way that you do not like. Once you tell them to stop, they should stop. If they do not, tell a parent or another trusted adult.

Health Journal

What are some of the qualities you really like in your good friends? In your Health Journal, write a list of some of your friends, and list some of the qualities you admire in each of them.

TABLE 2 Six Healthy Ways to Show Affection
saying kind words
offering a smile or a laugh
giving a high-five
writing a card or letter
patting someone on the back
being understanding, especially during hard times

Unhealthy Relationships

People change, and sometimes friendships turn bad. If you are in a relationship with someone who hurts you, threatens you, or encourages you to ignore your values, that relationship is unhealthy. In some unhealthy relationships, one person tries to control the actions of another person or to keep the other person away from other friends. Any unhealthy relationship can cause problems for you. An unhealthy relationship can also cause problems in your other relationships. If you or your parents are worried about any of your relationships, take a close look at how that relationship is affecting your life.

Resolving Unhealthy Relationships

If you are in an unhealthy relationship, first talk to your parents about resolving it. Sometimes, talking with the other person in the unhealthy relationship can also help. First, say why you are upset. For example, you could say, "I don't like to spend as much time with you anymore because you say mean things about my other friends." Next, say how you feel. For example, you could say, "When you make fun of my other friends, I get upset because I really like them." If the person continues to do things you find upsetting, you may need to say goodbye. You could say, "I don't think we can be friends anymore. I want the people around me to be good to all my friends." Honesty takes courage. But resolving unhealthy relationships gives you more time and energy for healthy ones.

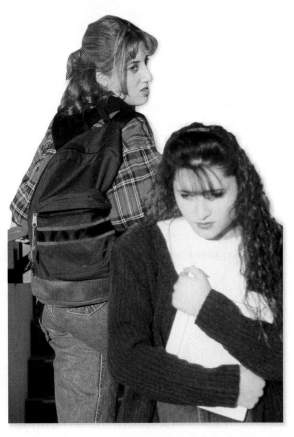

Figure 13 Sometimes, a relationship is unhealthy enough that you need to walk away.

Lesson Review

Using Vocabulary

1. Define *friendship*, and explain why healthy friendships are important.

Understanding Concepts

2. What is an unhealthy relationship? What is the first thing you should do if you find yourself in an unhealthy relationship?

3. What three messages does showing healthy affection send to your friends?

Critical Thinking

4. **Applying Concepts** Maria wants to run for class treasurer. She is very smart, good at math, and organized. But she is afraid to give speeches. What can her friends do to support her decision to run for office?

Practicing Abstinence

You are responsible for your own behavior. Decisions about your behavior affect your health and your relationships. Choosing sexual abstinence is one way to help protect yourself and others.

What You'll Do

- **Explain** how abstinence is a way to show that you care about yourself and others.
- **Describe** how refusal skills can help you maintain abstinence.
- **Identify** a sure way to prevent pregnancy and some diseases.

Terms to Learn

- sexual abstinence

Start Off
Write

How can you tell that someone cares about you?

Risky or harmful behavior puts you in danger. Refusing risky behavior helps keep you safe. For example, refusing to smoke helps you to stay healthy. Sexual activity is risky and harmful for teens, too. Sexual activity can lead to pregnancy and can expose you to deadly diseases. Refusing to take part in sexual activity is called **sexual abstinence** (SEK shoo uhl AB stuh nuhns). Practicing sexual abstinence is the best choice for teens.

Caring

Peer pressure to become sexually active can be very strong. People who pressure you to become sexually active are not looking out for your health or showing that they care about you. Choosing abstinence shows that you care about yourself and your future. It also shows that you care about the people around you. It shows that you want them to be safe from pregnancy and diseases. Maintaining abstinence in a relationship shows one of the highest levels of respect and love for someone.

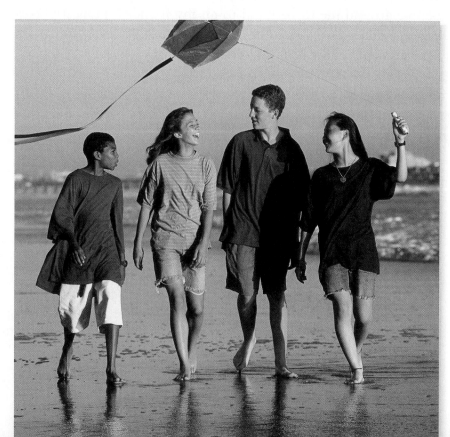

Figure 14 Friends have fun and take care of each other. Good friends never pressure you to risk your health.

Refusal Skills

Maintaining abstinence is easier when you are in healthy relationships. Good friends don't pressure you to change your values or risk your health. Refusal skills can also help. Try not to put yourself in risky situations. Say no whenever you need to. Stating your values can stop others from pressuring you. Remember: You always have the right to say no.

Risks

Teens who become sexually active risk harming themselves physically and emotionally. Sexually active teens risk pregnancy. They also risk getting diseases that are spread by sexual activity. Sexual abstinence prevents pregnancy and exposure to these diseases. Sexually active teens also risk feeling guilty and losing self-respect. Sexual abstinence helps avoid these problems, too. Being a teen is complicated enough without having the additional problems related to sexual activity. Teens who choose abstinence make their lives safer, healthier, and simpler.

Health Journal

During the next week, keep a record of how someone special to you has shown you affection in nonphysical ways. Keep a list of how you have demonstrated nonphysical affection to others.

TABLE 3 Six Benefits of Sexual Abstinence

preventing pregnancy with 100 percent certainty

avoiding exposure to diseases

knowing you made a healthy choice

avoiding emotional scars from being sexually active too soon

keeping your self-respect

making your life less complicated

Lesson Review

Using Vocabulary

1. Define *sexual abstinence*, and identify two benefits of sexual abstinence.

Understanding Concepts

2. How does abstinence show that you care for yourself and others?

Critical Thinking

3. Identifying Relationships Alcohol and drugs hurt your ability to make decisions. How does avoiding drugs and alcohol help you maintain sexual abstinence?

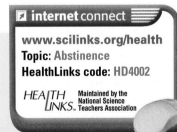

internet connect

www.scilinks.org/health
Topic: Abstinence
HealthLinks code: HD4002

HEALTH LINKS Maintained by the National Science Teachers Association

Chapter Summary

■ Healthy relationships require good communication skills, healthy behavior, and work. ■ Working together as a family requires taking roles seriously and supporting each member with nurture and respect. ■ When the family has problems, the family should work on those problems. ■ More serious problems, such as abuse and neglect, should be reported to a trusted adult as soon as possible. ■ Communities are made up of people who have something in common. Healthy communities also tolerate differences. ■ Friendships are healthy relationships between people who have similar interests and values. Friends support and care for each other. ■ Unhealthy relationships are risky. ■ Sexual abstinence prevents pregnancy and some diseases.

Using Vocabulary

1 Use each of the following terms in a separate sentence: *relationship, body language,* and *tolerance.*

For each sentence, fill in the blank with the proper word from the word bank provided below.

sexual abstinence	personal responsibility
community	behavior
friendship	nurturing
abuse	tolerance
neglect	body language

2 The way you choose to act or respond is called your ___.

3 ___ means not taking part in sexual activity.

4 Providing the things that people need in order to grow is called ___.

5 Treating someone in a harmful or offensive way is called ___.

6 People who have a common background or location or similar goals make up a(n) ___.

7 When you overlook differences and accept people as they are, you are showing ___.

8 A(n) ___ is a relationship between people who like and care for each other.

Understanding Concepts

9 Who makes up an extended family?

10 Explain how people communicate by using words and body language.

11 Explain how assertive behavior can help you learn and grow.

12 Describe two ways you can work through small family problems.

13 Describe the benefits of abstinence from sexual activity.

14 Describe three healthy ways to show affection to a friend.

15 What is a sure way to prevent pregnancy and other risks related to sexual activity?

16 Describe a way to cope with a serious problem, such as abuse or neglect.

17 Describe how refusal skills can help you maintain abstinence.

18 Describe how to identify and cope with an unhealthy relationship.

Critical Thinking

Applying Concepts

19 Teresa was dribbling a basketball in the house after her mother had asked her to stop. The ball took a bad bounce and knocked over a lamp. The lamp broke. How can Teresa respond in a way that shows personal responsibility?

20 Max wants to be a lifeguard when he is in high school. He knows how to swim, but he needs to learn rescue skills. How can Max use assertive behavior to learn what he needs to know to become a lifeguard?

21 Brianna's parents have asked Brianna to call home when she arrives at her friends' houses so that they know that Brianna has arrived safely. Most of the time, Brianna's friends understand. But Dominique teases Brianna and tells Brianna not to bother calling. This upsets Brianna and her parents. How could Brianna handle this relationship?

Making Good Decisions

22 You and your friend stop by a local store on your way home from school. You both buy a few things to eat and then leave the store. Your friend tells you that he shoplifted some candy. What would you do?

23 Brian borrowed Paul's guitar and broke a string. Brian dropped off the guitar at Paul's house while Paul was at soccer practice. Brian didn't tell Paul that the string was broken. When Paul asked Brian about the string, Brian said that it was no big deal and the guitar wasn't that nice anyway. How should Paul respond?

24 Lately, Clara has been lying to her friends a lot. Clara's friend, Denise, is angry with Clara and told her so. Clara thinks this criticism makes Denise a bad friend. Is Denise a bad friend? Explain your answer.

25 Use what you have learned in this chapter to set a personal goal. Write your goal, and make an action plan by using the Health Behavior Contract for your relationship skills. You can find the Health Behavior Contract at go.hrw.com. Just type in the keyword HD4HBC07.

Name _____ Class _____ Date _____

(Health Behavior Contract)
Encouraging Healthy Relationships

My Goals: I, _____, will accomplish one or more of the following goals:
I will identify three trusted adults with whom I could talk about a serious problem.
I will show support to a friend or family member.
I will use my refusal skills when someone tries to pressure me into doing something that I do not want to do.
Other: _____

My Reasons: By talking to an adult about a problem, I can help keep myself safe and healthy. By supporting my family and friends, I will learn better communication skills and how to improve my relationships with them. I will also develop assertive behavior when I use refusal skills.
Other: _____

My Values: Personal values that will help me meet my goals are
_____

My Plan: The actions I will take to meet my goals are
_____

Evaluation: I will use my Health Journal to keep a log of actions I took to fulfill this contract. After 1 month, I will evaluate my goals. I will adjust my plan if my goals are not being met. If my goals are being met, I will consider setting additional goals.

Signed _____

Date _____

Reading Checkup

Take a minute to review your answers to the Health IQ questions at the beginning of this chapter. How has reading this chapter improved your Health IQ?

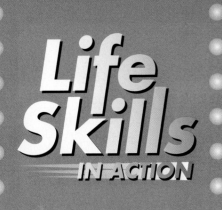

Evaluating Media Messages

You receive media messages every day. These messages are on TV, the Internet, the radio, and in newspapers and magazines. With so many messages, it is important to know how to evaluate them. Evaluating media messages means being able to judge the accuracy of a message. Complete the following activity to improve your skills in evaluating media messages.

Happy Family?

Setting the Scene

ACT 1

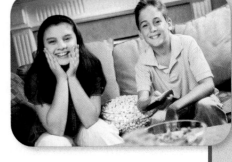

Elisa and her brother Brett love watching the TV show *Happy Family*. The two teenage characters on the show get into trouble a lot, and their parents are always yelling at them. Elisa and Brett think it is very funny when this happens. The best part of the show is when the teens talk their parents out of the punishment. In spite of all the trouble the teens cause, the show always ends with everyone being happy and laughing. Elisa and Brett wish that their family was like the family on the show.

The 5 Steps of Evaluating Media Messages

1. Examine the appeal of the message.
2. Identify the values projected by the message.
3. Consider what the source has to gain by getting you to believe the message.
4. Try to determine the reliability of the source.
5. Based on the information you gather, evaluate the message.

Guided Practice

Practice with a Friend

Form a group of three. Have one person play the role of Elisa and another person play the role of Brett. Have the third person be an observer. Walking through each of the five steps of evaluating media messages, role-play Elisa and Brett analyzing the *Happy Family* TV show. They should consider whether the interactions between the characters are realistic. The observer will take notes, which will include observations about what the people playing Elisa and Brett did well and suggestions of ways to improve. Stop after each step to evaluate the process.

Independent Practice

Check Yourself

After you have completed the guided practice, go through Act 1 again without stopping at each step. Answer the questions below to review what you did.

1. What audience is *Happy Family* trying to appeal to?

2. What values are projected by the behavior of the characters on *Happy Family*?

3. How realistic are the interactions between the characters on *Happy Family*?

4. Think about a TV show you like to watch. How do the characters on the show behave toward each other? Is their behavior similar to the behavior of people around you? Explain your answer.

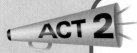

On Your Own

While watching *Happy Family* one evening, Elisa and Brett see a commercial for a new video game. Brett tells Elisa that he wants to buy that video game. Elisa tells Brett that one of the video games he already owns looks very similar to the new one. But Brett points out that the commercial says that the new video game is a big improvement over the one that he has. Make an outline showing how Brett could use the five steps of evaluating media messages to analyze the commercial for the video game.

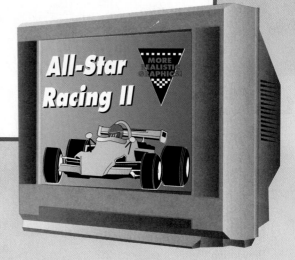

Conflict and Violence

Check out
Current Health
articles related to this chapter by
visiting **go.hrw.com**. Just type in
the keyword **HD4CH27**.

> **"** I got into a huge **fight** with my **mother** over my **curfew.** I got very angry and said some **terrible** things that I really didn't mean.
>
> My mother was upset. I think I hurt her feelings. I wish I could take it all back. **"**

PRE-READING

Answer the following true/false questions to find out what you already know about conflict and violence. When you've finished this chapter, you'll have the opportunity to change your answers based on what you've learned.

1. Violence appears in many places in our society.

2. Conflict does not happen in close relationships.

3. Bullies usually pick on people smaller than they are.

4. Body language is not a real form of communication.

5. People who tease others usually like to do so in front of an audience.

6. If a conflict gets out of control, the best thing to do is to keep working on the conflict until it is better.

7. To compromise is to give into another person's demands.

8. Anyone who is not part of a conflict can help to mediate that conflict.

9. Drinking or using drugs increases the chances that a person will become violent.

10. Violence and aggression are the same thing.

11. It is unnecessary to report threats of violence that sound like jokes.

12. The way you express yourself during conflict determines how a conflict ends.

ANSWERS: 1. true; 2. false; 3. true; 4. false; 5. true; 6. false; 7. false; 8. false; 9. true; 10. false; 11. false; 12. true

What Is Conflict?

Have you ever disagreed with somebody? Maybe you and your brother or sister wanted to watch different TV shows. Maybe your parents wanted you to do homework, but you wanted to go out with friends.

If you have had these types of disagreements, then you have experienced conflict. **Conflict** is any clash of ideas or interests. Everybody experiences conflict in his or her life. Conflict happens even in the closest relationships.

Recognizing Conflict

The first step toward solving any conflict is to recognize when conflict is happening or when conflict is about to happen. The following signs can tell you that a conflict is occurring or that a conflict is about to occur:

- **Disagreement** Every conflict starts with disagreement over an issue.
- **Emotions** If you find that a disagreement is causing emotions, such as anger or jealousy, the disagreement is becoming a conflict.
- **Other People's Behavior** If the other person or people in a disagreement begin ignoring you, raising their voices, or crossing their arms, a conflict is happening.

What You'll Do

- **Describe** three signs that a conflict is happening or is about to happen.
- **Identify** three reasons that conflicts happen.
- **Describe** how conflicts can happen at home, with peers, and at school.

Terms to Learn

- conflict
- bullying

Start Off
Write

What is the difference between teasing and bullying?

Figure 1 Conflict can arise anywhere, even when you are doing something fun, such as going on a vacation.

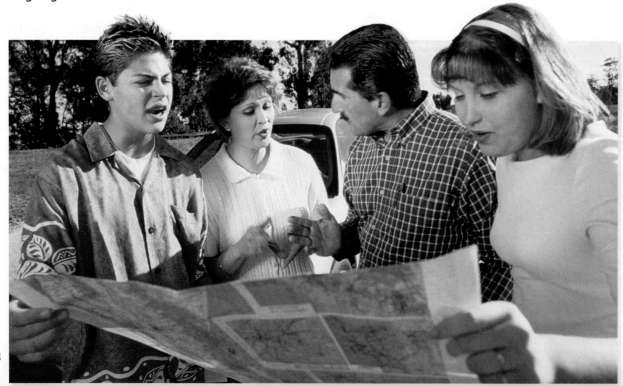

Why Does Conflict Happen?

Although conflict can happen over almost any issue, it usually happens for one of three reasons:

- **Resources** Conflicts can happen when two or more people want the same thing, but not all of them can have it.

- **Values and Expectations** Different things are important to different people. Many conflicts happen because people have different ideas about what is important or how things should be done.

- **Emotions** Conflicts can happen because people feel hurt or angry at the behavior of others.

Conflicts at Home

You and your family members usually spend a lot of time together. Because of this, there are many chances for conflict to arise at home. Conflicts can happen between you and your parents or caregivers because each of you has different expectations. For example, your parents may expect you to do certain chores, and you may feel that you shouldn't have to do as many chores. Conflict can also happen between you and your parents or caregivers because you disagree with their opinions or their rules for you.

You may also have conflicts with a brother or sister. For example, you may feel that you are asked to do more than your brother or sister. Or you may have conflict with a brother or sister over resources, such as the telephone or the computer. You may even feel that your brother or sister gets more attention than you do.

Conflicts in the home affect everyone in the family. For example, an unresolved conflict with your brother or sister may make your parents unhappy. When you have conflicts with members of your family or household, it is important to solve them quickly. Allowing conflicts at home to go on for too long can create a very difficult living situation.

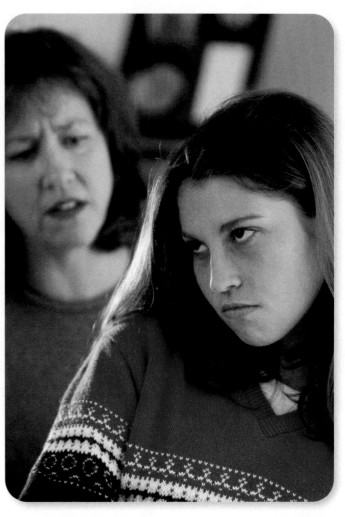

Figure 2 Conflict between you and your parents often occurs because they have different expectations than you do.

Myth & Fact

Myth: Conflict is bad, and it should always be avoided.

Fact: Conflict is a natural result of being around other people. Conflict itself is not bad, but the way in which people deal with conflict can be healthy or unhealthy.

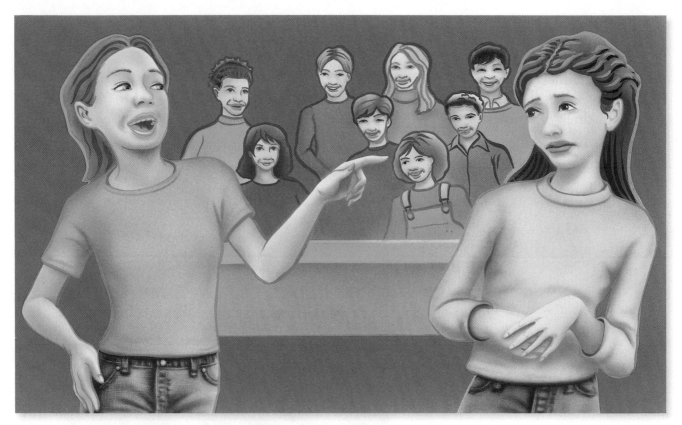

Figure 3 People who tease others often do so in front of an audience. Having an audience makes people who tease feel better about themselves.

Health Journal

Has anyone ever teased you? What happened? How did the teasing make you feel? Write about your experience in your Health Journal.

Conflicts with Peers

Often, conflicts happen with your peers. Your *peers* are people who are close to your own age with whom you interact. Many kinds of conflict can happen between peers. Some of these types of conflict are described below.

- **Conflicts with Friends** Even close friendships can face conflict. You and your friends may argue over what you want to do for fun. Or you may argue because you are jealous of other friendships. Whatever the reason for conflict between friends, these conflicts should be solved quickly before they destroy the friendship.

- **Teasing** You probably have been teased or have teased someone else before. It is important to realize that teasing can result in hurt feelings and emotional problems. Usually, people tease others in front of an audience to make themselves look better. You can deal with teasing by ignoring it, making a joke about it, or by confronting the teaser.

- **Bullying** Scaring or controlling another person by using threats or physical force is called **bullying.** Bullies almost always pick on people who are younger or smaller than they are. If a bully won't leave you alone or if any violence occurs, report the bully to an authority figure, such as a parent or teacher.

Conflicts at School

You spend a lot of time at school. While you are at school, you deal with different people, including friends, classmates, teachers, and other school authorities. Your relationships with these people are important for your social and mental development. But these relationships can also be sources of conflict. Some of the conflicts that can occur at school are listed below.

- **Conflicts with Peers** All of the conflicts with peers listed on the previous page can happen at school. In fact, these types of conflicts are the most common conflicts at school.

- **Competition with Classmates** Students often compete with one another in schoolwork or in sports. Some competition can be healthy, but if the competition begins to cause anger or hurt feelings, it may become a problem.

- **Conflicts with Teachers or Other School Authorities** Conflict can arise with teachers for many reasons. Sometimes, you may feel that a teacher is being too strict or unfair. A teacher may feel that you are causing trouble or are not doing your best.

Remember that you are at school to learn. It is very important to solve conflicts at school before they interfere with your education. If you need help with a conflict at school, you can ask a trusted adult, such as a parent, teacher, or counselor, for help.

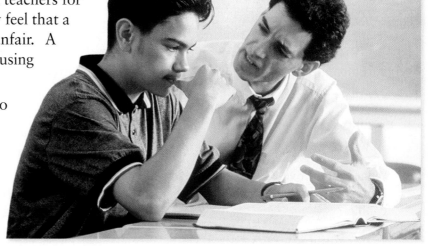

Figure 4 Conflict at school sometimes happens with school authorities. It is important to recognize and solve these conflicts quickly.

Lesson Review

Using Vocabulary

1. What is conflict?

Understanding Concepts

2. Describe three signs that a conflict is happening or is about to happen.

3. List three reasons that conflict happens.

4. Describe three types of conflict with peers.

5. What are three types of conflict that may occur at school?

Critical Thinking

6. Making Inferences Howard and his sister wanted to use the computer at the same time. Howard became angry and called his sister a hurtful name. Howard's sister became very angry, and Howard and his sister started fighting. Why did this conflict happen?

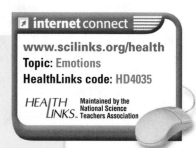

☑ **internet** connect

www.scilinks.org/health
Topic: Emotions
HealthLinks code: HD4035

HEALTH
LINKS. Maintained by the National Science Teachers Association

Communicating During Conflicts

What You'll Do

- **Describe** the importance of good communication.
- **Describe** body language and its importance.
- **Identify** five skills for good listening.
- **Describe** negotiation, compromise, and collaboration.

Terms to Learn

- body language
- negotiation
- compromise
- collaboration

Start Off
Write

What is a positive way to express yourself during a conflict?

> Pilar's sister was always using the phone. Pilar told her sister that she wanted to be able to use the phone, too. Pilar and her sister talked about the problem and worked out a schedule for using the phone.

Most conflicts can be solved easily by using good communication skills. By telling her sister how she felt and by working with her sister to solve the problem, Pilar was able to use the phone and to avoid fighting with her sister.

Expressing Yourself

The way you choose to express your emotions during a conflict will often determine whether the conflict is solved in a positive way or a negative way. When you are in a conflict, it is important to communicate honestly and openly. You must also avoid communicating in an angry or threatening way. Anger or threats almost always cause a conflict to end poorly. For example, in the situation above, if Pilar had started yelling at her sister or calling her sister names, the conflict would have ended differently. Pilar's sister could have become angry too, and the conflict may have ended in a screaming fight instead of a productive solution.

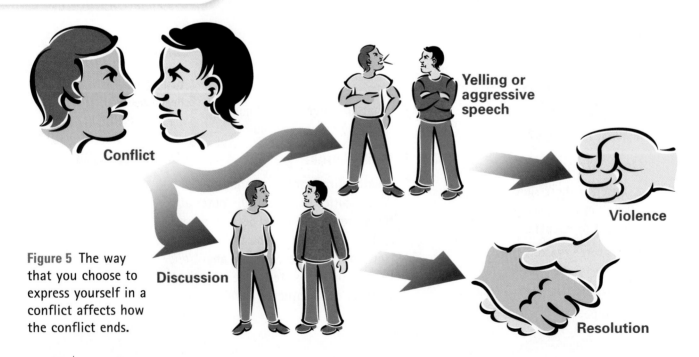

Conflict

Yelling or aggressive speech

Violence

Discussion

Resolution

Figure 5 The way that you choose to express yourself in a conflict affects how the conflict ends.

Choosing the Right Words

When you talk to another person during a conflict, choosing your words carefully is important. The words you choose should clearly describe how you feel in a way that is not hurtful, angry, or threatening. Do not call the other person names or make fun of his or her ideas. Instead, choose statements that accurately express your expectations and feelings about the situation. If possible, plan what you want to say ahead of time. By choosing the right words, you can make sure that the other person knows exactly how you feel. This understanding makes it possible to begin working on a solution to the conflict.

Body Language

Words are not the only way that you communicate your feelings to others. Your body often tells others a lot about how you feel. Communication that is done by the body rather than by words is called **body language.** You communicate with your body during a conflict in several ways.

- Facial expressions, such as frowns or smiles, communicate a lot about how you feel. In a conflict, make sure that the expression on your face is calm rather than angry or threatening.

- Gestures, such as pointing your finger at someone or shaking your fist at someone, can be very threatening or insulting. Avoid making these types of gestures in a conflict.

- Posture is very important in a conflict. Folding your arms tells the other person that you are not interested in what he or she is saying. Standing too close to someone can be very threatening. Try to keep a relaxed and open posture.

Figure 6 Body language can tell you a lot about how somebody feels. Can you tell how this teen feels in each of these pictures?

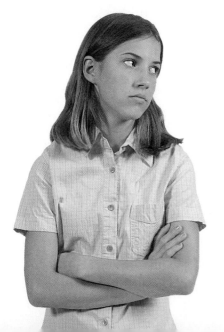
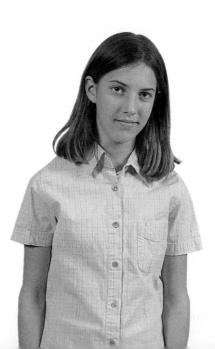
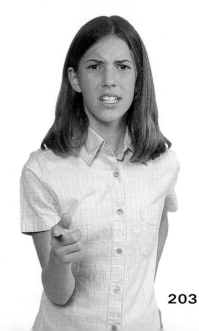

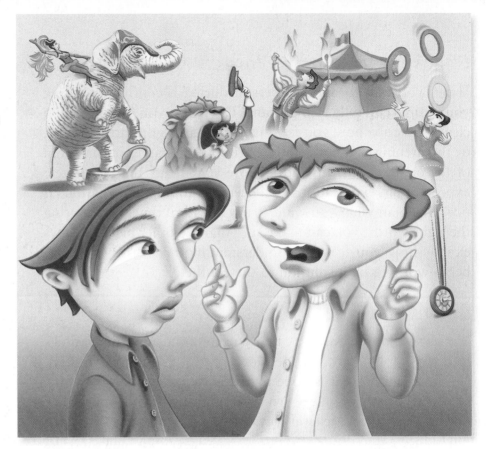

Figure 7 Good listening means focusing on the person who is talking, even if there are distractions.

Listening

When you are working to solve a conflict, good listening skills are just as important as good communication skills. By listening carefully to the other person's opinions, you can help to find a solution to the conflict that makes both sides happy. When you listen to another person, make eye contact. Do not become distracted by things that are going on around you. Keep your body relaxed and open. If you are unsure of what the other person said, repeat it to make sure you understand. Do not interrupt the person even if you disagree with him or her. Following these listening tips will let the other person know that you value his or her feelings. In addition, you will better understand the other person's opinions. When you understand the other person's opinions, solving the conflict will be much easier.

Negotiation

The most important tool for solving conflicts is negotiation. **Negotiation** is a discussion to reach a solution to a conflict. For negotiation to work, both sides must be willing to discuss their feelings and their needs openly and honestly. They must also be willing to listen carefully to the other person. Negotiation usually requires both sides to be willing to make sacrifices to reach a solution. If negotiation is used properly, it can solve conflicts positively and often quickly.

Compromise and Collaboration

Compromise and collaboration are two types of solutions to conflicts. **Compromise** is a solution in which each person gives up something to reach a solution that pleases everyone. For example, if you want to go to the park and your friend wants to go eat, you could compromise by going out to eat today and going to the park tomorrow. But an even better solution to conflict is collaboration. **Collaboration** is a solution to a conflict in which neither side has to give up anything to reach a solution that pleases everyone. Imagine again that your friend wants to eat, but you want to go to the park. Collaboration in this situation would be to have a picnic in the park. Unfortunately, not every conflict can be solved through collaboration. Most conflicts are solved by making sacrifices.

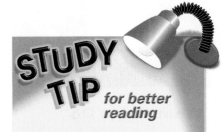

STUDY TIP *for better reading*

Reviewing Information
When you have finished reading this lesson, write every vocabulary term on a sheet of paper. Underneath each term, give an example of how it can affect a conflict.

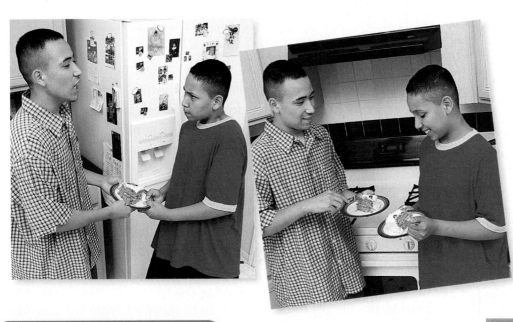

Figure 8 By cutting this piece of cake in half, these two brothers were able to solve their conflict through compromise.

Lesson Review

Using Vocabulary

1. What is body language and why is it important?

2. What is the difference between compromise and collaboration?

Understanding Concepts

3. Why is it important to use good communication skills in a conflict?

4. Name five things that you can do to be a good listener.

5. How can negotiation, compromise, and collaboration be used in a conflict?

Critical Thinking

6. **Applying Concepts** How can body language help you avoid a potential conflict? Explain.

internet connect

www.scilinks.org/health
Topic: Communication Skills
HealthLinks code: HD4022

HEALTH LINKS Maintained by the National Science Teachers Association

Getting Help for Conflicts

What You'll Do

- **Identify** five warning signs that a conflict may be out of control.
- **Describe** the use of mediation for solving out-of-control conflicts.
- **Identify** seven skills of a trained mediator.

Terms to Learn

- mediation

Start Off
Write

How do you know when to get help to solve a conflict?

Health Journal

Describe a time when you were in a conflict that you couldn't solve without help from another person. What did that person do to help solve the conflict?

Elena and her friend Toni were having an argument. Toni got so angry that she decided to stop talking to Elena. Elena can't solve the conflict now because Toni won't talk to her. Is there anything Elena can do?

Sometimes, a conflict gets to a point that the people cannot solve the conflict by themselves. When Toni stopped talking to Elena, she made it impossible for them to solve the conflict. With a little help, however, this conflict can be solved.

When Is a Conflict Out of Control?

There are many ways that a conflict can get out of control. By identifying the warning signs that a conflict is out of control, you can take steps to calm down and work toward a solution. A conflict may be out of control when communication becomes insulting or hurtful or when either person becomes very angry. If violence or threats are used, a conflict is definitely out of control. Sometimes, people in a conflict stop communicating, or they negotiate for a long time but cannot reach a solution. In these cases, the conflict is out of control because the people in the conflict cannot solve it. If a conflict that you are in gets out of control, take a break and return to the conflict later. The break will give you and the other person a chance to calm down. During the break, think about what you want from the conflict and what you are willing to give up. If you still cannot solve the conflict, you may need to talk to another person who is not part of the conflict.

TABLE 1 Signs That a Conflict Is Out of Control
Serious anger
Lack of communication
Hurtful or insulting speech
Inability to reach a solution after much negotiation
Violence or threats of violence

Mediation

The best way to solve a conflict that is out of control is to seek the help of somebody who is not part of the conflict. A third person can often think of solutions that neither side has considered. A third person can also help lower the level of anger in a conflict and can keep the discussion on track. This third party is called a *mediator*. A mediator is an uninvolved person who helps solve a conflict between other people. The process of using a mediator to solve a conflict is called **mediation.**

Not everyone can be a mediator. When selecting a mediator, you should select somebody who has special training in mediation. A person who is not trained in mediation can make a conflict worse or can become a part of the conflict. A good mediator

- sets ground rules, such as no name calling and no interrupting, and makes sure that everyone follows the rules
- keeps the conflict focused on finding a solution
- does not take sides
- listens carefully to both sides
- asks questions
- offers solutions
- does not allow the conversation to become angry

If you need to find a trained mediator to help solve a conflict, talk to a parent, teacher, or other trusted adult. He or she can help you find a trained mediator.

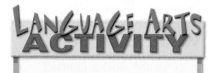

LANGUAGE ARTS ACTIVITY

Write a short story about two teens who seek the help of a mediator to solve a conflict.

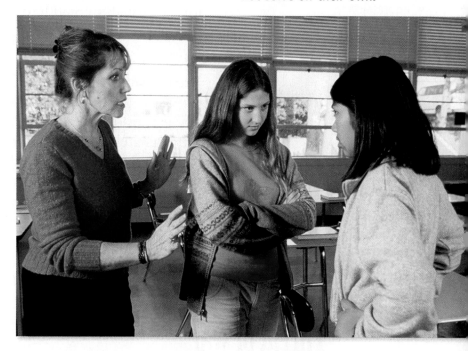

Figure 9 These two teens are using a mediator to help them solve a conflict that they could not solve on their own.

Lesson Review

Using Vocabulary

1. Define *mediation*, and give an example of when it may be used to solve a conflict.

Understanding Concepts

2. List five signs that a conflict may be getting out of control.

3. Why is it important for a mediator to have special training?

4. List seven skills of a trained mediator.

Critical Thinking

5. Applying Concepts Think of three rules not listed in the text that a mediator may set.

Violence: When Conflict Becomes Dangerous

What You'll Do

- **Describe** how a conflict becomes violent.
- **Identify** four signs that a conflict may become violent.
- **Explain** the importance of reporting all threats of violence.

Terms to Learn

- violence
- aggression

Start Off *Write*

How can you tell if a conflict is about to become violent?

Tom got in a fight at school. He was arguing with a classmate named Arman during lunch. The two teens got angrier and angrier until Arman hit Tom. Why did this conflict become violent? Could Tom have seen the violence coming?

Most conflicts will not become violent. However, if a conflict is handled poorly or is allowed to get out of control, it can become violent. Fortunately, there are signs that can warn you of violence before it happens. If Tom had known what signs to look for, he probably could have avoided violence.

What Is Violence?

You probably have an idea of what violence is. You may even have experienced violence. But what exactly is violence? **Violence** is the use of physical force to harm someone or something. Unfortunately, violence exists in many places in society. Movies and TV shows often include violence. Newspapers and news broadcasts report many stories of violence throughout the world. By knowing how and why conflicts become violent, you can avoid becoming a victim of violence.

Figure 10 You may often read about violent events in the newspaper. Unfortunately, violence is common in our world.

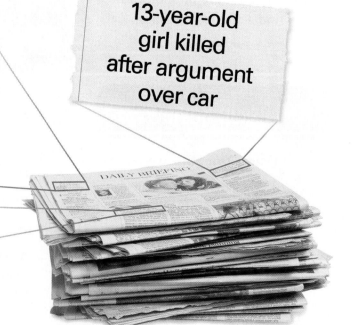

Threat of war looms over Colombia

13-year-old girl killed after argument over car

Man killed in gang fight at biker expo

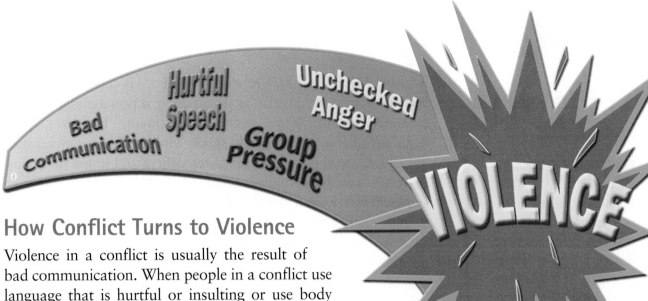

How Conflict Turns to Violence

Violence in a conflict is usually the result of bad communication. When people in a conflict use language that is hurtful or insulting or use body language that is threatening, anger increases. If anger continues to increase, the result can be violence. By knowing the signs to watch for, you can tell when violence is about to happen. If you see signs that a conflict is about to become violent, walk away. Walking away will give you and the other person a chance to calm down. Hopefully, you can solve the conflict later and can avoid a violent situation.

Figure 11 Several things, such as bad communication, anger, and group pressure, can cause a conflict to turn violent.

Watch for the Signs

Violence can happen quickly in a conflict. There are several signs that violence may happen. Recognizing these signs will help you avoid and prevent violent situations. The following signs can tell you that a conflict may become violent.

- **Bad Communication** When people in a conflict communicate in a negative way, violence can result. Bad communication can be hurtful speech—such as shouting, insults, and profanity—or can be refusal to listen to the other side.

- **Body Language** A person's body language can be a very good sign that the person is about to become violent. Examples of threatening body language include having clenched fists, standing too close, or having a clenched jaw.

- **Anger** People in a conflict often get angry. Anger is a normal emotion and can be expressed in positive and negative ways. If people are using negative expressions of anger, a conflict can turn to violence.

- **Group Pressure** People are more likely to become violent when other people are watching them. The group may be encouraging them, or they may want to look powerful in front of the group. Either way, be careful in conflicts that happen in front of an audience.

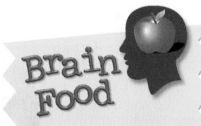

Brain Food

When a person is under a lot of stress, he or she is more likely to show violent behavior. Studies have shown that regular exercise can reduce stress significantly.

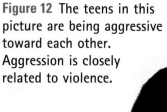
Aggression

Another behavior that is related to violence is called *aggression*. **Aggression** is any hostile or threatening action against another person. Violence is an aggressive behavior. However, most aggressive behavior is not physically violent. Some people, such as bullies, use aggression to frighten others and to get their way. A person can be verbally aggressive by teasing or humiliating someone else. Even a mean look can be a form of aggression. Even though aggression may not always cause physical harm, it can cause serious emotional damage. Aggression is also a good warning sign that violence may happen. A person who regularly uses aggression is likely to become violent in a conflict. If someone is being aggressive toward you, you should tell a trusted adult.

Threats

The most obvious sign that violence is about to happen is a threat. A *threat* is an expressed intention or plan to do harm to something or someone. Some threats are made in person. Other times, threats are sent in writing or are delivered by someone else. Sometimes, you may even hear someone threaten another person who is not present. People may use threats to get their own way, or threats may be a reaction to anger or other emotions. Whatever the reason for threats, all threats should be taken seriously. You cannot always tell whether a person is serious about a threat. Therefore, it is much better to be safe and to report the threat than to ignore the threat and find that the threat was real.

Figure 12 The teens in this picture are being aggressive toward each other. Aggression is closely related to violence.

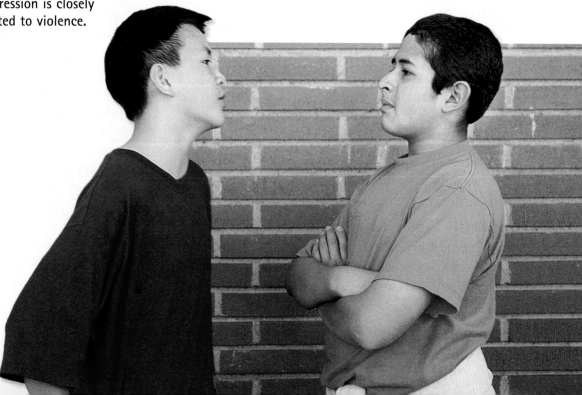

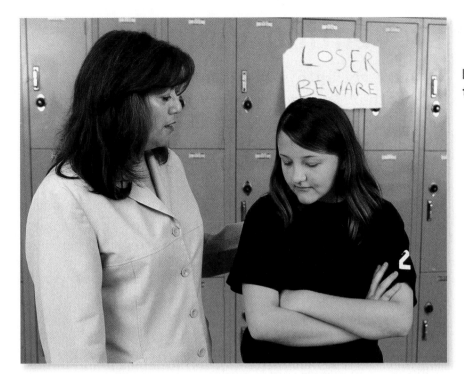

Figure 13 Report any threat to a trusted adult.

Reporting Threats of Violence

Reporting all threats of violence to a responsible adult is very important. If you know of a threat to yourself or to someone else, it is your responsibility to tell an authority or trusted adult of the danger. If you do not tell someone, violence that could have been avoided may happen. For example, many of the extremely violent events that have happened in schools recently could have been avoided if threats had been reported. In these cases, people heard threats but did not take them seriously. Even if you think that someone is joking, you must report any threat of violence. The possible consequences of not reporting threats are too great.

Health Journal

If you experienced acts or threats of violence, to whom could you report them? Make a list of 10 adults to whom you could report acts or threats of violence.

Lesson Review

Using Vocabulary

1. Define *violence*, and identify places where you might see violence.

Understanding Concepts

2. How does a conflict become violent?

3. Identify four signs that a conflict may become violent.

4. Why is it important to report all threats to a responsible adult?

Critical Thinking

5. Identifying Relationships Is all violence aggressive? Is all aggression violent? Explain your answers.

6. Making Inferences Do you need to report threats made against someone's property? Explain your answer.

Lesson 5

Preventing Violence

Luke got into a big fight with his little brother. Luke got so angry that he was about to hit his brother. Instead, Luke decided to go to his room to calm down. Later, Luke was very glad that he hadn't hit his brother.

Luke did the right thing by taking a break to control his anger. If Luke had hit his brother, the situation would have been much worse. Everybody has a responsibility to control his or her anger and to keep violence from happening.

Controlling Anger

Anger is like air filling a balloon. If the air is not allowed to escape, the balloon will eventually burst. To prevent anger from erupting into violence, use the following strategies:

- **Take a break.** Often, removing yourself from an angry situation for even a short time will allow you to calm down.

- **Focus on calming yourself.** Count to 10, and take deep, slow breaths.

- **Release your anger in a safe way.** Punching a pillow or a punching bag can allow you to release your anger without harming anyone or anything.

- **Exercise.** Physical activity can release anger and can allow you to focus on something else until you calm down.

- **Be creative.** Try drawing or writing in a journal. Creative activities can allow you to release your anger in a healthy and productive way. Some creative activities can also help you work through your problems.

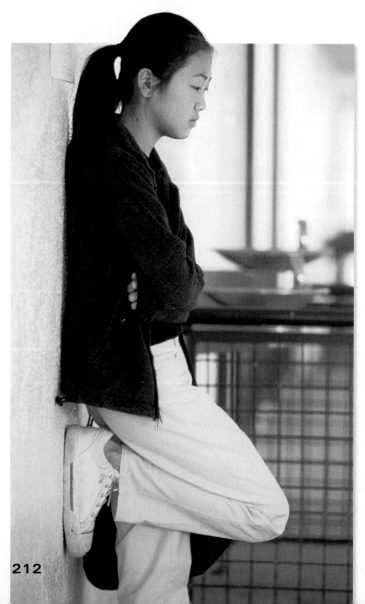

Figure 14 If you are getting too angry, take a break to calm down.

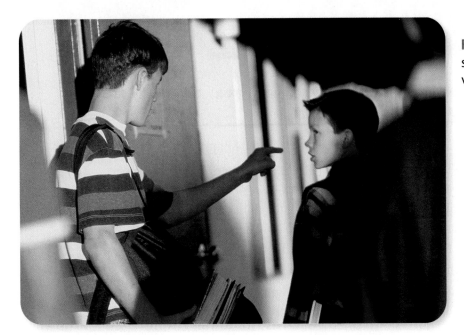

Figure 15 If you think a situation could become violent, walk away.

Protecting Yourself

Just as you have a responsibility to others to control your anger, you also have a responsibility to yourself to avoid violent situations. To lower your risk of becoming a victim of violence, do the following things:

- Pay attention to signs that violence might occur.
- Walk away from out-of-control conflicts.
- Take all threats seriously.
- Avoid people who carry weapons.
- Avoid conflict with people who have been drinking or using drugs. These behaviors increase the chance that a person will become violent.

Myth & Fact

Myth: If you avoid violent situations, you are a coward.

Fact: Violence does not solve anything. Avoiding violent situations is smart, not cowardly.

Lesson Review

Understanding Concepts

1. Name five things that you can do to control your anger.

2. Name five things that you can do to protect yourself from violent situations.

3. Why should you avoid conflict with people who have been drinking or using drugs?

Critical Thinking

4. **Applying Concepts** Steven is very angry at his brother, Eric. What is a positive way he can release his anger? What is a negative way he can release his anger? Explain.

Chapter Summary

■ Conflict is any clash of ideas or interests. ■ Most conflicts happen at home, with peers, or at school. ■ The way that you communicate during a conflict can often determine whether the conflict ends positively or negatively. ■ Communication by the body is called *body language*. ■ Tools for resolving conflicts include negotiation, compromise, collaboration, and mediation. ■ Watch for the signs that a conflict is out of control, and seek help for out-of-control conflicts. ■ Uncontrolled anger can lead to violence. ■ Watch for the warning signs that a conflict may turn violent. Walk away from conflicts that may turn violent. ■ Report any threats to authorities. ■ Controlling anger and avoiding violent situations are two ways to prevent violence.

Using Vocabulary

For each pair of terms, describe how the meanings of the terms differ.

1 negotiation/mediation

2 compromise/collaboration

3 aggression/violence

For each sentence, fill in the blank with the proper word from the word bank provided below.

mediator	body language
negotiation	threat
aggression	compromise

4 Communication by the body is called ___.

5 ___ is a discussion to reach a solution to a conflict.

6 An uninvolved person who helps solve a conflict between other people is called a(n) ___.

7 An expressed intention or plan to do harm to something or someone is called a(n) ___.

Understanding Concepts

8 How can you tell if a conflict is out of control?

9 Describe two types of conflict that can happen at home.

10 Why must a mediator be uninvolved in a conflict?

11 What is needed for negotiation to work?

12 Why is it important to resolve conflicts at school?

13 Why is collaboration better than compromise?

14 Give three examples of body language. Describe how each one could be used positively and negatively in a conflict.

15 How can bad communication increase the chance of violence?

16 How can group pressure increase the chance of violence?

17 Why should all threats be taken seriously?

18 How can exercise help you control your anger?

Critical Thinking

Making Inferences

19 How are bullies and people who tease others alike?

20 Even friends experience conflict with each other. In fact, in many cases, close friends experience more conflict than friends who aren't close. Why might close friends have more conflict?

21 Group pressure can cause a person to become violent in a situation in which he or she normally would not have become violent. Name two other situations in which group pressure may cause a person to do something that he or she normally would not do.

Making Good Decision

22 Imagine that you are in a conflict with a classmate. After arguing for a while, you both realize that you need the help of a mediator. Your classmate says that her mother is a trained mediator and can help you solve the conflict. Is your classmate's mother a good selection for a mediator in this case? Explain.

23 Imagine that you have a friend who is very angry at another boy at school. Your friend tells you how much he hates this other boy and tells you that he plans to bring a knife to school to threaten the other boy. When you tell your friend that bringing a knife to school is a bad idea, he says that he was joking. What should you do in this situation?

24 Imagine that you are very angry about a conflict that you are having with a friend. What is one physical way that you could control your anger? What is one creative way that you could control your anger? Which way do you think would work best for you? Explain.

25 Use what you have learned in this chapter to set a personal goal. Write your goal, and make an action plan by using the Health Behavior Contract for preventing violence and controlling your anger. You can find the Health Behavior Contract at go.hrw.com. Just type in the keyword HD4HBC08.

Name _____ Class _____ Date _____

Health Behavior Contract
Conflict and Violence _____

My Goals: I, _____, will accomplish one or more of the following goals:
I will use good communication skills to avoid conflicts.
I will control my anger.
I will avoid situations that could become violent.
Other: _____

My Reasons: By expressing myself clearly and calmly, using good body language, and listening well, I will increase my chances of avoiding conflicts. By controlling my anger and by avoiding dangerous situations, I can prevent violence.
Other: _____

My Values: Personal values that will help me meet my goals are _____

My Plan: The actions I will take to meet my goals are _____

Evaluation: I will use my Health Journal to keep a log of actions I took to fulfill this contract. After 1 month, I will evaluate my goals. I will adjust my plan if my goals are not being met. If my goals are being met, I will consider setting additional goals.

Signed _____

Date _____

Reading Checkup

Take a minute to review your answers to the Health IQ questions at the beginning of this chapter. How has reading this chapter improved your Health IQ?

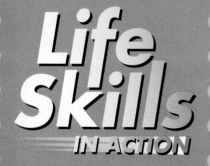

Communicating Effectively

Have you ever been in a bad situation that was made worse because of poor communication? Or maybe you have difficulty understanding others or being understood. You can avoid misunderstandings by expressing your feelings in a healthy way, which is communicating effectively. Complete the following activity to develop effective communication skills.

The Threat

ACT 1

Setting the Scene

Ramón and his friend Jonas are joking around as they walk down a hallway in school. Jonas accidentally bumps into an older student named Kevin and causes Kevin's books and schoolwork to scatter across the hallway. Jonas apologizes and helps Kevin pick up his things, but Kevin is furious. "You're going to pay for this!" growls Kevin.

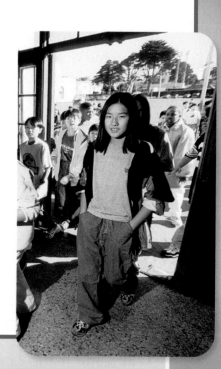

The 4 Steps of Communicating Effectively

1. Express yourself calmly and clearly.
2. Choose your words carefully.
3. Use open body language.
4. Use active listening.

Guided Practice

Practice with a Friend

Form a group of three. Have one person play the role of Ramón and another person play the role of Jonas. Have the third person be an observer. Walking through each of the four steps of communicating effectively, role-play Ramón and Jonas talking about the situation. In the conversation, Ramón should try to convince Jonas to report Kevin's threat. Jonas should explain why he doesn't want to report the threat. The observer will take notes, which will include observations about what the person playing Ramón did well and suggestions of ways to improve. Stop after each step to evaluate the process.

Independent Practice

Check Yourself

After you have completed the guided practice, go through Act 1 again without stopping at each step. Answer the questions below to review what you did.

1. Why should Ramón express himself calmly and clearly when talking to Jonas?

2. What should Ramón say to Jonas to convince him that it is important to report the threat?

3. Why is it important for Ramón to use active listening when Jonas is talking?

4. Why is it important to report all threats of violence?

ACT 2

On Your Own

Over the next few days, Kevin threatens Jonas whenever he sees Jonas. Jonas is unhappy about the threats, and Ramón is finally able to convince Jonas to report them. Jonas goes to talk with one of his teachers about the threats. Draw a comic strip showing how Jonas could use the four steps of communicating effectively to tell his teacher about the threats.

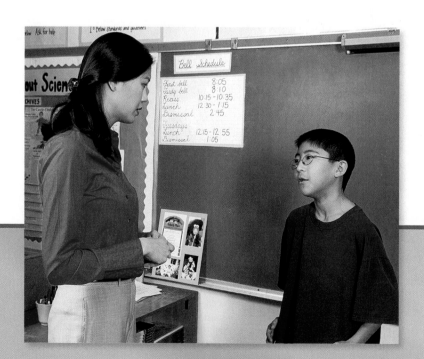

CHAPTER 11

Teens and Tobacco

Lessons

Check out
Current Health
articles related to this chapter by
visiting go.hrw.com. Just type in
the keyword **HD4CH26.**

> **"** I promised both **my parents** and **myself** that I would **never try smoking.**
>
> There are a couple of kids that I hang out with who have just started smoking. And they have been bugging me lately to give it a try. I'm not going to start smoking, but I wish I knew how to get them to quit. **"**

Health IQ

PRE-READING

Answer the following true/false questions to find out what you already know about tobacco. When you've finished this chapter, you'll have the opportunity to change your answers based on what you've learned.

1. As long as someone remains a light smoker, that person will not experience the harmful effects of smoking.

2. You have to use tobacco products for many years before the tobacco has harmful effects on you.

3. The smoke that comes from the tip of a burning cigarette is not as dangerous to your health as the smoke that is inhaled by the smoker.

4. It is against the law to sell any form of tobacco product to someone under the age of 18.

5. Nicotine is a drug.

6. Young people do not get hooked on cigarettes as easily adults do.

7. Most people can quit smoking without any help.

8. Chewing tobacco does not cause cancer.

9. More women die from breast cancer than from lung cancer.

10. Cigarettes are as addictive as heroin and cocaine.

11. The only way to successfully quit smoking is to just go "cold turkey."

12. Cigar and pipe smoking are safer than cigarette smoking because people rarely inhale smoke from cigars and pipes.

ANSWERS: 1. false; 2. false; 3. false; 4. true; 5. true; 6. false; 7. false; 8. false; 9. false; 10. true; 11. false; 12. false

Tobacco: Dangerous from the Start

Approximately one in two people who smoke throughout their lifetime will die prematurely!

Smoking has many harmful effects. Yet, many people continue to smoke and eventually become ill or die from a smoking-related illness. In this lesson, you will learn about the different types of tobacco products and how they affect your health.

What's in a Tobacco Product?

The tobacco plant has grown naturally in this country for centuries. But tobacco products are far from natural. When tobacco is processed, the leaves of the tobacco plant are combined with hundreds of other ingredients called additives. **Additives** are the chemicals that help keep the tobacco moist, help it to burn longer and taste better. One example of an additive is ammonia. Ammonia is also found in urine and in cleaning products.

When you light a cigarette, the burning tobacco produces smoke that contains thousands of chemicals. One of these chemicals is benzene, which is known to cause cancer. Other chemicals that are produced by the burning smoke are tar and carbon monoxide. Carbon monoxide is a gas that enters the bloodstream and starves your body of oxygen. Tar is a solid, sticky substance. When tar is inhaled, it coats the airways and lungs, blocking small air sacs. Chronic bronchitis, lung cancer, and other lung diseases can eventually result from smoking.

What You'll Do

- **List** three chemicals that are produced when a cigarette is lit.
- **List** five effects of tobacco on your body that appear early in a cigarette habit.
- **Describe** health problems associated with smokeless tobacco use.
- **Identify** four types of tobacco products other than cigarettes.
- **Explain** why environmental tobacco smoke is harmful.

Terms to Learn

- additive
- nicotine
- environmental tobacco smoke (ETS)

Start Off *Write*

What are some of the dangerous effects of tobacco?

Figure 1 Cigarettes and other tobacco products contain many ingredients other than just tobacco.

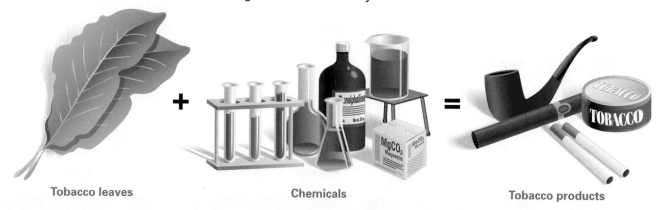

Tobacco leaves + Chemicals = Tobacco products

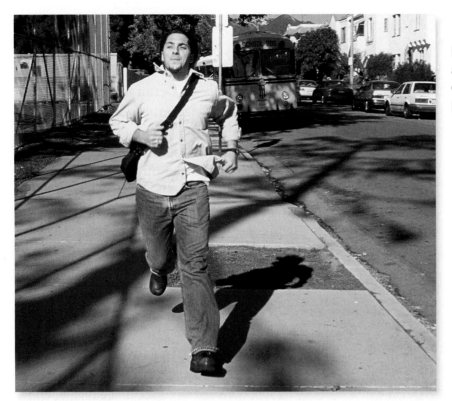

Figure 2 Even things as simple as running to get to school on time become difficult for people who smoke.

Cigarettes: Effects Appear Early

You do not have to be a heavy or lifelong smoker to feel the harmful effects of cigarettes. The harm begins with the first puff, when nicotine enters the lungs. **Nicotine** is a highly addictive drug that occurs naturally in the leaves of the tobacco plant. Some early effects of tobacco on your body are as follows:

- Nicotine travels from the lungs into the bloodstream and into the brain, where the nicotine raises the heart rate and blood pressure.

- Skin, breath, hair, and clothing will immediately smell of smoke. And other people usually notice the odor first.

- Most people feel nauseated and dizzy when they begin smoking because they are not used to the chemicals that enter their bloodstream and brain.

- Your senses of smell and taste usually suffer. As a result, foods no longer smell or taste the same.

- Even light smokers report shortness of breath and increased coughing. Smokers are unable to run as long or as fast as they did before they started smoking.

- Smokers are sick more frequently and stay sick longer.

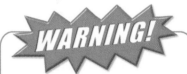

Contents of Smoke

Carbon monoxide is found in car exhaust fumes, tar is used to pave roads, and cyanide is found in rat poison. These chemicals are also found in tobacco smoke, and they enter your body when you smoke!

Smokeless Tobacco Products

Tobacco products are not always smoked or burned. *Smokeless tobacco* includes chewing tobacco and snuff. *Chewing tobacco* is coarsely chopped tobacco leaves that contain flavorings and additives much like the tobacco in cigarettes. Chewing tobacco is placed in the mouth and chewed. Nicotine enters the bloodstream through the lining of the mouth. Chewing creates brown-stained saliva that must be spit out often. *Snuff* is also put in the mouth, but it is a flavored powder. It is placed between the cheek and gum. Snuff doesn't need to be chewed for the nicotine to be absorbed into your body. If saliva from either chewing tobacco or snuff is swallowed, the user can become very sick. First-time users of these products often become nauseated and dizzy. Long-term effects include bad breath, yellowed teeth, and an increased risk of oral cancer.

Other Tobacco Products

Pipe tobacco, cigars, and clove cigarettes are other common tobacco products that are smoked. The way that tobacco in pipes and cigars is processed allows the nicotine to be absorbed more easily than the nicotine from cigarettes is. Cigars can contain seven times more tar and four times more nicotine than cigarettes do.

Bidis (BEE deez) are unfiltered cigarettes that are wrapped in tobacco leaves. Bidis are flavored to make them attractive to teens. But with their high levels of nicotine, tar, and carbon monoxide, bidis may be more dangerous to your health than cigarettes are.

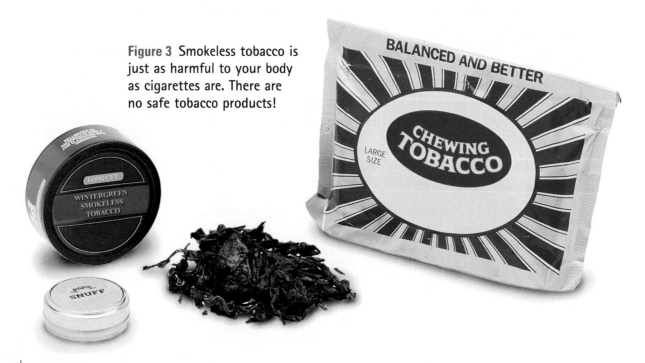

Figure 3 Smokeless tobacco is just as harmful to your body as cigarettes are. There are no safe tobacco products!

Environmental Tobacco Smoke

Smokers are not the only ones who are exposed to the dangerous chemicals found in tobacco products. Smoke that comes from the tip of a lit cigarette and the smoke that is exhaled from a smokers' mouth are called **environmental tobacco smoke,** or **ETS.** ETS is also called secondhand smoke. People who are around smokers breathe second-hand smoke and are sometimes called *passive smokers*. The same chemicals that are found in the smoke inhaled by smokers are also found in ETS—sometimes in higher concentrations. Therefore, it is harmful to be near a person who is smoking even if you are not smoking.

Until recently, smoking was allowed in most public places, which exposed nonsmokers to ETS. More laws are now in place to protect nonsmokers. These laws may differ from state to state. Some states have stricter laws than other states do. For example, some states have laws that require a nonsmoking section in restaurants. But this area of the restaurant is not protected from ETS unless it is in a completely separate room. Other cities forbid smoking anywhere in restaurants.

Nonsmokers who breathe ETS are at risk for the same health problems that smokers are. And many of these nonsmokers will die each year from smoking-related illnesses.

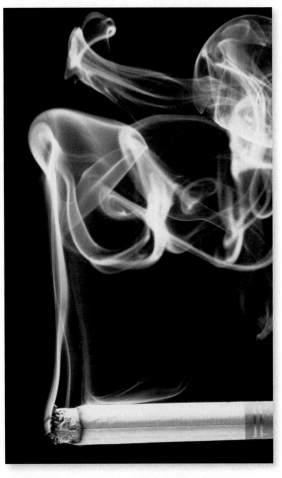

Figure 4 Smoke from a cigarette tip may contain a higher concentration of chemicals than inhaled smoke does because the filter traps a small portion of the chemicals.

Lesson Review

Using Vocabulary

1. Define *additive*.

2. What is nicotine?

3. Define *ETS*, and explain why it is dangerous.

Understanding Concepts

4. What are three chemicals produced by a burning cigarette?

5. What are five health problems that occur early in a smoking habit?

6. What are three long-term effects of smokeless tobacco?

7. What are four forms of tobacco other than cigarettes and smokeless tobacco?

Critical Thinking

8. Making Inferences What is one way that you think advertisers make smoking appealing to kids?

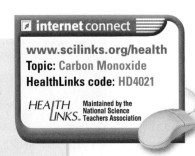

internet connect
www.scilinks.org/health
Topic: Carbon Monoxide
HealthLinks code: HD4021

HEALTH LINKS. Maintained by the National Science Teachers Association

Tobacco Products, Disease, and Death

What You'll Do

- **Describe** two respiratory diseases associated with smoking.
- **Explain** how smoking affects the cardiovascular system.
- **Describe** the relationship between smoking and cancer.
- **Identify** five other health problems associated with using tobacco products.

Terms to Learn

- chronic bronchitis
- emphysema
- cardiovascular disease

Start Off *Write*

How can smoking affect your respiratory system?

Bradley was worried about his mother because she had smoked cigarettes for a long time. And Bradley knew that smoking could cause terrible diseases and even death. Bradley was hoping that his mom would quit smoking soon.

It's never too late to quit smoking. Many of the effects of smoking can be reversed after a person quits. In this lesson, you will learn about the diseases that are caused by smoking. You will also learn why it is so important to never start smoking.

Respiratory Problems

Shortness of breath and coughing are common signs of chronic respiratory disease which affects most smokers. A *chronic disease* is a disease that, once developed, is always present and will not go away. Two chronic respiratory diseases are chronic bronchitis and emphysema. **Chronic bronchitis** is a disease that causes the airways of the lungs to become irritated and swollen. This irritation causes the person to produce a lot of mucus in the lungs. As a result, the person coughs a lot. **Emphysema** destroys the tiny air sacs and the walls of the lung. The holes in the air sacs cannot heal. Eventually, the lung tissue dies, and the lungs can no longer work.

Cigarette smoke causes more than 80 percent of all cases of chronic bronchitis and emphysema. Death from heart failure follows. Usually, the more cigarettes people smoke each day, the more serious the respiratory disease is.

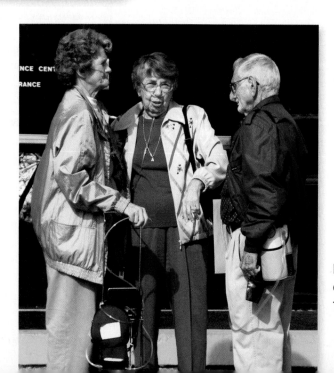

Figure 5 People who have emphysema often have to take oxygen tanks with them so they can get enough oxygen.

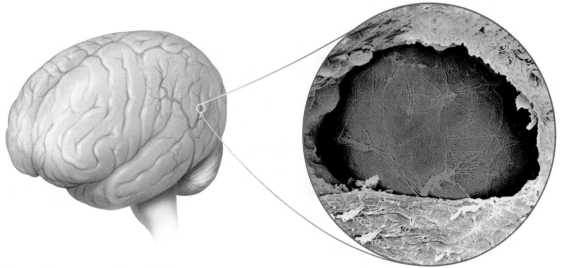

Cardiovascular Disease

Scientific research has shown a direct link between smoking and cardiovascular disease. A **cardiovascular disease** is a disorder of the circulatory system. This type of disorder includes high blood pressure, heart disease, and stroke. These diseases prevent organs and limbs from getting the amount of blood they need. Cardiovascular disease is the leading cause of death for adults in the United States.

Smoking also damages the inside lining of the arteries. This damage allows solid material to build up inside the artery. Eventually, the artery becomes blocked. When the arteries that supply oxygen to the heart become blocked, a heart attack results. A stroke results when the arteries that supply blood to the brain become blocked. Blocked arteries that supply blood to limbs of the body can cause severe pain. Sometimes, the need for an amputation, which is the surgical removal of an arm or leg, can result from blocked arteries that can no longer supply blood to the arms or legs. The younger people are when they start smoking and the more they smoke, the higher their risk for stroke and heart attack.

Figure 6 Blood clots in the brain can block the flow of blood through a blood vessel. This blockage can cause a stroke.

Hands-on ACTIVITY

HOW MUCH TAR?

1. The teacher will pass out the outer paper wrappings of cigarettes that have been laminated. These papers are from regular and low-tar brands of cigarettes.

2. Compare the paper wrapper from a regular brand of cigarettes to the low-tar wrapper by holding the papers up to the light. Count the number of holes in each paper wrapper.

Analysis

1. Which paper had more holes? Why do you think the holes are present in the wrapping papers? Do you think the holes in the cigarette papers do what they are intended to do? Explain your answer.

2. Do these increased number of holes make low-tar cigarettes safer than regular cigarettes? Explain your answer.

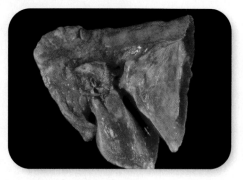
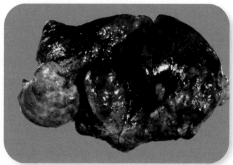

Figure 7 A normal, healthy lung is shown in the left photo. The right photo shows a lung that has been damaged from cigarette smoke.

Lung Cancer

Smoking causes cancer. *Cancer* is a disease in which damaged cells grow out of control. All tobacco products contain chemicals that cause cancer. Smoking can cause cancer of the bladder, kidneys, throat, mouth, and lung. But lung cancer is the leading cause of cancer deaths among both men and women who smoke. Finding lung cancer early is difficult because it spreads very quickly. Also, symptoms usually don't appear until the disease is advanced. If a smoker quits, then the risk of cancer decreases. But it usually does not decrease to the level of someone who has never smoked.

Surprisingly, the risk of lung cancer is just as high for people who smoke light and low-tar cigarettes as it is for those who smoke regular brands. Because smoke from light cigarettes is made to feel smoother, smoke is usually inhaled more deeply into the lungs. This increases the damage done to the lungs.

Figure 8 Smokeless tobacco can cause the formation of lesions, which can become cancerous.

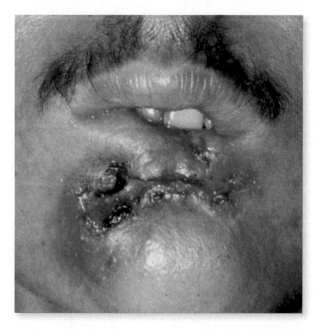

Mouth Cancer

Smokeless tobacco causes cancers of the mouth, head, and neck. In fact, a person that uses smokeless tobacco has a higher risk of getting mouth cancer than a cigarette smoker does. Sores form in the mouth of one-half to three-quarters of smokeless tobacco users. These sores may develop into cancer. When the user quits, these sores can disappear. The risk of oral, or mouth cancer depends on how long and how much smokeless tobacco was used. Quitting smokeless tobacco lowers the risk of getting oral cancer. And if a person does get oral cancer, he or she has a better chance of surviving if he or she has quit using smokeless tobacco.

Other Health Problems

Not surprisingly, the ingredients and additives in tobacco can lead to many different illnesses. The following list contains more reasons to avoid tobacco products.

- Cigarette smokers catch the flu and colds more often. And they do not recover from them as quickly as nonsmokers do.

- Smokers take longer to heal from wounds and surgeries than nonsmokers do.

- All tobacco products increase the risk for gum and dental diseases.

- Cigarette smoking has been associated with many eye diseases.

- Smoking can cause premature signs of aging. Smoke has negative effects on certain tissues in the skin, which causes premature wrinkling.

- Smoking is harmful to a fetus. When a pregnant woman smokes, she is more likely to have a miscarriage.

- Babies born of mothers who smoked during pregnancy are often smaller and may suffer from health complications as well. These babies are also at a higher risk for sudden infant death syndrome, or SIDS.

The list could go on and on. There are NO good effects of smoking.

Figure 9 Smoke does more than just harm the person who is smoking; it has negative effects on other people, too.

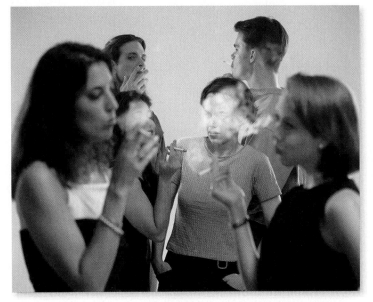

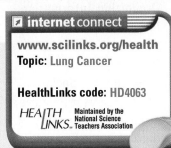

Lesson Review

Using Vocabulary

1. Define *chronic bronchitis*.

2. Define *emphysema*.

Understanding Concepts

3. Describe four health problems other than respiratory problems, cardiovascular problems, and cancer that are caused by tobacco use.

4. Explain how smoking affects the cardiovascular system.

5. What is the relationship between smoking and cancer?

Critical Thinking

6. **Making Inferences** Explain why a person who has a respiratory disease, such as asthma, should not be around people who are smoking.

7. **Analyzing Ideas** Explain whether you agree or disagree with the following statement: If a smoker already has chronic bronchitis, it's too late to quit smoking.

internet connect

www.scilinks.org/health
Topic: Lung Cancer

HealthLinks code: HD4063

HEALTH LINKS. Maintained by the National Science Teachers Association

Social and Emotional Effects of Tobacco

What You'll Do

- **Describe** laws and school policies regarding teen tobacco use.

- **Explain** how using tobacco can lead to social strain.

Terms to Learn

- social strain

Start Off
Write

How can underage smoking lead to strain within the family?

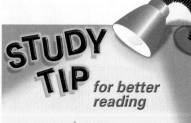

STUDY TIP *for better reading*

Organizing Information

Make a chart that has two columns. Title one column "Breaking rules" and the other column "Social strain." List as many rules about smoking as you can think of in the first column. In the second column, list social problems caused by smoking.

Greg felt guilty about avoiding his father lately. But he didn't want his father to smell the cigarette smoke on his clothes or breath. Now, whenever Greg comes home, he goes directly to his room.

There are other consequences for smoking than health problems. For example, lying to family or friends, feeling weak about giving in to peer pressure, and sneaking around to avoid getting caught are just a few of the problems that teen smokers face.

Breaking Rules

As the public learned about the dangers of tobacco products, more laws were developed to decrease the use of tobacco. Governments want to reduce the number of people who get sick and die because of tobacco use. So, many states are writing new policies about tobacco use. For example, it is against the law to sell tobacco products to anyone under the age of 18. Schools forbid smoking on school grounds and at school events. And most parents have their own rules regarding tobacco products. So, deciding to smoke means breaking rules on many different levels. Smoking also means hiding tobacco use from others, which is not always an easy thing to do. Cigarette smoke makes your skin, hair, and clothing smell bad. And tobacco products give you bad breath and yellow teeth.

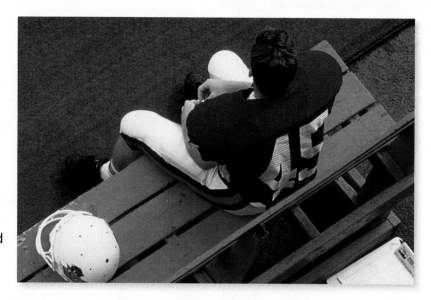

Figure 10 If you are caught smoking, you may not be allowed to participate in certain school activities and sporting events.

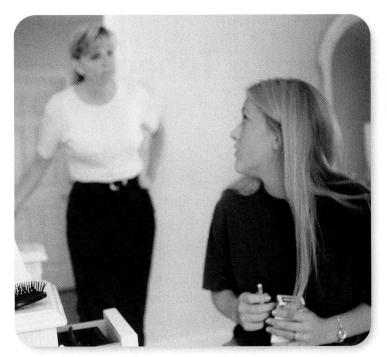

Figure 11 It is difficult to hide your smoking habit from other people.

Social Strain

Imagine being with someone who is underage when that person is trying to break the law and buy cigarettes. Even though you have done nothing wrong, you may be considered guilty because you are with that person. Or how about being around a group of people who insist on smoking even when it bothers other people? These people may not intend to hurt others but may simply find it too difficult to quit. These situations describe social strain. **Social strain** is when the use of tobacco causes awkward or risky situations and creates tension among family and friends. It is difficult for both parents and children to watch a loved one increase his or her chances of dying from a deadly disease. It is especially hard when that disease could have been prevented in the first place. Social strain also arises when pressure is placed on people to use tobacco even if they do not want to.

Lesson Review

Using Vocabulary

1. What is social strain?

Understanding Concepts

2. What is the law regarding teen tobacco use?

3. Why does using tobacco lead to social strain?

Critical Thinking

4. Making Inferences Describe a specific example of how smoking may cause social strain.

5. Making Predictions How could the current law prohibiting smoking for people under 18 years of age be better enforced?

Forming a Tobacco Addiction

Among middle school students, about 15 percent currently smoke. Of these smokers, 55 percent said they want to stop smoking.

Nicotine: The Addictive Drug

Nicotine is a poisonous substance. After a person puffs on a cigarette, nicotine goes from the lungs into the bloodstream. It only takes seconds for the nicotine to reach the brain. Once in the brain, nicotine attaches to special structures on nerve cells. These structures are called *receptors*. When nicotine attaches to these receptors, chemical messages are sent throughout the body. These messages cause your heart to beat faster and your blood pressure to rise. The brain has to adapt to the nicotine by increasing the number of nicotine receptors in the brain. Therefore, tobacco users need more nicotine to fill these receptors.

The body gradually becomes used to the nicotine and cannot feel normal without it. This is because using nicotine causes an addiction. **Addiction** is a condition in which a person can no longer control his or her need or desire for a drug. The more a substance is used, the more it is needed. And people who try cigarettes are more likely to become addicted than people who try alcohol, cocaine, or heroin are.

Figure 12 The more nicotine that enters the body, the more nicotine that the body needs to satisfy the addiction.

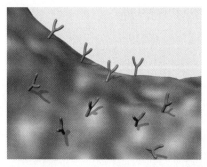

Exposure to nicotine over a long time

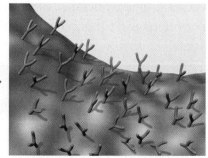

Nicotine receptors in the brain

When a person uses tobacco products for a long time, the brain develops more binding sites, or receptors, for nicotine.

Increased number of nicotine receptors in the brain

When blood carries nicotine through the brain, these receptors catch the nicotine. With more receptors, the brain needs more nicotine to fill them.

Figure 13 Facts About Smoking

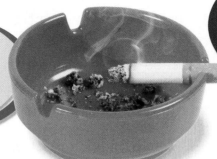

Fact
Studies have shown that once people are hooked on smoking their tolerance to nicotine never declines, even after years of not smoking.

Fact
More than 90 percent of young people who use tobacco daily experience at least one symptom of nicotine withdrawal, such as difficulty concentrating and irritability.

Fact
Three-fourths of young people who use tobacco daily report that they continue to use tobacco because they find it hard to stop using tobacco.

Tolerance, Dependence, and Withdrawal

Most long-time smokers smoke more cigarettes than beginning smokers do. This is because they have developed a tolerance to nicotine. **Tolerance** is a condition in which a user needs more of a drug to get the same effect. So, long-time smokers experience smaller and smaller effects, even with more cigarettes. As tolerance develops, smokers begin to feel more normal when using nicotine than when not using it. This is called physical dependence. *Physical dependence* on a drug is when the user relies on the drug to feel normal. A person can also be psychologically dependent on a drug. People who rely on tobacco products as an emotional crutch are psychologically dependent. If tobacco users have to go for a very long time without nicotine, they begin to feel sick, nervous, and irritable. These symptoms are examples of withdrawal. **Withdrawal** is the way in which the body responds when a dependent person stops using a drug. Withdrawal is the sign that a person has become physically dependent on tobacco products. Withdrawal usually includes uncomfortable physical and psychological symptoms. A major reason that it is hard for long-time smokers to quit smoking is the discomfort of withdrawal.

Myth & Fact

Myth: I'm too young to get addicted. That only happens to adults.

Fact: Young people can get addicted to tobacco products just as easily as adults can.

Lesson Review

Using Vocabulary

1. What is addiction?

2. Define *tolerance*.

Understanding Concepts

3. What is the difference between physical and psychological dependence?

4. Explain how tolerance to nicotine leads to dependence.

Critical Thinking

5. Making Inferences What would be the best way to overcome psychological dependence on nicotine? Explain your answer.

internet connect
www.scilinks.org/health
Topic: Nicotine
HealthLinks code: HD4069
HEALTH LINKS. Maintained by the National Science Teachers Association

What You'll Do

- **Explain** how peer pressure can cause adolescents to try tobacco.
- **Explain** how advertisements can influence someone's attitude toward tobacco.

Terms to Learn

- peer pressure
- targeted marketing

Start Off
Write

Why do most young people start using tobacco?

Why People Use Tobacco

Bonnie was very hurt that Sue had laughed at her in front of a group of people just because she didn't want to try a cigarette. Bonnie couldn't believe that there could be so much pressure to use tobacco!

Pressure from friends is one of the main reasons teens begin to smoke. Having to say no to your friends is very difficult to do. In this lesson, you will learn about different influences on teens and why some teens eventually give in to smoking.

Influence from Others

Why would someone begin a habit that could cause serious health problems or death and is a very difficult habit to break? Experimenting with tobacco and risking addiction makes little sense—so why do people do it? There are many forces at work that influence people's decision to start using tobacco.

One of the most powerful forces comes from your peers. *Peers* are people of about the same age as you with whom you interact every day. **Peer pressure** is the feeling that you should do something because your friends want you to. Influence from peers is one of the main reasons that teens first try cigarettes. Most teens smoke because they want to be accepted by their peers. And they want to experiment with an "adult activity."

Sadly, most teens do not think they will become addicted. Nor do teenagers believe that they will have any serious tobacco-related health problems. Studies show that most teen smokers wish they could quit. And quitting is just as difficult for adolescent smokers as it is for adult smokers. Because adolescents are still growing and developing, they can seriously hurt their bodies by smoking.

TABLE 1 Reasons Why Kids Smoke	
Why kids smoke	**Why that reason is bad**
My friends smoke.	Just because your friends smoke doesn't make it a good idea!
It's cool to smoke.	Smoking doesn't make you cool—it makes you smell bad.
Smoking is fun.	Respiratory disease is not fun.

The Power of Advertising

Tobacco companies spend nearly $1 million *an hour* to advertise their products. Ads often use targeted marketing. **Targeted marketing** is advertising aimed at a particular group of people. Teenagers, sports fans, and outdoor enthusiasts are especially good targets. The ads make the companies' products and brands appealing to people in these groups. For example, most cigarette ads show very attractive people doing something very exciting while smoking their brand of cigarettes. Laws have been passed to ban tobacco advertising on TV, on billboards, and in certain magazines. But most people everywhere still recognize the name and packaging of popular cigarette brands.

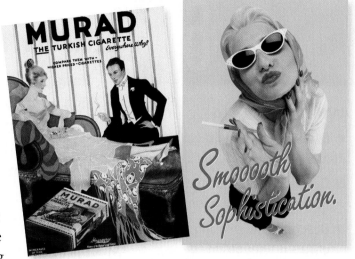

Figure 14 Tobacco companies create ads to make cigarette smoking look glamorous and accepted, but these ads are misleading.

Feeling Tempted

Peer pressure, family members who smoke, advertising, TV, and movies all influence your attitude about smoking. The movies and TV often make smoking look very glamorous. And, even though you know the dangers of tobacco use, it is difficult not to be curious about a product that is made to look so attractive. But people need to learn to see through these messages because once people begin to use tobacco, they will probably become addicted to nicotine.

Once people are addicted, the glamour of smoking quickly fades. Most smokers develop a nasty cough. And their clothes, hair, and breath smell of smoke. So, the next time you see ads that make smoking look cool, remember that this is what the advertisers want to emphasize, not the negative effects of smoking.

Health Journal

In your Health Journal, write about a time in which you saw an advertisement that made you want to buy something. Describe that ad, and explain why the advertisement appealed to you.

Lesson Review

Using Vocabulary

1. Define *peer pressure*.

2. Define *targeted marketing*.

Understanding Concepts

3. Describe three different influences that cause teens to try smoking.

4. Describe how advertisements influence your attitude about smoking.

Critical Thinking

5. **Applying Concepts** Using the power of peer pressure, write a convincing argument to another student about why he or she should quit smoking.

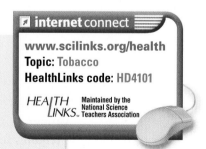

internet connect

www.scilinks.org/health
Topic: Tobacco
HealthLinks code: HD4101

HEALTH LINKS. Maintained by the National Science Teachers Association

Quitting

Pawan hated smoking. He hated that he could not control his habit. Pawan had tried quitting before by gradually decreasing the number of cigarettes he smoked, but it hadn't worked.

What You'll Do

- **Explain** why it is difficult to quit using tobacco.
- **Describe** three strategies for quitting a tobacco habit.
- **Describe** how smoking causes disruptions in everyday life.

Terms to Learn

- nicotine replacement therapy (NRT)

Start Off
Write

What can a person do if he or she wants to quit smoking?

It's Tough to Quit

Most people who use tobacco products wish they didn't. Every year, about 70 percent of adult smokers say they want to quit. Of the 50 percent of all adult smokers who try to quit, only about 7 percent of them are successful. By age 18, about two-thirds of teens who smoke say they regret having started smoking. And about half of these teens will try to quit but fail. Still, that means that many teens do successfully quit.

The younger a person is when they quit, the more that person's body can recover. Often, quitting takes several attempts. So, why is quitting so difficult? Once tobacco users quit using tobacco, withdrawal begins. They get headaches, become dizzy, have trouble sleeping, and get depressed. Withdrawal symptoms make it difficult to stay tobacco free. Even when withdrawal ends, many people still miss using tobacco. Some people crave tobacco products years after they've quit. But quitting has major health benefits even if the person is already sick with a smoking-related disease.

Figure 15 Quitting often requires several attempts, but it can be done.

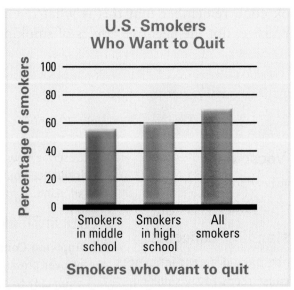

Source: Centers for Disease Control and Prevention.

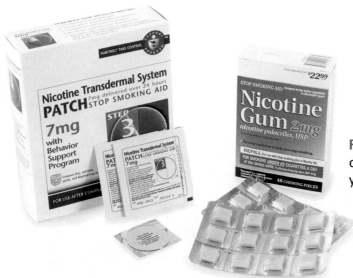

Figure 16 Many products on the market can help you quit smoking.

Tools That Can Help

For years, there was little help for people who wanted to quit using tobacco. Today, there are many tools to help smokers quit. Listed below are some of the tools that can help people who want to stop smoking.

- Support groups and counseling programs can provide encouragement for people who want to quit using tobacco.

- Nonprescription **nicotine replacement therapy,** or NRT, is a safe medicine that delivers a small amount of nicotine to the body. Many withdrawal symptoms are caused by a lack of nicotine in the body, so NRT was developed to help ease the symptoms. Nonprescription NRT is available as nicotine gum and nicotine patches.

- Prescription NRT can also help a person quit smoking. The latest prescription nicotine replacement therapies are nicotine inhalers and nicotine nasal sprays.

- A regular exercise program has helped many people quit smoking because it helps the person focus on his or her health. It also takes the person's mind off of the unpleasant side effects of quitting smoking.

Most of the prescription and nonprescription medicines available as aids to quit using tobacco have been tested only on adults. So, teens under 18 should talk to their doctor. It is important for smokers to know that a technique that works for one person may not always work for another person.

Sometimes, a combination of more than one method will work. For example, some people may use the nicotine patch while going to a support group. The nicotine patch can help with the physical addiction. The support group may help the person adjust mentally to not smoking. Anyone who really wants to quit will have to find the method that works best for him or her.

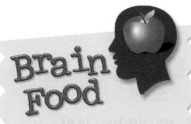

Brain Food

In one year, more than 800,000 cigarette butts were among the millions of pounds of debris collected along the U.S. coastline. These butts are responsible for the death of many birds and marine animals.

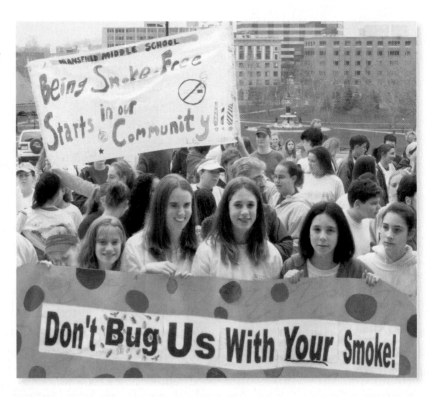

Figure 17 Teens across the country have joined organizations to show support for smoke-free youth.

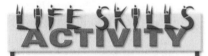

USING REFUSAL SKILLS

Work in a group of three or four people to write a skit about refusing tobacco. Think of multiple endings to the skit that show different ways to refuse tobacco.

Relaxing Without Tobacco

Hanging out with friends and enjoying life is much easier without tobacco. It's hard to relax and have fun when you know that you're breaking the law, becoming addicted to nicotine, and damaging your health as well as the health of others around you. Many everyday activities, such as playing sports, going to the movies, or shopping at the mall become a hassle when you're a tobacco user. Smokers often worry about what they will do in situations in which they can't smoke. It is difficult to travel on trains, buses, or planes now that smoking has been banned on them. Tobacco users face disruptions in their everyday lives because they have to find a place and time to smoke so that they won't have withdrawal symptoms.

Being addicted to nicotine means that if you don't get your nicotine fix you don't feel right. And that can be quite a problem. There are many times when you can't light up a cigarette or take a dip of snuff. Getting used to a tobacco-free life means making some changes in your lifestyle. You have to learn how to relax without tobacco. Some people need to stay away from places where other people will be using tobacco. It's hard to stay tobacco free when others around you are using tobacco. But over time, people find that they enjoy life more without tobacco. There is no more worrying about hiding your habit from parents or figuring out when and where you can smoke.

Finding Healthy Habits

Many teens are first offered tobacco during middle and high school. Many of these teens will try it, get hooked, and ultimately die because of it. Understanding the dangers of tobacco and being prepared to refuse tobacco are the best ways to ensure a healthy life. The lifestyle choices that you make now will affect your future health and happiness. Make the right decisions about diet, exercise, and caring for your body—it's never too early to start practicing healthy habits. There are many fun, healthy things that you can do rather than use tobacco. A newfound feeling of physical health will come after the nicotine leaves your body. And you will also feel a well-deserved sense of accomplishment.

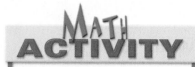

Calculate how much it costs to smoke for one year if a pack of cigarettes cost $4.00, and a person smokes 1 pack a day.

How much would smoking cost over a lifetime if this same person started smoking at 16 years of age and lived to be 70? Assume that the price of cigarettes stays the same and this person keeps smoking 1 pack a day.

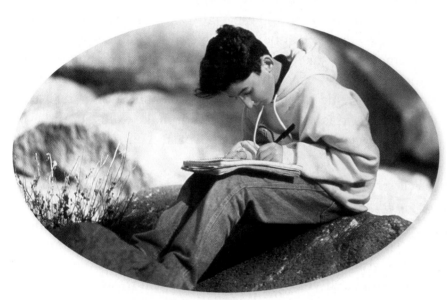

Figure 18 Plan ahead. Think of ways to say no when peers offer you tobacco, and write these ideas in your journal.

Lesson Review

Using Vocabulary

1. Define *NRT*. Explain how NRTs work.

Understanding Concepts

2. Describe withdrawal symptoms that make it difficult to stop smoking.

3. Identify three methods that can help a person quit smoking.

4. Identify three ways that smoking disrupts everyday life.

Critical Thinking

5. Making Inferences Do you think it is likely that a person could become addicted to nicotine gum or patches? Explain your answer.

6. Making Predictions Doug is a smoker and is flying across country. What problems may he face on the plane?

Lesson 7

Choosing Not to Use Tobacco

What You'll Do

- **Demonstrate** three ways to refuse tobacco.
- **Explain** the difference between positive and negative peer pressure.
- **Identify** four reasons to stay tobacco free.

Start Off
Write

How can positive peer pressure help you refuse tobacco?

Lee knew that he didn't want to try chewing tobacco. When his friend Chris asked him if he wanted to try it, all Lee said was, "No, thanks," and Chris left him alone.

Refusing Tobacco

Most people will probably be offered tobacco at some time in their lives. Sometimes, it may be easy to refuse. However, other times it can be stressful, especially if peer pressure is used. Learning to say no can be a valuable tool. Your response could be a simple "No" or "No, thanks." Or you could reply, "Smoking is too dangerous—especially if my parents find out!" Whichever way you decide to handle the situation, don't feel that you have to explain why you refused or make excuses. And even if you've accepted tobacco in the past, you can still say no this time.

Peer pressure is not always a bad thing. If your friends do well in school, enjoy a particular sport, or choose not to use tobacco, you probably behave in a similar way. This is positive peer pressure. Positive peer pressure influences you to do something that benefits you. It is easier to stay tobacco free if none of your friends smoke. If your friends try to get you to smoke, they are using negative peer pressure. Negative peer pressure can harm you if you let it. You will want to avoid this kind of pressure.

Figure 19 You can refuse tobacco products in many ways.

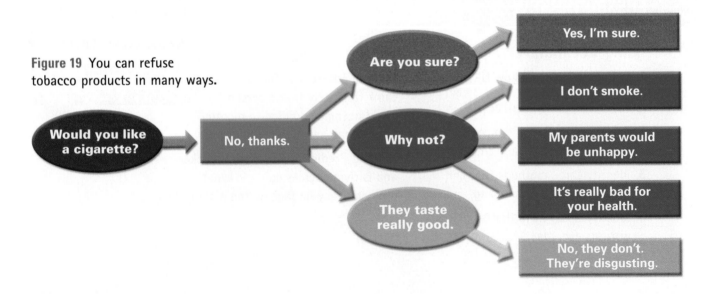

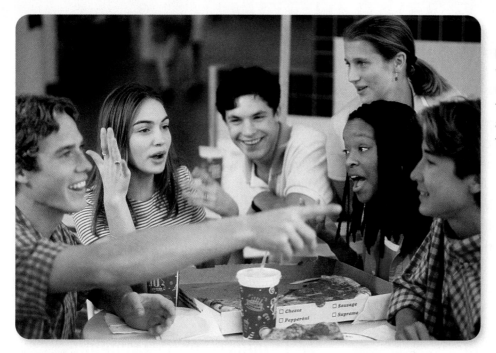

A Tobacco-Free Life

If you have never used tobacco, don't start! The following is a list of reasons not to smoke.

- It is very easy to become addicted to nicotine. In fact, it is easier to become addicted to tobacco than to most other drugs.

- Using tobacco is deadly. Smoking is the leading preventable cause of death in the United States.

- Tobacco makes your skin, hair, breath, and clothing smell bad. It also makes your teeth yellow.

- Tobacco in any form is expensive, and it is getting more expensive every day.

Make a healthy choice to stay tobacco free. You won't regret it!

Health Journal

Write in your Health Journal five reasons why you will not start using tobacco products.

Lesson Review

Understanding Concepts

1. What are three ways to tell a friend that you don't want to try tobacco?

2. What is the difference between positive and negative peer pressure?

3. What are four reasons to never start using tobacco?

Critical Thinking

4. **Making Inferences** If tobacco has so many negative effects, explain why most people don't quit using it.

5. **Analyzing Ideas** Why do you think there are more people addicted to cigarettes and other forms of tobacco than are addicted to illegal drugs?

Chapter Summary

■ Tobacco products contain hundreds of chemicals. Additives make cigarettes more appealing to the user. ■ All tobacco products produce harmful health effects as soon as people start to use them. ■ ETS is harmful to people who are near someone who is smoking. ■ Respiratory diseases, cardiovascular diseases, and cancer are some of the major classes of illnesses caused by tobacco use. ■ Most smokers want to quit, but few can stop on the first try. ■ Using tobacco can create strain and tension between friends and family. Smoking is also against the law if you are under the age of 18. ■ Peers often influence a person's decision to use tobacco.

Using Vocabulary

For each sentence, fill in the blank with the proper word from the word bank provided below.

additives	tolerance
marketing	cancer
NRT	nicotine
peer pressure	environmental
dependent	tobacco smoke
targeted	

1 Many ___ are put in cigarettes during processing to make them taste better.

2 ___ helps people quit smoking by providing nicotine.

3 ___ describes the smoke that is exhaled from the mouth of the smoker and comes from the tip of a burning cigarette.

4 Many of the chemicals in tobacco products are responsible for causing ___.

5 People can become physically and psychologically ___ on tobacco.

6 ___ is the substance in tobacco products to which people become addicted.

7 ___ is a feeling that you should do something because your friends want you to do it.

Understanding Concepts

8 How does nicotine enter the body when someone smokes a cigarette, and where does the nicotine go?

9 Why is it harmful to be near someone who is smoking even if you are not?

10 List three activities that are made more difficult by being a tobacco user.

11 Explain how smoking can damage the cardiovascular system.

12 Explain how nicotine replacement therapy helps people quit smoking.

13 What has the government done to try to control death and disease caused by tobacco?

14 List at least three reasons someone would choose to start using tobacco.

15 Explain why light cigarettes are just a dangerous as regular cigarettes.

16 Name five types of tobacco products.

17 List two common respiratory diseases.

18 What is the most common type of cancer caused by smokeless tobacco?

Critical Thinking

Analyzing Ideas

19 When Mary began smoking cigarettes, she promised she would limit herself to one a day, because she thought that would be less dangerous. She is now smoking a pack each day. Why wasn't she able to keep her original promise?

20 Yi-tee is a tobacco user and has just noticed some white sores on his gums and on the inside of his mouth. What product does Yi-tee likely use, and what has happened to his gums and mouth?

21 Antonio and his best friend, Dean, had been smoking for almost a year when they both decided to quit. Antonio quit without too much trouble. But Dean relapsed twice and is now smoking again. What may have caused Antonio and Dean to have different experiences with quitting?

22 Imagine that you find your younger sister smoking bidis with her friends. What can you tell her about bidis to help her decide not to use them?

Using Refusal Skills

23 Shari's family had just moved, and she was eager to make friends in her new school. One group of girls invited her to meet them after school so that they could get together, smoke some cigarettes, and chat. What should Shari do?

24 Some friends are thinking about going to a convenience store that they know sells cigarettes to teens without checking IDs. What should you say to your friends?

25 You and your best friend, Joe, play baseball for the same team. One night at a baseball game Joe tells you he has started using chewing tobacco, and he asks you if you want to try it. Joe also tells you that chewing tobacco won't cause lung cancer or any of the other diseases that smoking can cause. What should you tell your friend?

26 Use what you have learned in this chapter to set a personal goal. Write your goal, and make an action plan by using the Health Behavior Contract for ways to refuse tobacco. You can find the Health Behavior Contract at go.hrw.com. Just type in the keyword HD4HBC09.

Name _____ Class _____ Date _____

(Health Behavior Contract)
Teens and Tobacco

My Goals: I, _____, will accomplish one or more of the following goals:
I will not use tobacco products.
I will help a friend who is being pressured to try tobacco products.
I will encourage friends or family members who smoke to quit smoking.
Other: _____

My Reasons: By refusing to use tobacco products, I will decrease my risk of tobacco-related illnesses. I will also be a positive influence to other people who may be tempted to use tobacco or who are trying to break the habit.
Other: _____

My Values: Personal values that will help me meet my goals are _____

My Plan: The actions I will take to meet my goals are _____

Evaluation: I will use my Health Journal to keep a log of actions I took to fulfill this contract. After 1 month, I will evaluate my goals. I will adjust my plan if my goals are not being met. If my goals are being met, I will consider setting additional goals.

Signed _____

Date _____

Reading Checkup

Take a minute to review your answers to the Health IQ questions at the beginning of this chapter. How has reading this chapter improved your Health IQ?

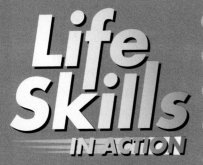

Making Good Decisions

You make decisions every day. But how do you know if you are making good decisions? Making good decisions is making choices that are healthy and responsible. Following the six steps of making good decisions will help you make the best possible choice whenever you make a decision. Complete the following activity to practice the six steps of making good decisions.

Tobacco Troubles

ACT 1

Setting the Scene

Owen and his friend Curtis are playing baseball in the park. During a break in the game, Curtis takes out a can of chewing tobacco and puts some in his mouth. Curtis offers some to Owen and says, "Try it, you will be like a real baseball player. Chewing tobacco isn't dangerous like smoking cigarettes." Owen is not sure what to do.

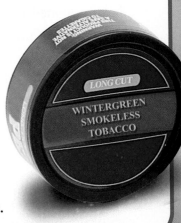

The 6 Steps of Making Good Decisions

1. Identify the problem.
2. Consider your values.
3. List the options.
4. Weigh the consequences.
5. Decide, and act.
6. Evaluate your choice.

Guided Practice

Practice with a Friend

Form a group of three. Have one person play the role of Owen and another person play the role of Curtis. Have the third person be an observer. Walking through each of the six steps of making good decisions, role-play Owen deciding whether or not to try the chewing tobacco. When Owen reaches step 5, he should tell Curtis his decision and explain his reasoning behind it. The observer will take notes, which will include observations about what the person playing Owen did well and suggestions of ways to improve. Stop after each step to evaluate the process.

Independent Practice

Check Yourself

After you have completed the guided practice, go through Act 1 again without stopping at each step. Answer the questions below to review what you did.

1. What values should Owen consider before making his decision?

2. What options does Owen have in this situation?

3. What are the positive consequences and negative consequences of each of Owen's options?

4. How can Owen evaluate his choice?

ACT 2 On Your Own

Owen and Curtis are walking home after the game. Curtis tells Owen that he wants to get some more chewing tobacco. Curtis explains that he plans to shoplift the tobacco from a convenience store and he needs Owen to distract the cashier while he does it. Make a flowchart that illustrates how Owen could use the six steps of making good decisions to decide what to do in this situation.

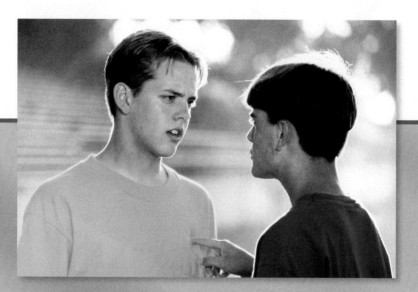

CHAPTER 12

Teens and Alcohol

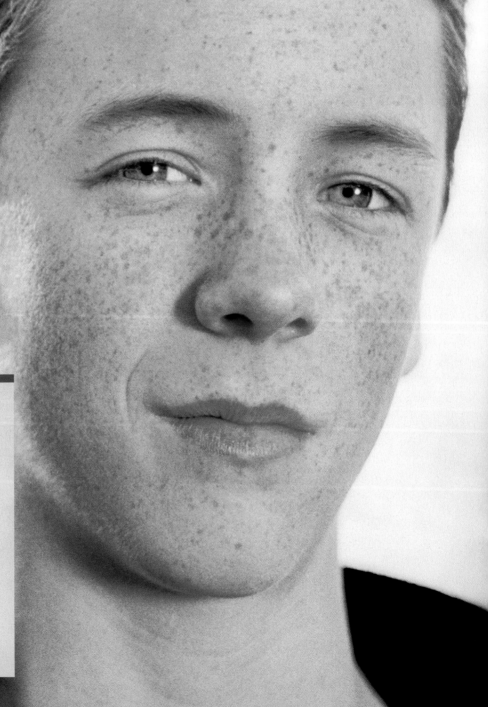

Check out
Current Health
articles related to this chapter by
visiting **go.hrw.com**. Just type in
the keyword **HD4CH27**.

Lessons

> "My uncle is **addicted** to alcohol. When he drinks, he acts **stupid** and **crazy.** Sometimes he gets **violent.**
>
> In the last year, he has had to go to the hospital a couple of times, and he lost his job. I'm not going to drink."

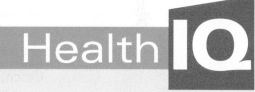
Health **IQ**

PRE-READING

Answer the following multiple-choice questions to find out what you already know about alcohol. When you've finished this chapter, you'll have the opportunity to change your answers based on what you've learned.

1. Reasons that teens drink alcohol include
  a. wanting to fit in.
  b. curiosity.
  c. wanting to look more adult.
  d. All of the above

2. Which is NOT an effect of drinking alcohol?
  a. relaxed, clear thinking
  b. reduced coordination
  c. poor concentration
  d. blurry vision

3. Your blood alcohol concentration measures
  a. the number of drinks you've had in an hour.
  b. the percentage of alcohol in your blood.
  c. the relationship between your weight and the number of drinks you have had.
  d. the amount of alcohol in the beverages you have drunk.

4. Alcoholism is an illness that
  a. can be completely cured with medicine.
  b. is treatable if the alcoholic wants treatment.
  c. only certain kinds of people get.
  d. lasts only a few weeks or months.

5. One way to avoid the pressure to drink is to
  a. have an interesting hobby.
  b. hang around with people who don't drink.
  c. recognize that alcohol can cause permanent damage to your brain.
  d. All of the above

ANSWERS: 1. d; 2. a; 3. b; 4. b; 5. d

Understanding Teens and Alcohol

Pascal loves to watch sports on TV. He thinks that some of the beer commercials are really cool. Pascal sees his dad drink beer, so Pascal decides to try it.

What things in Pascal's home encourage him to drink? What else in Pascal's life may tempt him to drink?

Why Teens Drink

There are many reasons why teens may drink. Many social settings encourage drinking. Beer ads showing images of people drinking and having a good time seem to be everywhere. Alcoholic beverages are often sold in grocery stores and convenience stores. And some adults may make alcohol easy to get or may even offer teens a drink.

Often, teens drink because they are curious about what other people are doing. They may see drinkers enjoying themselves, and want to try it. It is common for teens to see older family members, relatives, or family friends drinking alcoholic beverages after work, on the weekends, at parties, and on holidays. And it is perfectly normal for teens to be curious about drinking.

Some teens drink because of peer pressure. A *peer* is someone about your age with whom you interact every day. **Peer pressure** is a feeling that you should do something because your friends want you to. Teens do not want to feel left out. If friends are drinking and seem to be having a good time, it can be a challenge to resist the pressure to join in.

Some teens may think that drinking makes them look and feel like adults. They feel more mature with a drink in their hand. Some teens are unhappy and hope that alcohol will make them feel better. But there are no good reasons for teens to drink.

Figure 1 Beer and wine are often displayed in ways that encourage purchases.

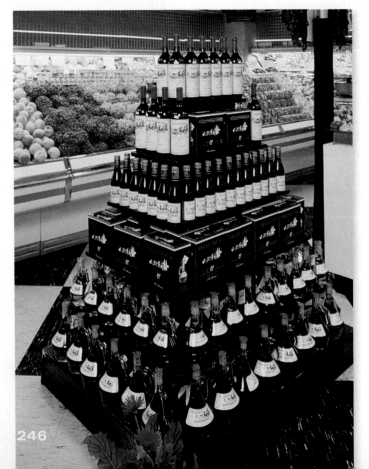

Teens and Alcohol

Why is alcohol bad for teens? One reason is because teens are still growing. Teens' bodies may continue to grow until they are in their early twenties. Teens' brains are still developing, and alcohol can have serious effects on a brain that is growing and changing.

Another reason is that teens' emotional responses are changing. Teens are making the change from being a child to being a young adult. Sometimes the emotional part of growing up is the hardest part of all. And alcohol may affect emotions in many ways. Alcohol may produce conflicting, unexpected, or even uncontrollable feelings. You can't predict what these feelings will be, or whether they will be pleasant or unpleasant.

But you do not have to drink. The truth is that most adults have less than one alcoholic drink a month or don't drink at all. People have a variety of reasons for not drinking. For some people, not drinking is a personal choice. Other people do not drink because they feel better able to meet their personal duties and responsibilities if they do not drink. Other people do not drink because of their religious beliefs, family values, or health problems. Any reason for not drinking is a good reason.

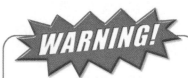

Drunk Is Disgusting

Being drunk can make you very unpopular with your friends and family. No one enjoys being around someone who is vomiting, violent, or out of control.

Figure 2 Some teens use alcohol to overcome sadness. But drinking can make sadness even worse.

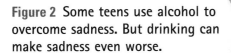

Lesson Review

Using Vocabulary

1. What is peer pressure?

Understanding Concepts

2. What are three reasons that teens may drink alcohol?

3. What are three reasons teens should not drink?

Critical Thinking

4. Using Refusal Skills What advice should you give to a friend who tells you he or she wants to start drinking?

5. Analyzing Ideas How may different social settings affect the feelings of a person who is drinking?

Alcohol and Your Body

What You'll Do

- **Describe** what happens to alcohol in the body.
- **Identify** three short-term effects of alcohol.
- **Describe** two effects of alcohol abuse.

Terms to Learn

- drug
- depressant
- blood alcohol concentration (BAC)
- intoxication
- reaction time
- alcohol abuse

Start Off
Write

How does alcohol affect the body and the brain?

Trisha was confused—her aunt had gotten silly and sick from drinking alcohol at the family picnic. However, Trisha's uncle drank the same amount and he didn't seem to be affected by it at all.

How can people have such different reactions to the same amount of alcohol?

Alcohol in Your Body

Alcohol is a drug. A **drug** is any substance that changes how the mind or body works. And alcohol does have powerful effects on how your mind and body work.

As you drink alcohol, it goes from the mouth to the stomach and then to the intestines. Most alcohol quickly enters the bloodstream through the stomach and the intestines. Blood carries alcohol to every tissue and organ. Alcohol in the blood quickly reaches the brain, where its effects begin immediately. Blood also carries alcohol to the liver, where alcohol is converted into harmless waste products.

Even though alcohol is processed in your body as if it were food, alcohol has almost no nutritional value. In fact, when your body breaks down alcohol, your body stops making and storing glucose. Glucose is the sugar that your body uses as a source of energy. So, if you drink too much alcohol, your body cannot process your other food properly.

In addition to affecting your digestion, alcohol also is a depressant. A **depressant** is a drug that slows brain and body functions. Drinking too much alcohol is a drug overdose and may slow your bodily functions so much that they stop. This overdose and collapse is called *alcohol poisoning*.

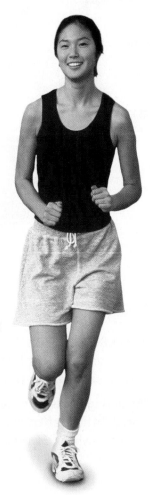

Figure 3 Alcohol affects all parts of your body. Drinking too much alcohol will make your central nervous system stop working.

Alcohol and the Brain

As a depressant, alcohol slows the activities of your body's central nervous system (CNS), which is made up of your brain and your spinal cord. Alcohol slows your thinking, your reactions, and your breathing. It slurs your speech, blurs your vision, and interferes with your muscle coordination. Alcohol also has negative effects on brain functions such as learning, motivation, and emotions. And the more alcohol in the blood, the more serious the effects on the CNS and all the things it controls. For example, alcohol slows the nerves that control your heart and your breathing. A fatal dose of alcohol will stop these functions.

How much alcohol is a fatal dose? That depends on the person and how much alcohol is in his or her blood. Generally, a blood alcohol concentration of 0.40 or above will be fatal to most people. **Blood alcohol concentration (BAC),** also called *blood alcohol level,* is the percentage of alcohol in a person's blood. For example, a BAC of 0.10 percent means that you have 10 parts of alcohol per 10,000 parts of blood in your body. A drinker's BAC is affected by a number of factors, such as his or her weight, how many drinks he or she has had, and whether he or she has eaten recently. But even one drink in an hour produces effects on the brain in many drinkers. The figure below shows how BAC, the number of drinks in one hour, and the effects of those drinks are related. For example, the BAC of a person who has three drinks in an hour will be about 0.10 to 0.12. At that level, the person's muscle coordination, reaction time, vision, and balance are all significantly impaired. A person with a BAC of 0.10 is legally drunk in all states.

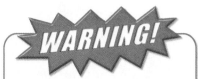

Brain Changes

Even with as few as two drinks in an hour, recognizable changes in the brain occur. A person may feel lightheaded and giddy. Their coordination may be slightly altered, and driving becomes significantly more dangerous.

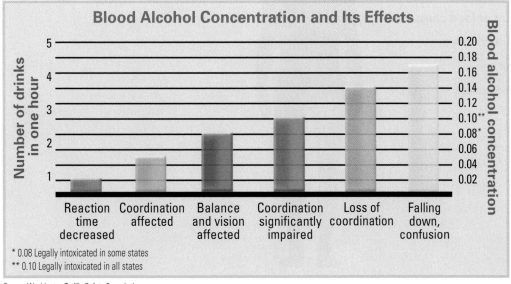

Blood Alcohol Concentration and Its Effects

* 0.08 Legally intoxicated in some states
** 0.10 Legally intoxicated in all states

Source: Washington Traffic Safety Commission.

Figure 4 This graph shows alcohol's effects on a body after a number of drinks in one hour. The approximate BAC caused by those drinks is also shown.

Short-Term Reactions to Alcohol

Each body reacts differently to alcohol. As BAC rises, intoxication occurs. **Intoxication** is the physical and mental changes produced by drinking alcohol. At lower BAC levels—after one or two drinks—some people experience increased energy, positive feelings, and less anxiety. Other people feel less shy or cautious. But other people are more quiet and calm. They may feel sad or negative. And some people, after one or two drinks, feel few effects at all.

Several factors affect the way a body reacts to alcohol. For example, a person who has several drinks in a short time is likely to be affected more than a person who has a single drink in the same time. Food in a drinker's stomach can also slow alcohol absorption into the blood. Finally, women absorb and process alcohol differently from men. Women achieve a higher BAC than do men who drink the same amount.

As BAC increases, mental and physical abilities decline. Moods are affected first, then physical abilities, then memory. Muscle coordination, especially important for walking and driving, decreases. Vision becomes blurred. Speech and memory are impaired. Reaction time slows. **Reaction time** is the amount of time that passes from the instant when your brain detects an external stimulus until the moment you respond.

At higher BAC levels, your central nervous system slows down so much that you might pass out or even die. And nothing speeds the process to sober you up—not coffee, cold showers, or exercise.

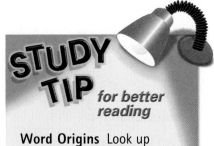
Figure 5 The smaller a person is, the more affected he or she will be by drinking a given amount of alcohol.

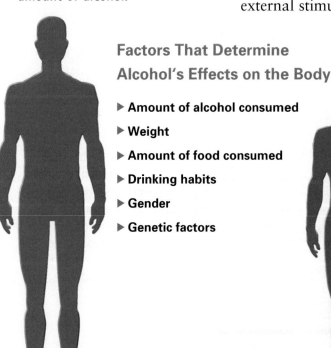

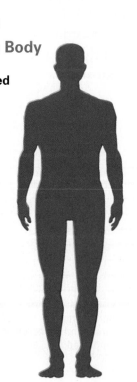

Factors That Determine Alcohol's Effects on the Body

▶ **Amount of alcohol consumed**

▶ **Weight**

▶ **Amount of food consumed**

▶ **Drinking habits**

▶ **Gender**

▶ **Genetic factors**

Alcohol Abuse

Young people who start drinking alcohol at an early age or who drink regularly are more likely to abuse alcohol later in life. **Alcohol abuse** is the failure to drink in moderation or at appropriate times. And regular alcohol use causes drinkers to develop tolerance to alcohol's effects. *Tolerance* for alcohol means that a person needs more alcohol to produce the same effects. Tolerance may be a sign of a drinking problem.

Young people who drink alcohol may damage their brain and nervous system. Young drinkers are likely to show impaired memory and to perform poorly in school. Their verbal skills may be reduced and never catch up. And long-term alcohol abuse increases the risk of illnesses such as stroke, heart disease, cancer, and liver diseases such as hepatitis and cirrhosis.

Alcohol abuse doesn't only mean drinking too much. It also means drinking at the wrong time. Even one drink at the wrong time or wrong place may be alcohol abuse. Alcohol abuse can lead to car crashes, or to death through drowning or overdose. Your risk of injury or permanent disability grows with every drink. As your mental and physical abilities are impaired, you are less able to protect yourself and others. You are more likely to become a victim of physical or sexual assault. The consequence of an assault may be pregnancy or sexually transmitted diseases, including HIV infection. Alcohol abuse also makes depression, family problems, and violence more likely.

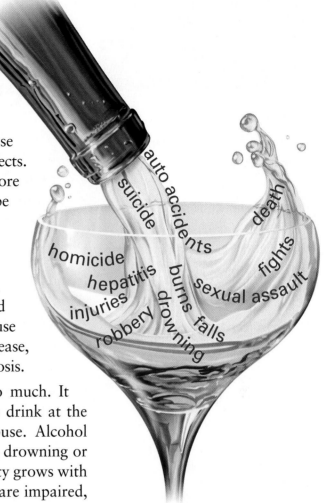

Figure 6 Alcohol abuse contributes to a wide range of social and personal problems.

Lesson Review

Using Vocabulary

1. What is a depressant?

2. What does BAC measure?

Understanding Concepts

3. What happens to alcohol in the body?

4. Describe three short-term effects of alcohol.

Critical Thinking

5. Making Good Decisions After drinking several beers at the picnic, Tricia's aunt said she wanted to go swimming. She wanted Tricia to walk down to the lake and swim with her. What should Tricia do? Why?

6. Analyzing Ideas Describe two results of alcohol abuse that might affect a young person differently from an adult.

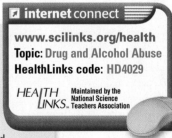

⚹ internet connect

www.scilinks.org/health

Topic: Drug and Alcohol Abuse

HealthLinks code: HD4029

HEALTH LINKS. Maintained by the National Science Teachers Association

Alcohol, You, and Other People

Sarah has noticed that when her college-age brother is with his friends, they are usually friendly and fun. But, when they have been drinking, they argue more, have more fights, and sometimes get violent.

Does everyone behave the way that Sarah's brother and his friends do when they drink? Why would they behave this way?

Alcohol and Decision Making

Alcohol makes it more difficult to think clearly about your choices. It makes remembering all your options less likely. For example, if you have had a couple of drinks, you may get into a car with a drunk driver. You may not even think about all the safer ways you could get home.

Alcohol affects your memory. You may forget what you said or did. Alcohol also affects your ability to process information. As a result, you may ignore, misunderstand, or not recognize a dangerous situation. You may not notice that the driver of the car is drunk, or you may not care. Either way, alcohol has affected your ability to make a good decision.

Alcohol harms your coordination, slows your reactions, and changes the way you see situations. As a result, low risk situations may become high risk ones. For example, activities such as swimming or cycling become more difficult and dangerous. You may take risks you usually do not take and increase your chances of having a serious, or even deadly, accident.

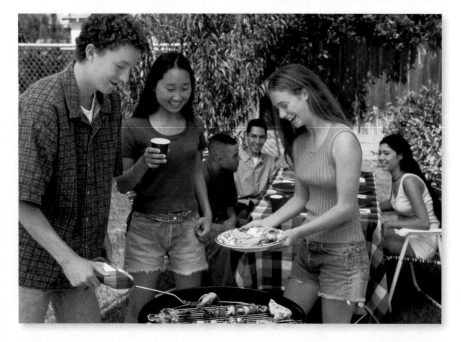

Figure 7 If alcohol harms a person's ability to make a good decision, even a small amount of alcohol may indirectly cause harm to others.

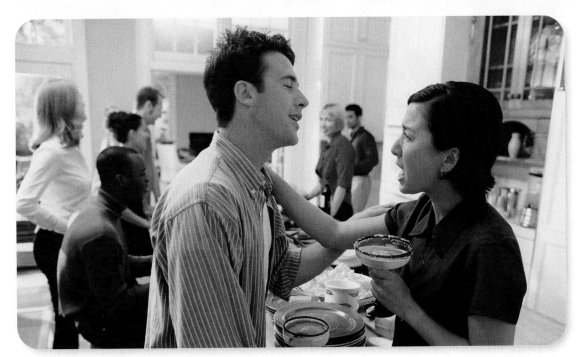

Figure 8 Alcohol affects your emotions and your relationships with other people.

Alcohol and Social Decisions

Alcohol also affects the decisions you make in social situations. What's fun for a drinker may be seen as obnoxious to those nearby. Intoxicated people are less likely to think about how their decisions will influence their lives. Intoxication can easily lead to dangerous decisions and dangerous behaviors. For example, drinking makes you less careful about your sexual behaviors. The chances increase for unplanned, unprotected, and unwanted sex. And with the increased chances of sexual activity, the chances for getting sexually transmitted diseases (STDs) or for becoming pregnant also increase. Such consequences can be life changing.

Alcohol may change your feelings. You may become very happy and silly. Or you may become very sad, very angry, or even violent. Alcohol may make you forget your values. As a result, you may say or do things that you regret later on. For example, drinking is often associated with fights, arguments, and injuries. You may start a fight with a friend, someone you would usually never fight with. Or you may start a fight with someone you do not even know.

Alcohol's social effects are even stronger in people who binge drink. **Binge drinking** for men is drinking five or more drinks in one sitting, and for women is drinking four or more drinks in one sitting. Binge drinking increases the chances that the drinkers will be involved in violence or other harmful behavior. But even one drink can lead to unpleasant and unhappy results.

Myth & Fact

Myth: It is safer to drink beer than it is to drink whiskey or wine.

Fact: Any kind of alcohol can make you drunk, sick, and at risk for serious problems. A beer may affect you just as much as a glass of wine or a drink that contains whiskey does.

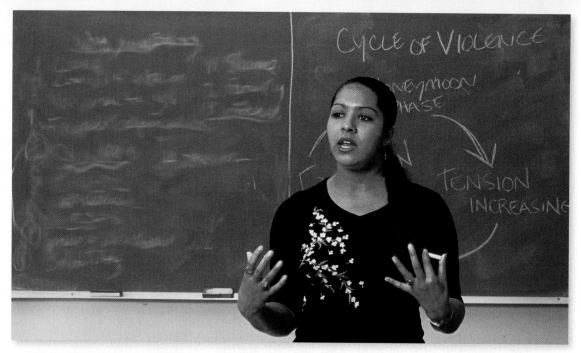

Figure 9 Alcohol can affect family life. When violence occurs in the home, the family may need counseling or other help.

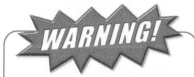

Alcohol Harms Everyone

Drinkers are not the only ones who may be harmed by alcohol use. Those around them, such as family and friends, are at increased risk for alcohol-related harm.

Alcohol and Violence

Alcohol and violence often go together because alcohol can reduce a drinker's self-control. In fact, some people think drinking causes their behaviors. And some people use alcohol as an excuse for their actions. For example, some people drink so that they can lose control and act in ways that they normally wouldn't. But silliness, rude behavior, fighting, and sexual aggression are not caused by drinking. The way that you behave when you are drunk is heavily influenced by your personal values, your expectations of what will happen, and the social setting where you are drinking. Drinking is never an excuse for violence.

Alcohol does not cause violence, but it does make violence more likely. Alcohol makes conflict more difficult to control by making emotions and behaviors seem stronger. Some people who drink become upset or angry easily. They become rude or want to argue. Insults, careless threats, arguments, and fights become more likely. Someone who is drinking may have trouble understanding what other people are trying to say. He or she may imagine an insult or feel threatened. He or she may want to start a fight without worrying about who gets hurt. And in some cases, an intoxicated person who is depressed or unhappy may even try to harm himself or herself.

Someone who is drinking is also more likely to become a victim of violence. That's because intoxication reduces your ability to defend yourself. Drinking also reduces your alertness to danger signs or risky situations. When you are intoxicated, you become an easier target for assault, battering, robbery, or rape.

Alcohol and Pregnancy

Alcohol poses special risks for a fetus. A fetus has its own blood supply. But when a pregnant woman drinks alcohol, the alcohol in the mother's blood passes into the fetus's blood. **Fetal alcohol syndrome (FAS)** is a group of birth defects that can happen when a pregnant woman drinks alcohol. The child's birth defects range from mild, such as small size at birth, to severe. The more-severe effects may include brain damage, mental retardation, and severe emotional problems as the child grows up. Individuals with FAS often have difficulties with learning, memory, attention, problem solving, and interacting with other people in social situations. There is no known safe level of drinking during pregnancy. Not drinking totally prevents FAS.

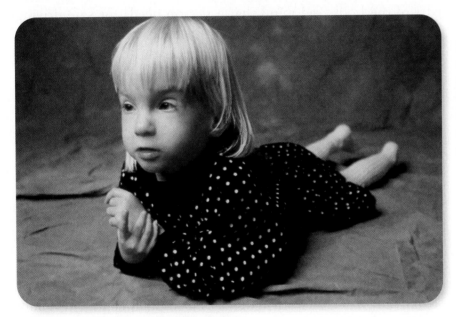

Figure 10 The little girl has fetal alcohol syndrome. Her condition causes her small size and distinct facial characteristics. But the condition's greatest effects are on behavior and mental development.

Lesson Review

Using Vocabulary

1. What is binge drinking?

Understanding Concepts

2. What are three effects of fetal alcohol syndrome?

3. Explain how alcohol can lead to bad decisions and violence.

4. How can a person's decision to drink alcohol affect other people?

5. How does drinking alcohol make a person more likely to become a victim of violence?

Critical Thinking

6. **Analyzing Ideas** Why is drinking alcohol never an excuse for rude, dangerous, or violent behavior?

Drunk Driving

In a recent year, 14 percent—about 1 out of 7—of 16- to 20-year-old drivers involved in fatal crashes were legally drunk.

What You'll Do

- **Explain** how alcohol affects a person's ability to drive.
- **Identify** two ways that you can prevent drinking and driving.

Terms to Learn

- driving under the influence (DUI)

Start Off
Write

How does drinking impair a person's ability to drive?

And 26 percent—more than 1 out of every 4—of 21- to 24-year old drivers were legally drunk. *Legally drunk* means that the driver's BAC is higher than the limit set by the state.

Drinking and Driving Is Dangerous!

Alcohol makes driving and other activities, such as skateboarding and riding a bike, so dangerous because alcohol affects every part of the body and mind that a person needs for safe driving or riding. Alcohol makes driving mistakes and crashes more likely. These often lead to injuries and death.

After a single drink, a driver may not feel or look drunk, but he or she already can't drive as safely as before having the drink. His or her vision and muscle coordination may be impaired. Even one drink slows a driver's reaction time. For example, one drink increases the time between when a driver sees the light turn red and when the driver moves to put on the brakes.

Every state has laws that make driving under the influence of alcohol illegal. **Driving under the influence (DUI)** happens when a person who is legally intoxicated or who is using illegal drugs drives a motor vehicle. In most states, a person is legally intoxicated when his or her BAC is greater than 0.08. A few states set the limit at 0.10. In all states, a person under age 21 is legally intoxicated if his or her BAC is above 0.00. People convicted of DUI, whatever their age, may lose their driver's license or permit. A DUI conviction may mean no more driving for months or years.

Figure 11 The combination of alcohol and motor vehicles can be deadly. A drunk driver is not the only one who may be hurt.

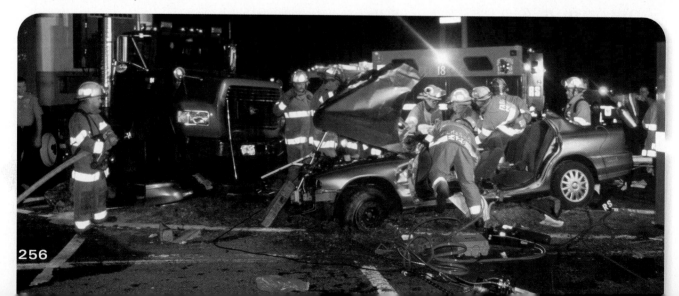

Alcohol-Related Highway Deaths

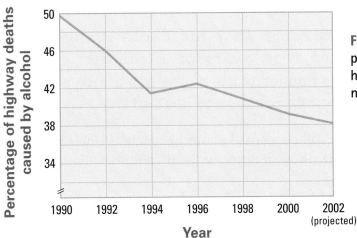

Source: Washington Traffic Safety Administration FARS data

Figure 12 Efforts by many people in the last few years have helped reduce the number of deaths due to DUI.

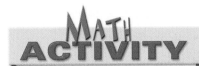

Have students research the latest statistics on alcohol-related highway deaths. Then have them copy the graph in the figure above and revise it to incorporate the latest information. Ask students to make a second graph that shows their state's information on alcohol-related deaths.

What Can You Do About Drunk Driving?

Would you walk in front of a car steered by a drunk driver? Probably not. You can't always control what other people do, but you can control and protect yourself. Don't ride with a drunk driver. Get home some other way, or try to arrange a ride beforehand. Avoid situations in which there might be drinking. You can help protect others, too. If a friend is about to drive after drinking, try to stop him or her. Do not ride along. And if someone is drinking, don't let him or her skateboard or bike ride. No matter what you hear, there is no way for anyone to sober up quickly. So be safe, not sorry.

What else can you do to prevent drunk driving? You can join others in a group to prevent DUI, such as SADD (Students Against Destructive Decisions) or MADD (Mothers Against Drunk Driving). Stay away from people who drink and drive. Take control of your life and stay safe.

Lesson Review

Using Vocabulary

1. What is DUI?

Understanding Concepts

2. Why is driving after drinking so dangerous?

3. How can a reaction time that is slowed by alcohol cause problems?

4. What are two ways that you can prevent drinking and driving?

Critical Thinking

5. Making Inferences What do you think are the reasons that some state DUI laws make 0.00 the BAC limit for people under 21?

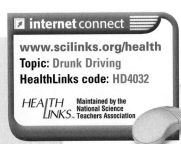

🔲 internet connect

www.scilinks.org/health
Topic: Drunk Driving
HealthLinks code: HD4032

HEALTH LINKS Maintained by the National Science Teachers Association

Alcoholism

Bobby is happy that his Uncle Frank has recovered from years of alcoholism. But Bobby is concerned because his uncle still has a lot of problems to deal with.

Why is Bobby still concerned about his uncle if Uncle Frank has recovered? Is alcoholism different from an illness such as the flu?

What Is Alcoholism?

Alcoholism is an illness. **Alcoholism** is a physical and psychological dependence on alcohol. Like other illnesses, alcoholism has certain symptoms. Alcoholism's main symptoms are a strong need for a drink, an inability to stop or limit drinking, an increasing tolerance for alcohol, and a physical dependence on alcohol. *Physical dependence* means that your body needs alcohol to function normally. Like other illnesses, alcoholism may get worse if it is not treated. Alcoholism may eventually lead to death.

Alcoholism has different causes. Frequent heavy drinking will change your body's reactions to alcohol and result in dependence. Alcoholism may partly be hereditary, because certain genes seem to make alcoholism more likely. But family environment, especially in childhood, and your choice of friends may be stronger influences. For example, friends and relatives may offer you alcohol and encourage drinking.

But alcoholism is not automatic. It occurs in families with and without a history of alcoholism. And not all children whose parents have alcoholism become alcoholics. People who start drinking as adults are less likely to develop alcoholism than people who start drinking in their teens are.

Alcoholism is an illness that affects individuals. But alcoholism also affects everyone in an alcoholic's life. A person with alcoholism may become violent and hurt other family members, or may be moody and unpredictable. Family members don't know what to expect from their loved one. Parents with alcoholism cannot meet their duties or provide emotional support to their children. They may lose their job and create serious financial problems for the family.

What You'll Do

- **Identify** three factors that can contribute to a person developing alcoholism.
- **Explain** how alcoholism may affect an alcoholic's family.

Terms to Learn

- alcoholism
- recovery

Start Off
Write

How can alcoholism affect a family?

Figure 13 Alcoholism is a lifelong illness. But many people with alcoholism can recover and live productive, happy lives.

Overcoming Alcoholism

There is no cure for alcoholism, but alcoholism is treatable. Not drinking at all, or *abstinence from alcohol,* is the best treatment. When a person with alcoholism stops drinking, he or she may experience withdrawal. *Withdrawal* is the reaction the body goes through when it does not get a drug that it is dependent on. A person with alcoholism going through withdrawal may experience severe headaches, extreme nervousness, shaking, or seizures (SEE zuhrz). Medical help may be needed to get through withdrawal.

A person with alcoholism will always be addicted to alcohol. But many people with alcoholism do recover and stay sober by seeking treatment and help. **Recovery** is learning to live without alcohol. Recovery means that the drinker—not alcohol—is in control. But recovery from alcoholism requires that the person wants to stop drinking. Recovery is possible with medication, and with the support and help of other people. Treatment consists of medical help and counseling. Groups, such as Alcoholics Anonymous, may provide help and support for the person with alcoholism.

Counseling also helps families affected by alcoholism. Alanon and Alateen help families cope with alcoholism's effects. Teenage children whose parent has alcoholism can ask a trusted adult for help. Together, they can find a program that provides assistance for teens.

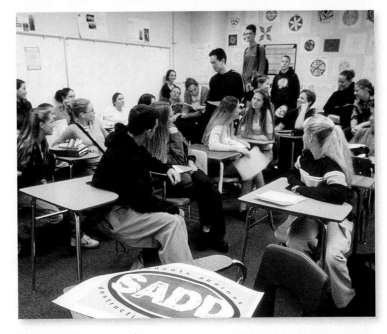

Figure 14 Every member of the family is affected by the disease of alcoholism. But help is available for every family member.

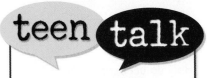

Teen: I've heard that once you start drinking, nothing you do will stop you from becoming a person with alcoholism.

Expert: One drink does not cause alcoholism. But alcoholism is a lot less likely if you don't drink until you are an adult. If you think you are at risk for alcoholism, avoid it by not drinking.

Lesson Review

Using Vocabulary

1. Define *alcoholism.*

Understanding Concepts

2. What are three factors that can contribute to a person developing alcoholism?

3. Can alcoholism be cured? Explain.

Critical Thinking

4. **Making Inferences** Explain how alcoholism may affect many people other than the alcoholic.

5. **Identifying Relationships** How might the recovery of a person who has alcoholism benefit his or her family?

internet connect

www.scilinks.org/health

Topic: Alcoholism

HealthLinks code: HD4007

HEALTH LINKS™ Maintained by the National Science Teachers Association

Lesson 6 Resisting the Pressure to Drink

What You'll Do

- **Identify** three pressures to drink that teens face.
- **Explain** how people can be influenced by advertisements for alcohol.
- **Identify** three questions that can help you resist the pressures to drink.

Start Off
Write

How do beer commercials try to convince you to drink?

> Rudy was angry with his friend Shanna. Rudy knew that Shanna didn't drink alcohol, but then he saw Shanna drinking beer at a party.

What should Rudy do? He doesn't know why Shanna decided to drink. What may have made Shanna change her mind?

Pressures to Drink

Society provides all kinds of pressures to drink. For teens, peer pressure may be the strongest pressure of all. Peers may make you feel that if you don't drink, you'll be left out and alone. You want to be accepted by groups that have the same interests you do. So, if some of the people you are with start drinking, you may feel pressure to drink, too. That peer pressure is what Shanna felt at the party. Resisting peer pressure is one of the hardest things for teens to do. That is why choosing friends who do not drink is so important.

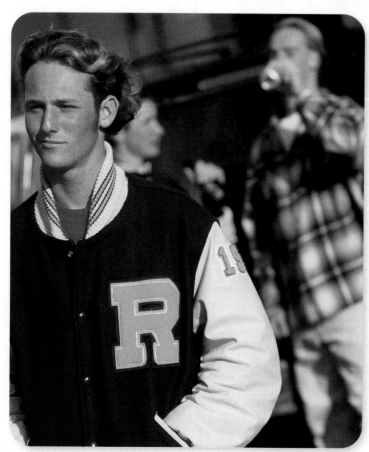

Another source of pressure to drink is advertisements for alcohol. Alcohol advertising is in magazines and on TV and radio. There are ads at sports arenas and on buses and trucks. Drinking is shown in movies and on TV. The message in the ads is that alcohol is a normal part of life. The ads want to convince you that drinking is fun. That's why they never show sick, unhappy, injured, or lonely drinkers. People in the ads are good-looking, smart, happy, athletic, and popular. Sometimes, teens hope that drinking will make them look like the adults in the ad. Some teens may actually think that drinking is the only way to have a good time.

Figure 15 Social and peer pressures influence many people to take a drink.

Knowing What You Want

Sometimes, messages in ads for alcohol may make knowing what you really want more difficult. After all, alcohol advertising targets parts of you that you may not feel good about, such as appearance or popularity. The ads aim for your fears or your hopes. Or, if you're bored, the ads make drinking seem exciting and fun. How can you make it through all the messages about drinking that you get? You can start by knowing what is right for you.

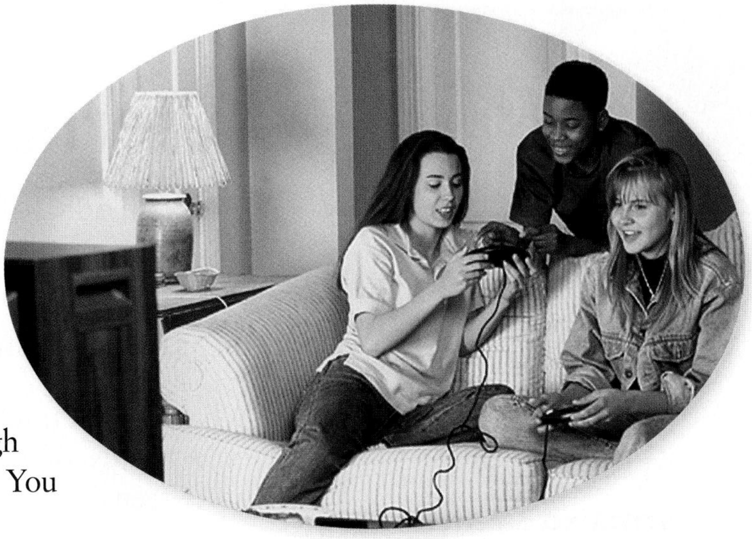

Figure 16 Friends can support your decision not to drink by joining you in healthy alternatives.

Knowing what you want is a lot easier if you take some time to think about it. Try to sort it out with the help of someone you trust. Remember, no matter what the ads tell you, most adults and teens either don't drink at all or drink very rarely.

To drink or not to drink is only one of thousands of choices that teens have to make. Knowing what's best for you helps you make smart choices. Ask yourself the following questions, and write down your answers.

- What makes you happy?
- What do you do to feel good or to feel adult and in charge?
- How can drinking hurt you or get you in trouble?
- What pressures to drink do you feel?
- How can you avoid or stop those pressures?

If you've already decided not to drink, or not to drink again, good for you. But answer the questions anyway. The answers will help you focus on the important things in your life and will help you make good decisions about many different things.

Health Journal
In your Health Journal, write why your decision about whether or not to use alcohol should be based only on your own ideas rather than on what someone else thinks.

Lesson Review

Understanding Concepts

1. What are three questions that might help you resist pressures to drink?

2. Identify three kinds of pressure to drink that teens face.

3. Identify two steps that you would take in making the decision about whether to drink or not.

Critical Thinking

4. **Analyzing Viewpoints** Explain why you should be very careful about believing advertisements for alcohol.

5. **Making Good Decisions** Brandi was eating dinner at her best friend's house. Brandi's friend offered her a glass of wine with dinner. Brandi doesn't drink. What should Brandi do?

Alternatives to Alcohol

SuLinda left her first rock-climbing lesson with a huge smile on her face. She was thrilled by the chance to try something new and exciting outdoors.

What You'll Do

■ **Describe** two ways to have fun without using alcohol.

■ **Identify** three sources of help for drinking problems.

Terms to Learn

• hobby

Start Off
Write

How might a hobby or other interest help you avoid using alcohol?

What do you think SuLinda liked about rock climbing? What other kinds of activities would be exciting for SuLinda or other teens?

Friends and Fun

If you are struggling with a decision about drinking alcohol, one of your best sources of help may be your friends. Friends are usually people you like, trust, talk to, and have a good time with. Your real friends will not pressure you to drink. And you will want to go with your friends to places where you can do things you enjoy. Being with friends who do not drink will keep the pressure to drink off of you. So, pick your friends carefully.

Many activities, such as sports teams, school and religious groups, and community volunteering, provide fun ways to avoid alcohol. Join a group that does things you enjoy, and you may not have time to worry about drinking. Every community has fun things to do, so look around.

Another way to prevent the pressure to drink from getting to you is to find a hobby. A **hobby** is something you like to do or to study in your spare time. Only you can say what interests you and what bores you. If physical challenges, such as rock climbing, excite you, look for places to learn these skills and do them safely. Or maybe you like astronomy or painting. Look for clubs or groups focused on an activity that you enjoy. These are good places to meet new friends.

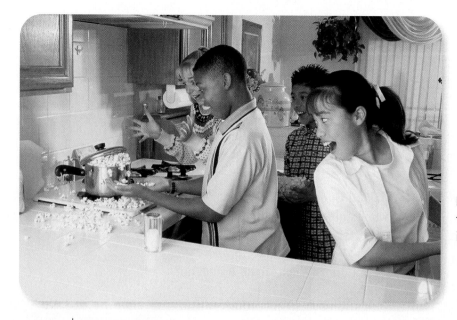

Figure 17 Having fun with friends who share your values is a way to avoid alcohol.

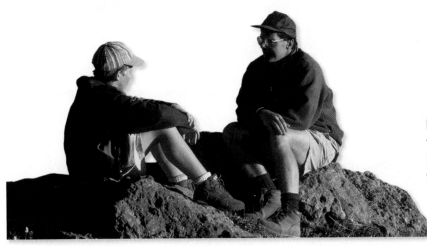

Figure 18 Sometimes, just talking to someone can help you find alternatives to alcohol.

Resources for Emotional Problems

If you have a problem with alcohol, talking to someone you trust may help. Major problems may require more help than your friends can provide. But there is help around you. Adults may have some experience and suggestions about help for drinking problems that they can offer you. A trusted teacher, coach, or guidance counselor can help. You can also talk to your parents, a relative, or another adult you trust. For many teens, talking with a religious or spiritual leader about the mental and emotional problems related to alcohol is best. And for any physical problems related to alcohol, seek help from a parent, school nurse, or family doctor. Don't wait. If you need help, ask someone you trust.

Sometimes, it is a friend who needs help. Be a good listener. Don't judge him or her. And if the alcohol problems are too difficult for you or your friends to handle, help your friend find someone who can help. Seeking professional help is especially important for problems involving alcohol. If you don't know where to start, ask a trusted adult for suggestions.

LIFE SKILLS ACTIVITY

MAKING GOOD DECISIONS

Make a list of the top ten fun things you like to do that don't involve alcohol. With your classmates, make a class list of fun activities on the board. Put a star by any new ideas that appeal to you. Try new activities when you are bored or tempted to drink alcohol.

Lesson Review

Using Vocabulary

1. What is a hobby? Name a few examples.

Understanding Concepts

2. What are two ways to have fun without drinking?

3. List three sources of help for drinking problems.

Critical Thinking

4. **Identifying Relationships** Why is it important to have friends who have the same interests and values that you have?

5. **Using Refusal Skills** Describe two realistic ways to avoid alcohol in the next week.

Chapter Summary

■ Teens drink alcohol for a variety of reasons, including to fit in and to feel more adult. ■ Alcohol is a depressant drug that affects the central nervous system. ■ Blood alcohol concentration (BAC) is a measure of the amount of alcohol in the blood. ■ Alcohol's effects on the brain may make a person more likely to be involved in violence. ■ Alcohol's long-term effects include alcohol abuse and liver diseases, such as hepatitis and cirrhosis. ■ Alcohol's effects on the body and brain make it extremely dangerous to drink and drive or do any other complex activity. ■ Alcoholism is an illness in which a person is physically and psychologically dependent on alcohol. ■ You can resist the pressure to drink by considering your options and by understanding the dangers of drinking alcohol.

Using Vocabulary

1 Use each of the following terms in a separate sentence: *blood alcohol concentration (BAC)* and *depressant*.

2 In your own words, write a definition for the term *alcoholism*.

For each sentence, fill in the blank with the proper word from the word bank provided below.

binge drinking	hobby
alcohol abuse	intoxication
blood alcohol concentration	recovery
fetal alcohol syndrome (FAS)	reaction time

3 The physical and mental changes produced by drinking alcohol are ___.

4 Frequent or excessive drinking is ___.

5 ___ is learning to live without alcohol.

6 Something you like to do in your spare time is a(n) ___.

7 The possible physical and mental effects on a fetus that has been exposed to alcohol are called ___.

8 Drinking several drinks in one sitting is ___.

Understanding Concepts

9 Describe how alcohol acts as a depressant.

10 How does alcohol affect a person's ability to drive?

11 Explain the statement, "There is no cure for alcoholism, but alcoholism is treatable."

12 Give three reasons that teens drink alcohol, and three reasons for not drinking.

13 How can you prevent someone from drinking and driving?

14 Why might drinkers become involved with violence more easily than nondrinkers?

15 Why is it dangerous for a pregnant woman to drink alcohol?

Critical Thinking

Inferring Conclusions

16 Marie's uncle is an alcoholic, and Marie's father drinks a lot. Marie's college-age brother also seems to drink quite a bit, but usually only on the weekends. Would you predict that Marie will become an alcoholic? Why or why not?

17 Brian's older brother, David, is a binge drinker. David drinks heavily on Friday nights on his way home from work, and on Saturday nights at home with his family. The rest of the time, David doesn't drink. Brian thinks that David abuses alcohol. Explain why you agree or disagree with Brian.

18 Imagine that you are at a family reunion and see your cousin have a couple of drinks in a very short time. About half an hour later, your cousin seems a bit clumsy and a little sleepy. Is it possible the alcohol has anything to do with your cousin's condition? Explain.

Making Good Decisions

19 Imagine that you see a very funny beer commercial on TV. Using the steps for making good decisions, describe how you would react to the ad.

20 At the family reunion, you run into some cousins and their spouses, all in their twenties and thirties. Some of them have been drinking. They have decided to go shopping at a nearby mall, then stop and get some ice cream. They invite you to go with them. Discuss in detail how you would decide whether to go or not.

Interpreting Graphics

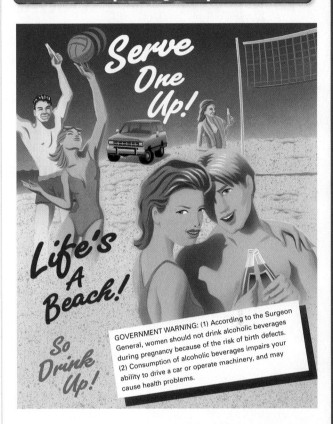

Use the figure above to answer questions 21–24.

21 Who is this ad trying to reach?

22 Why do you think a company would make an ad like this to advertise an alcoholic beverage?

23 Is this ad misleading? Why or why not?

24 What information should an ad for an alcoholic beverage contain?

Reading Checkup

Take a minute to review your answers to the Health IQ questions at the beginning of this chapter. How has reading this chapter improved your Health IQ?

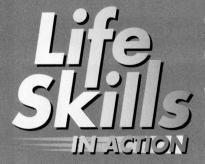

Using Refusal Skills

Using refusal skills is saying no to things you don't want to do. You can also use refusal skills to avoid dangerous situations. Complete the following activity to develop your refusal skills.

Sophie and the Secret Alcohol

Setting the Scene

Sophie is at a high school football game with her friend Faith and Faith's older brother. During the game, Faith and her brother go to buy snacks and drinks. When they return, Faith tells Sophie that her brother managed to sneak in some alcohol. He poured some alcohol into each of the soda cups so that no one would know. Faith hands Sophie a cup and laughs as she tells Sophie to enjoy her soda.

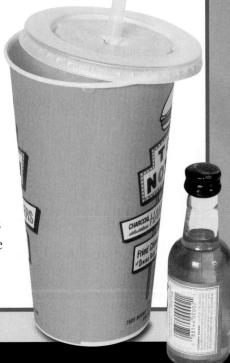

The 5 Steps of Using Refusal Skills

1. Avoid dangerous situations.
2. Say "No."
3. Stand your ground.
4. Stay focused on the issue.
5. Walk away.

Guided Practice

Practice with a Friend

Form a group of three. Have one person play the role of Sophie and another person play the role of Faith. Have the third person be an observer. Walking through each of the five steps of using refusal skills, role-play Sophie telling Faith that she does not want to drink alcohol. Faith should try to convince Sophie that drinking alcohol is okay. The observer will take notes, which will include observations about what the person playing Sophie did well and suggestions of ways to improve. Stop after each step to evaluate the process.

Check Yourself

After you have completed the guided practice, go through Act 1 again without stopping at each step. Answer the questions below to review what you did.

1. Which refusal skill will not work in this situation? Explain.

2. What could Sophie say to Faith when she is standing her ground?

3. What plan could Sophie have to get out of this situation?

4. How would you say no to your friends if they offered you alcohol?

ACT 2

On Your Own

The next weekend, Faith calls Sophie to invite her over to her house. Faith says that her parents went out for the evening and her brother is having a few of his friends over to hang out. Sophie doesn't want to go to Faith's house because she thinks Faith's brother and his friends will be drinking. Write a skit about the conversation between Sophie and Faith. Sophie should use the five steps of using refusal skills during the conversation.

CHAPTER 13 Teens and Drugs

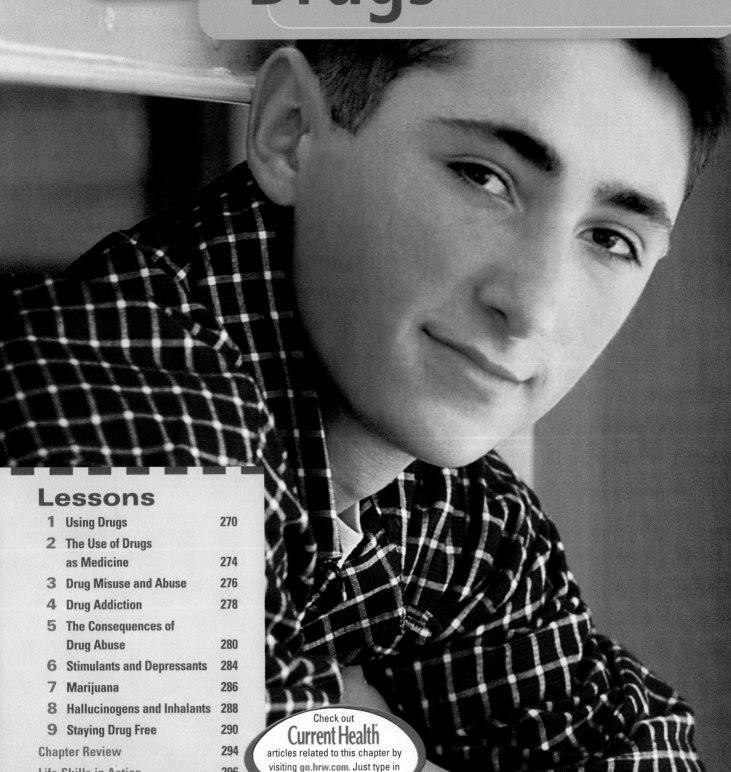

Lessons

Check out **Current Health** articles related to this chapter by visiting **go.hrw.com**. Just type in the keyword **HD4CH28**.

> " I used to be the **best player** on my school's **basketball** team. Then, I started **smoking marijuana.** Before long, I got out of breath whenever I played. I also started skipping practice to go smoke marijuana with my friends. Last week, the coach told me that I was off the team. I wish I had never started using drugs. "

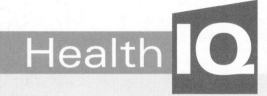

PRE-READING

Answer the following multiple-choice questions to find out what you already know about drugs. When you've finished this chapter, you'll have the opportunity to change your answers based on what you've learned.

1. **Which of the following statements about drugs is true?**
   a. Food is a drug.
   b. A medicine is not a drug.
   c. Drugs do not provide your body with any nutrients that you need to live.
   d. All drugs can be purchased legally with a prescription.

2. **Which statement about prescription drugs is NOT true?**
   a. You need a doctor's approval to use prescription drugs.
   b. Prescription drugs should never be shared with another person.
   c. People can get addicted to prescription drugs.
   d. Prescription drugs are always legal, even if they are used improperly.

3. **When a person's body has a chemical need for a drug, the person has**
   a. a physical dependence.
   b. a psychological dependence.
   c. a drug prescription.
   d. used a stimulant.

4. **Marijuana is**
   a. made in a laboratory.
   b. a plant.
   c. harmless if it is used properly.
   d. a relatively new drug.

5. **Which of the following statements is a good reason to avoid drugs?**
   a. Drugs are illegal.
   b. Using drugs can damage your relationships.
   c. Drugs can damage your health.
   d. all of the above

6. **Ways to refuse drugs include**
   a. saying, "No, thank you."
   b. giving a reason.
   c. suggesting another activity.
   d. All of the above

Using Drugs

What You'll Do

■ **Explain** what a drug is.

■ **Describe** five different ways in which drugs can enter the body.

Terms to Learn

• drug

Start Off
Write

What are some ways that drugs can be taken?

Jamal's head was pounding. Jamal had a math test and a big soccer game that day. He was afraid that with the headache, he wouldn't be able to pass the test or run well. Jamal's mother gave him a painkiller, and his headache went away. Did Jamal use a drug?

When he took the painkiller, Jamal used a drug. A **drug** is any substance other than food that changes a person's physical or psychological state. When many people think of drugs, they think of harmful, illegal drugs that can cause serious problems. But there are many different kinds of drugs. Some, such as aspirin and other painkillers, are legal. Others, such as marijuana and cocaine, are illegal. It can also be easy to forget that many drugs, such as the painkiller that cured Jamal's headache, are used to treat diseases and pain. So, what exactly is a drug?

Is It a Drug or Not?

Not everything you take into your body is considered a drug. Food and water provide your body with chemicals, vitamins, and nutrients that your body needs to live. Without food and water, you cannot survive. Unlike food, drugs do not provide your body with any nutrients that are necessary for life. But many foods do contain drugs, although food itself is not a drug. For example, chocolate and cola both contain the drug caffeine.

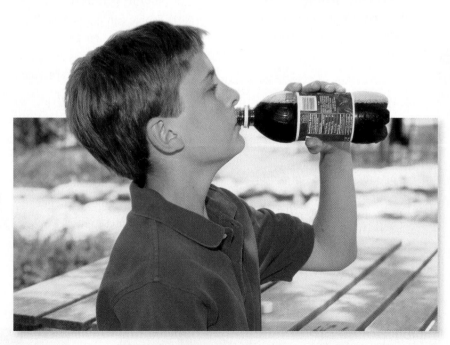

Figure 1 Drugs are contained in many products, including the soft drink that this teen is drinking.

Taking Drugs Orally

The painkiller that Jamal took was taken *orally*, which means that it was taken through the mouth. Swallowing, chewing, and drinking are all ways of taking drugs orally. These are the simplest ways to take drugs. Drugs taken orally may be pills, capsules, or liquid. Pills, sometimes called *tablets*, are medicine in a solid form. Capsules are tiny containers that hold a drug in powdered or liquid form.

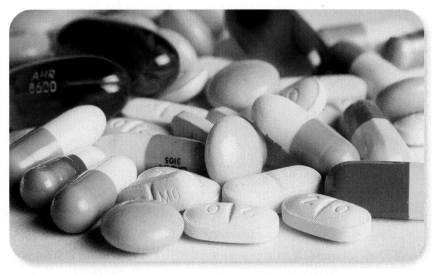

Figure 2 Many drugs can be taken orally.

After a pill or a capsule is swallowed, it is dissolved in the stomach. The medicine is absorbed by the stomach and the small instestine into the bloodstream. The blood carries the drug to the body's cells, where it begins to take effect.

Some capsules have a coating that makes them dissolve more slowly. These capsules are called *controlled-release capsules*. A controlled-release capsule allows the body's cells to take in the medicine over a long period of time, rather than all at once. These capsules enter the small intestine. There, as the container dissolves, the medicine is absorbed slowly into the bloodsteam.

Taking Drugs by Injection

At some point in your life, you have probably gotten a shot—and you probably didn't like it. A shot is an injection of a drug into the body through a special needle called a *hypodermic needle* (HIE poh DUHR mik NEED'l). A doctor often gives an injection when he or she wants a drug to act quickly or when a drug won't work properly if it is taken orally. Drugs are usually injected into a muscle in the thigh, upper arm, or buttocks. On some occasions, drugs are injected directly into a vein.

Some illegal drugs are taken by injection. Injection is the fastest and most powerful way for the drug to reach the body and the brain. People who abuse injected drugs usually inject the drugs directly into a vein to get a greater effect from the drug. They also often share hypodermic needles. If one person has an infectious disease, he or she can pass the disease to others who use the same needle.

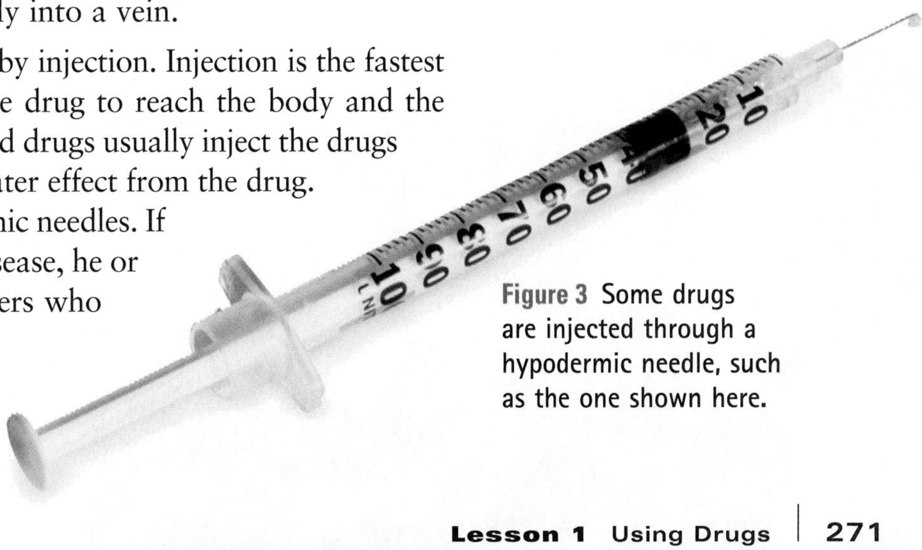

Figure 3 Some drugs are injected through a hypodermic needle, such as the one shown here.

Taking Drugs by Smoking

Nicotine, which is found in tobacco, is the most common drug that is smoked. Some illegal drugs, such as marijuana and crack cocaine, are also smoked. When a person smokes, the chemicals in the drug enter the lungs and pass through tiny blood vessels into the bloodstream. From there, they are carried throughout the body.

All smoke contains poisonous substances. Tobacco smoke contains nicotine, carbon monoxide, and tar. Tar increases the smoker's chance of getting lung diseases, such as cancer and emphysema (EM fuh SEE muh). Carbon monoxide increases the likelihood of heart disease and blood vessel disease. Regular use of marijuana has effects on the lungs that are similar to those caused by tobacco.

Myth & Fact

Myth: Using tobacco in the form of chewing tobacco or snuff is much safer than smoking.

Fact: Although chewing tobacco doesn't cause lung diseases like smoking does, it does cause other serious diseases, such as mouth cancer.

Inhaling Drugs

If you or a friend has asthma, you are probably familiar with taking a drug by inhaling, which means breathing in the drug. Some drugs, such as those used to treat asthma, are stored in air or gas and are then breathed in through a device called an *inhaler*. Each time the inhaler is pumped, a certain amount of the drug is released. The drug is inhaled into the lungs, where it acts directly on cells in the lungs. Other drugs, such as those used to relieve nasal congestion, are dissolved in water and inhaled through the nose. In an operating room or a dentist's office, anesthetics (AN es THEHT iks)—drugs used to numb patients during medical procedures—are sometimes given by having the patient inhale the drugs.

Inhaling drugs is different from taking in drugs by smoking. When a drug is inhaled, the user breathes the drug directly into the lungs. In smoking, the drug is burned, and the resulting smoke is then inhaled.

Many drugs, such as nitrous oxide, are abused by inhaling. Inhaling substances to get "high" is extremely dangerous. In fact, it can cause heart failure, brain damage, suffocation, and instant death.

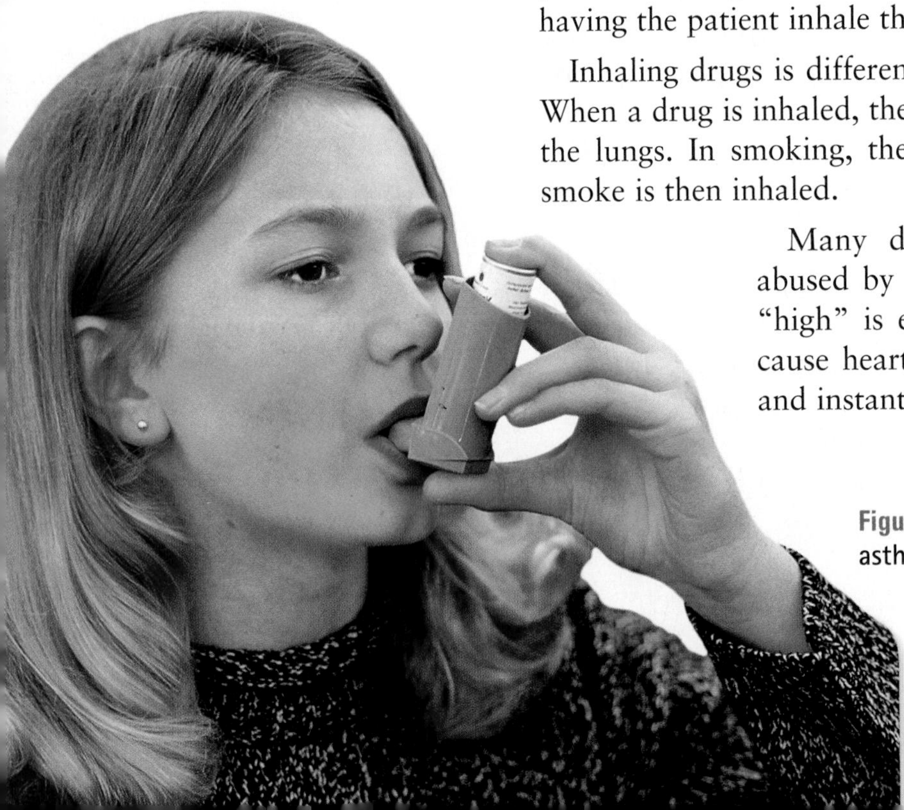

Figure 4 This teen is treating her asthma by using an inhaled drug.

Other Ways That Drugs Are Taken

There are many other ways to take drugs. One way is called a *transdermal patch* (tranz DUHR muhl PACH). A transdermal patch sticks to the skin like a bandage. The medicine contained in the patch is slowly released into the skin and absorbed into the bloodstream.

Some drugs do not need to enter the bloodstream to be effective. For example, ointments are applied directly to the skin and do not enter the bloodstream. Drops of medicine used for infections in the ears or eyes also do not enter the bloodstream.

Same Drug, Different Forms

Some drugs can be taken in more than one form. The way in which a drug is taken can change the effects it has. For example, the antibiotic drug penicillin may be taken orally in either pill or liquid form, or it may be injected. When penicillin is injected, it has a much stronger and faster effect than when it is taken orally. Another example is nicotine, which is generally taken by smoking cigarettes or is taken orally in the form of chewing tobacco. People who are trying to stop smoking may take nicotine orally by chewing nicotine gum. Or they may use a transdermal patch, which releases nicotine slowly through the skin. Nicotine gum and transdermal patches do not hurt the body as much as tobacco does because they do not contain many of the poisons that tobacco contains.

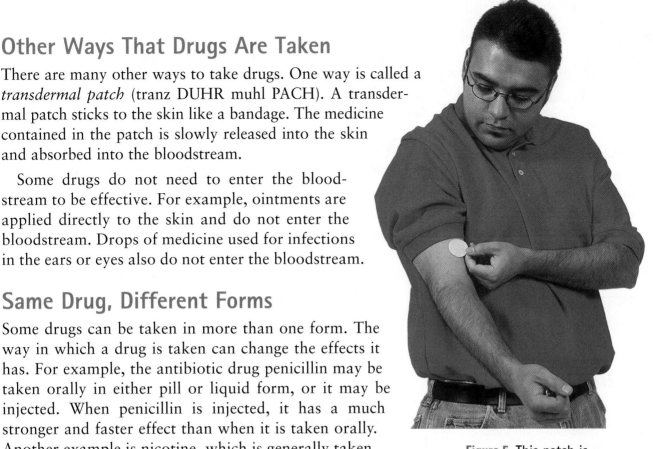

Figure 5 This patch is delivering medicine to the body through the skin.

Lesson Review

Using Vocabulary

1. What is a drug?

Understanding Concepts

2. What are five different ways that drugs can be taken?

3. How do medicines and other drugs get to the body's cells?

4. Do all drugs enter the bloodstream? Explain.

Critical Thinking

5. **Analyzing Ideas** Chocolate contains caffeine, but chocolate is also food. If you eat chocolate, are you taking a drug? Explain your answer.

6. **Making Good Decisions** Imagine that you have a bad headache. Your father offers you a choice between medicine in a liquid form and medicine in a controlled-release capsule. Which would you choose? Explain your answer.

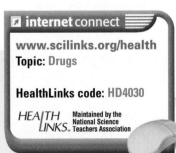

internet connect

www.scilinks.org/health
Topic: Drugs

HealthLinks code: HD4030

HEALTH LINKS. Maintained by the National Science Teachers Association

The Use of Drugs as Medicine

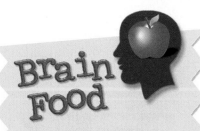

Brain Food

The R$_X$ symbol that often appears on prescription medicine labels stands for the word *recipe*, which means "to take" in Latin. Pharmacists now use the symbol to indicate that a medicine can be bought only with a prescription.

Melissa had a bad cough. She took cough medicine from the drugstore, but it didn't help. When Melissa went to the doctor, he gave her a different cough medicine. Melissa soon started to feel better.

Many drugs are used as medicine. A **medicine** is any substance used to treat disease, injury, or pain. Different kinds of medicine are used to treat different problems. As Melissa discovered, treating an illness or a disease requires finding the right medicine.

Prescription Medicine

Medicine that can be bought only if a doctor orders its use is called **prescription medicine.** To get prescription medicine, you must have written instructions from your doctor, known as a *prescription* (pree SKRIP shuhn). A prescription contains the patient's name, the medicine's name, and the doctor's signature. It also contains information on the proper dosage (DOHS ij), or how much of the medicine to take and when to take it. As with any medicine, taking prescription medicine exactly as instructed is important. Taking too much of the drug can be harmful. Taking too little of the drug or taking it incorrectly can keep it from working.

Figure 6 Reading a Prescription Medicine Label

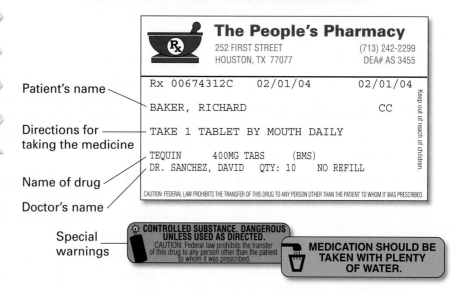

Figure 7 Reading an Over-the-Counter Medicine Label

List of ingredients

Directions for taking the medicine

Special warnings

COUGH SUPPRESSANT/EXPECTORANT

ACTIVE INGREDIENTS (in each 5 mL tsp): Dextromethorphan HBr, USP 10 mg; Guaifenesin, USP 100 mg. See carton for complete list of inactive ingredients.

USES: Temporarily relieves cough due to minor throat and bronchial irritation as may occur with a cold; helps loosen phlegm (mucus) and thin bronchial secretions to make coughs more productive.

DIRECTIONS: Do not take more than 6 doses in any 24 hour period. Adults and children 12 years and over — 2 teaspoonfuls every 4 hours as needed. Children 6–12 years of age —1 teaspoonful every 4 hours as needed.

WARNINGS: Do not take if you are now taking a prescription monoamine oxidase inhibitor (MAOI) (certain drugs for depression, psychiatric, or emotional conditions, or Parkinson's disease), or for 2 weeks after stopping the MAOI drug. If you do not know if your prescription drug contains MAOI, ask a doctor or pharmacist before taking this product.

Keep this and all drugs out of reach of children. In case of accidental overdose, get medical help or contact a poison control center immediately. Store at 20-25°C (68-77°F), alcohol free, dosage cup provided. Made in U.S.A. 8685-22/21A

LOT 011954
Exp 5 2004

Over-the-Counter Medicine

Any medicine that can be purchased without a prescription is called **over-the-counter medicine.** These drugs are most often used for minor problems, such as headaches or mild allergy symptoms. Thousands of over-the-counter medicines exist, including pain relievers and cold and cough medicines.

If used improperly, over-the-counter medicines can be harmful. You should take over-the-counter medicines just as carefully as you take prescription medicines. Following the medicine's instructions is important. Make sure you take the right dosage at the right time. Taking too much of any medicine, even an over-the-counter medicine, can be very dangerous.

Health Journal
Write about a time when you used an over-the-counter medicine to treat pain or an illness. How did you feel after taking the medicine?

Lesson Review

Using Vocabulary

1. What is a medicine?
2. What is the difference between prescription medicines and over-the-counter medicines?

Understanding Concepts

3. What information is included in a prescription?

Critical Thinking

4. **Making Inferences** Some medicines are sold in both prescription and over-the-counter forms. What might be the difference between these forms?

5. **Analyzing Ideas** Why is it important for a prescription to contain a doctor's signature?

Drug Misuse and Abuse

Tyla had allergies and she took an allergy medicine to stop her symptoms. But she also liked the way the medicine made her feel. Pretty soon, she was ignoring the instructions and taking the medicine whenever she felt like it. Before long, she was taking it all the time.

When Tyla started ignoring the instructions that came with her medicine, she began misusing the medicine. Pretty soon, this misuse turned into abuse.

Using Medicines Improperly

Any use of a medicine that is different from the intended use is **drug misuse.** This includes not following the directions. Whenever you take any kind of medicine, take it exactly as instructed. Misuse can sometimes lead to overdose, drug abuse, or addiction. If you're not sure how to take a medicine, talk to your doctor or pharmacist. When taking medicine, follow these rules:

● Follow all instructions, not just the ones that are convenient.

● Never increase the amount of the medicine that you take without your doctor's permission.

● Don't stop taking a prescription medication without your doctor's permission, even if your symptoms are gone.

● Never take someone else's prescription medicine.

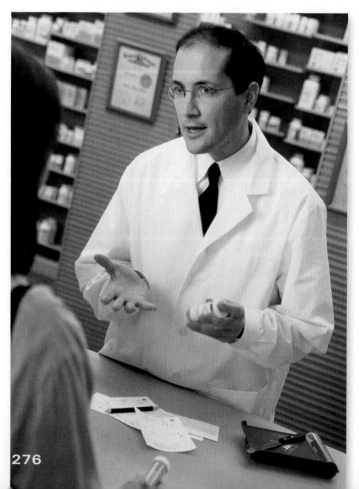

Figure 8 If you have questions about how to take a medicine properly, you may talk to a pharmacist.

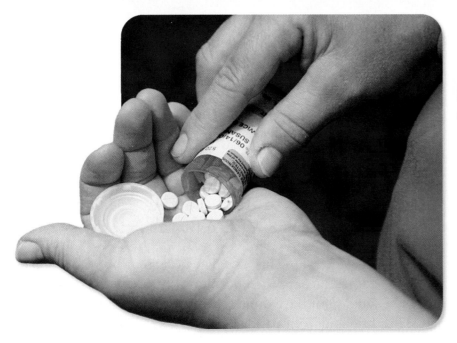

Figure 9 Misusing a drug can sometimes lead to drug abuse.

When Does Misuse Become Abuse?

When Tyla started taking her allergy medicine to feel good rather than to treat her symptoms, she started abusing the drug. **Drug abuse** is misusing a legal drug on purpose or using any illegal drug. Misuse of a drug often involves taking too much of the drug. The person becomes used to the higher dosage and craves more of the drug when he or she takes the correct dosage. The person begins to take more of the drug more often. This is how drug abuse often starts.

People abuse drugs for many reasons. Often, like Tyla, they like how the drug makes them feel. Sometimes, people abuse a drug because they feel that the drug helps them perform better or helps them forget problems. All drugs are dangerous if misused or abused. If you think you have been misusing or abusing a drug, talk to a doctor or a trusted adult right away.

LIFE SKILLS ACTIVITY

PRACTICING WELLNESS

Find an over-the-counter medicine at your home. Read the instructions for taking this medicine. How much should be taken? How often? Are there any special warnings?

Lesson Review

Using Vocabulary

1. What is drug misuse?

2. In your own words, explain the difference between drug misuse and drug abuse.

Understanding Concepts

3. What kinds of medicines can be misused or abused?

4. Describe how drug misuse can lead to drug abuse.

Critical Thinking

5. Making Inferences Steven lost the label from his bottle of prescription medicine. How could this lead to drug misuse?

internet connect

www.scilinks.org/health
Topic: Medicine Safety
HealthLinks code: HD4066

HEALTH LINKS. Maintained by the National Science Teachers Association

Drug Addiction

What You'll Do

- **Describe** what drug addiction is, and explain how it happens.
- **Describe** the difference between physical dependence and psychological dependence.

Terms to Learn

- drug addiction
- withdrawal
- physical dependence
- psychological dependence

Start Off
Write

Why is it difficult for some people to stop abusing drugs?

Tom had knee surgery and was given a prescription painkiller. At first, he liked the way the medicine relieved his pain. But soon, he found that he had to take more of the medicine to feel better and would become anxious if he didn't take it.

Tom couldn't stop taking his medicine because he was addicted to it. Tom's addiction happened very quickly, and it made him do things he would not have done before, such as misusing the medicine. But how did Tom's addiction happen?

What Is Addiction?

The effects that some drugs produce can cause people to want to use the drug over and over. When a person cannot control his or her use of a drug, that person has a drug addiction. **Drug addiction** is the uncontrollable use of a drug. Someone who is addicted to a drug continues to take it even if the drug is harming his or her health and relationships.

A person with an addiction cannot control his or her use of a drug because he or she has become dependent on the drug. *Dependence* on a drug means needing the drug in order to function properly. If the person stops taking the drug, he or she will experience withdrawal. **Withdrawal** is the negative symptoms that result when a drug-dependent person stops taking a drug. There are two types of dependence: physical dependence and psychological dependence.

Figure 10 The path to drug addiction may be easy, but recovery can be difficult.

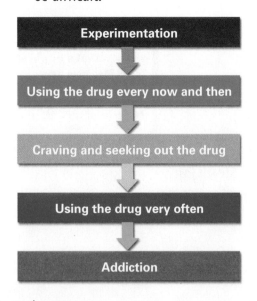

Experimentation

↓

Using the drug every now and then

↓

Craving and seeking out the drug

↓

Using the drug very often

↓

Addiction

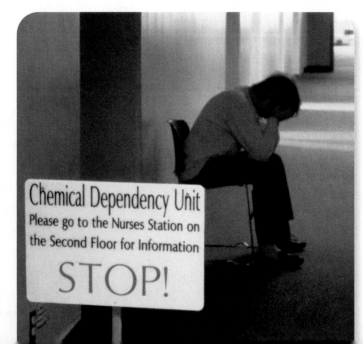

Chemical Dependency Unit
Please go to the Nurses Station on the Second Floor for Information
STOP!

Physical Dependence

When a person abuses a drug long enough, his or her body gets used to the drug. In fact, chemical changes take place in the body. These changes make the body need a regular supply of the drug to keep functioning normally. This type of dependence is called physical dependence. **Physical dependence** is the body's chemical need for a drug. If a person with a physical dependence suddenly stops taking the drug, he or she will quickly go into withdrawal. A person in physical withdrawal may experience vomiting, muscle and joint pain, fever, chills, anxiety, and many other symptoms.

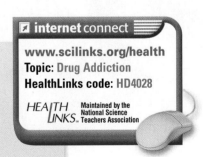

Figure 11 Even psychological dependence can lead to withdrawal symptoms, such as being unable to sleep.

Psychological Dependence

Some people also have a psychological need for a drug. This type of addiction is called psychological dependence. **Psychological** (SIE kuh LAHJ i kuhl) **dependence** is a person's emotional or mental need for a drug. A person with psychological dependence craves the drug and feels that he or she can't get along without the drug. Psychological dependence is sometimes even harder to overcome than physical dependence.

Psychological dependence can also cause physical withdrawal symptoms. These symptoms may include sleeplessness, nervousness, irritability, and depression.

Lesson Review

Using Vocabulary

1. What is drug addiction?

2. Describe the difference between physical and psychological dependence.

3. What is withdrawal? When does it happen?

Understanding Concepts

4. How does physical dependence happen?

Critical Thinking

5. **Analyzing Ideas** Is it possible to be addicted to a legal drug? Explain your answer.

🔲 internet connect

www.scilinks.org/health

Topic: Drug Addiction

HealthLinks code: HD4028

HEALTH LINKS... Maintained by the National Science Teachers Association

The Consequences of Drug Abuse

What You'll Do

■ **Describe** five types of problems that can arise because of drug abuse or addiction.

Start Off Write

How can drug abuse affect your performance in school?

Trish and her brother Doug used to talk about everything, but lately Doug has been acting strangely. Then, after Trish's last baby-sitting job, all the money was gone from her purse. Trish suspects that Doug stole the money to buy drugs, and she isn't sure she can trust him anymore.

When a person abuses or becomes addicted to drugs, his or her relationships usually suffer. But damaged relationships, such as the one between Trish and Doug, are just one of the consequences of abusing drugs.

Problems with Family and Friends

Drug abuse does not affect just the people using drugs. It also affects the people in their lives. Drug abuse causes changes in a person's behavior, which can lead to problems at home. Teens who use drugs are likely to show anger toward family members. People who abuse drugs often have serious mood swings, which can make them difficult to talk to. They may have violent outbursts and become verbally or even physically abusive. Because they need money for drugs, people who abuse drugs often steal from family members. All of these behaviors can permanently damage family relationships.

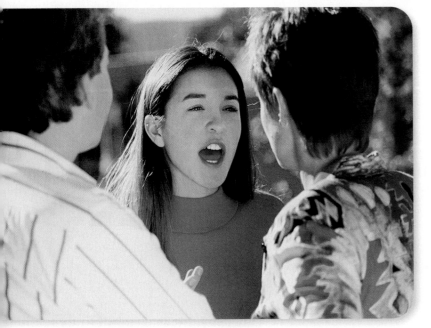

Figure 12 This teen's moods are affected by drug abuse. Her behavior is seriously damaging her family relationships.

Problems with other people aren't limited to the family. Teenagers who abuse or become addicted to drugs lose interest in activities that were once important to them. They also may begin to care less about the friends with whom they shared these activities. Friendships fall apart. At first, people who abuse drugs will spend time with new friends who share their interest in drugs. Eventually, they may find that they do not have any friends at all.

REPORT CARD

Subject	Grade
Mathematics	F
English	D
Social Studies	F
Science	F
Foreign Language	F
Music	D
Physical Education	D

Teacher Comments

William has difficulty concentrating and sticking to the task at hand. Without the ability to focus, his study habits are poor at best. I think it would be helpful for us to have a conference to discuss his behavior and study problems.

Parent Signature

x _____

Figure 13 A teen who abuses drugs will usually do poorly in school.

Problems at School

Most teens who abuse drugs begin to have serious problems at school. Most people who abuse drugs do not think or care about the future, and they lose their interest in education. In addition, learning becomes difficult for a person who abuses drugs. A person who abuses drugs will have difficulty concentrating, and he or she may forget from one day to the next what happened in class. Teens who abuse drugs usually stop doing homework, and their grades drop. They often skip school and school-related activities. When they are in school, they may interfere with the learning of others by disrupting classes. Teens who abuse drugs often get in trouble with school authorities. Many teens who abuse or become addicted to drugs eventually drop out of school.

Money Problems

Abusing drugs is expensive. Drugs cost a lot of money. As a person's drug problem gets worse, he or she will need more and more money. People who abuse or are addicted to drugs will often do anything to get money. Sometimes, the things they do are harmful to other people. They will lie or cheat. They will borrow or steal money or property from family members, friends, strangers, and even stores. A person who abuses drugs doesn't think about the possible consequences of these acts. To a person with a drug problem, respecting others' property is less important than getting drugs.

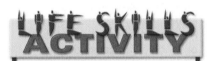

LIFE SKILLS ACTIVITY

MAKING GOOD DECISIONS

Research on the Internet or in the library how much money a person with a drug addiction spends on drugs each month. Then write a paper about how the money could be better spent. Give examples of other things that the money could be spent on.

Health Problems

Drug abuse and addiction are very harmful to the body. The abuse of certain drugs may cause sores on the mouth and skin. Many drugs cause damage to internal organs, such as the liver, kidneys, heart, and brain. Drugs that affect the brain can cause brain damage and memory loss. Abusing some drugs can lead to dangerous infections. For example, using dirty needles to do drugs can lead to HIV infection, which causes AIDS.

Drug abuse can also cause many mental and emotional problems. People who abuse drugs run a high risk of depression. Emotional problems, such as nervousness and fear, are also common. The chances of suicide or attempted suicide increase with drug abuse.

Figure 14 The Effects of Drug Abuse on the Body

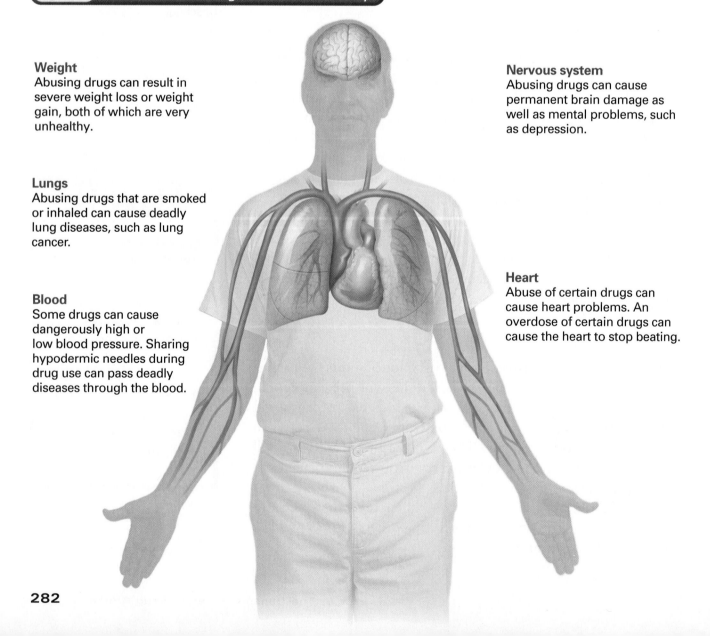

Weight
Abusing drugs can result in severe weight loss or weight gain, both of which are very unhealthy.

Lungs
Abusing drugs that are smoked or inhaled can cause deadly lung diseases, such as lung cancer.

Blood
Some drugs can cause dangerously high or low blood pressure. Sharing hypodermic needles during drug use can pass deadly diseases through the blood.

Nervous system
Abusing drugs can cause permanent brain damage as well as mental problems, such as depression.

Heart
Abuse of certain drugs can cause heart problems. An overdose of certain drugs can cause the heart to stop beating.

Problems with the Law

Some drugs are illegal. Even legal prescription drugs can be illegal if they are used improperly. Developing a problem with drug abuse or addiction can quickly lead to problems with the law. Getting arrested and going to court can affect a person's entire life. For example, if you have been convicted of a crime, it may be harder to find a job because many employers do not want to hire someone with a criminal record. A conviction for illegal drug use or a drug-related crime can also result in a jail sentence. Sentences for having or using illegal drugs are becoming more and more serious. And when it comes to illegal drugs, you have to get caught only once to go to jail. Time spent in jail not only means a loss of freedom. It can also mean the loss of dreams for the future.

Drug abuse can lead to other crimes as well. People with drug problems often steal to get drug money. They may begin by stealing from family members, but later they may steal from others. Theft and burglary are very serious crimes, and they carry very harsh punishments.

Another type of crime associated with drug abuse is driving under the influence, or DUI. When a person under the influence of drugs operates a car, he or she puts everyone on the road in danger. The law takes this action very seriously, especially if anyone is hurt or killed in a car accident.

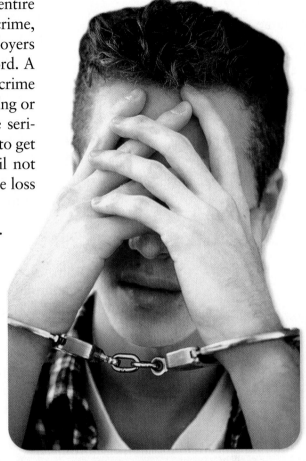

Figure 15 This teen has been arrested for having illegal drugs.

Lesson Review

Understanding Concepts

1. What types of problems can arise as a consequence of drug abuse?

2. How can drug abuse damage family relationships?

3. Why do people who abuse drugs have problems with money?

4. What are three ways that a person who uses drugs can get into trouble with the law?

Critical Thinking

5. **Making Inferences** Imagine that your dream is to become a professional athlete. Describe how drug abuse could affect these plans.

6. **Making Inferences** Driving under the influence puts others in danger. Describe another situation in which one person's drug use could put other people in danger.

Stimulants and Depressants

What You'll Do

- **Describe** the effects of stimulants.

- **Identify** dangers associated with the use of stimulants.

- **Describe** the effects of depressants.

- **Identify** dangers associated with the use of depressants.

Terms to Learn

- stimulant

- depressant

Start Off
Write

Why do people drink coffee in the morning? How does this relate to stimulants?

Dorie drank a can of cola at dinner. After dinner, she found that it was easier to pay attention to her homework. But when it was time to go to bed, Dorie couldn't sleep.

Dorie was experiencing the effects of caffeine, a drug found in the cola she drank. Caffeine is one drug in a group of drugs called *stimulants*. Stimulants (STIM yoo luhnts) and another group of drugs called *depressants* (dee PREHS uhnts) include some of the most commonly used and abused drugs.

Stimulants

Any drug that speeds up the activity of the heart and the brain is a **stimulant.** Stimulants increase blood pressure and heart rate and tighten blood vessels. Stimulants also raise the level of sugar in the blood. All of these changes make a user feel more awake and alert. Dangers of using stimulants include heart failure, brain damage, and stroke. Stimulants include legal drugs, such as caffeine and nicotine, and illegal drugs, such as cocaine and methamphetamine.

TABLE 1 Common Stimulants

Name	How it is taken	Effects	Dangers
Caffeine	found in many foods, such as chocolate and cola, and in some over-the-counter medicines; taken orally	alertness, energy, and ability to think more clearly	causes users to experience a "crash," or a feeling of illness or lack of energy after the drug has worn off
Nicotine	found in all tobacco products; can be smoked or taken orally	alertness, feeling of calm, mild *euphoria* (yoo FOR ee uh), or a sense of well-being	is very addictive; people addicted to nicotine abuse tobacco products, which can cause cancer and heart disease
Cocaine	taken by *snorting*, (inhaling through the nose), by injection, or by smoking	euphoria, alertness, or feeling of increased strength; causes users to crash and to crave more of the drug	is very addictive; can cause increased heart rate, anxiety, paranoia, or sudden death
Methamphetamine (crystal meth)	can be snorted, smoked, or injected	euphoria, alertness, or feeling of increased strength; effects last several hours	is very addictive; can cause increased heart rate, violent behavior, strokes, or death

Depressants

Any drug that causes activity in the body and brain to slow is called a **depressant.** The effects of depressants are opposite of the effects of stimulants. Depressants reduce heart rate, blood pressure, and breathing. People who take depressants become relaxed or sleepy and react slowly.

Many depressants are prescription drugs, such as Valium™ (VAL ee uhm) and Xanax™ (ZAN aks), that doctors use to treat problems with nervousness and sleeplessness. These drugs are all extremely addictive. Taking too much of a depressant can cause brain damage, heart failure, or death.

The most commonly used depressant is alcohol. Heavy alcohol use increases the risk of health problems such as heart disease, cancer, and liver damage. When taken with another depressant, alcohol is very dangerous. Misuse or abuse of any depressant can lead to both physical and psychological dependence.

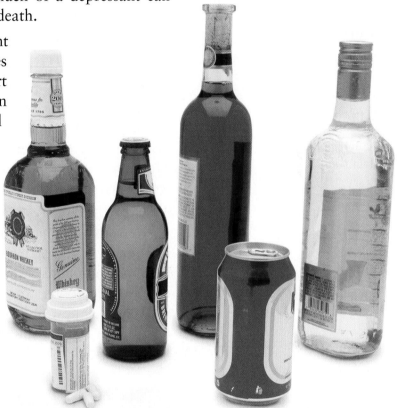

Figure 16 Depressants include different drugs, including alcohol, which is the most commonly used depressant.

Lesson Review

Using Vocabulary

1. What is a stimulant?

2. What is a depressant?

Understanding Concepts

3. Compare the effects of stimulants and depressants.

4. Describe three dangers of using stimulants and three dangers of using depressants.

Critical Thinking

5. **Making Inferences** How could you tell the difference between somebody who was using stimulants and somebody who was using depressants?

6. **Applying Concepts** Why is it dangerous to drive a car or operate heavy machinery while under the influence of alcohol?

Lesson 7

Marijuana

What You'll Do

- **Describe** the effects of marijuana.
- **Identify** the dangers of using marijuana.

Terms to Learn

- marijuana
- THC

Start Off *Write*

Is marijuana harmless? Explain your answer.

Ben wanted Samuel to smoke marijuana with him. Ben said he'd done it dozens of times and it was great. He told Samuel not to worry, nothing bad would happen. Samuel didn't know what to do.

Samuel needed more information about marijuana. Many people, such as Ben, will tell you that marijuana is totally harmless. But anyone who tells you that isn't telling you the whole truth.

What Is Marijuana?

Of all illegal drugs, marijuana may be the most widely used. But what is marijuana? **Marijuana** (mar uh WAH nuh) is the dried flowers and leaves of the *Cannabis* plant. Marijuana has a long history of use and now grows almost everywhere in the world. Marijuana has more than 200 slang names, including pot, grass, weed, green, and Mary Jane. Marijuana is usually smoked, although it can also be eaten.

The active chemical in marijuana is called **THC.** The way marijuana affects a person depends on how much THC the marijuana contains, how the marijuana is taken, and what the user's expectations are. Some people feel nothing. Others feel relaxed or happy. Still others have severe panic attacks or feel unable to move. Drinking alcohol or using other drugs at the same time increases the effects of marijuana.

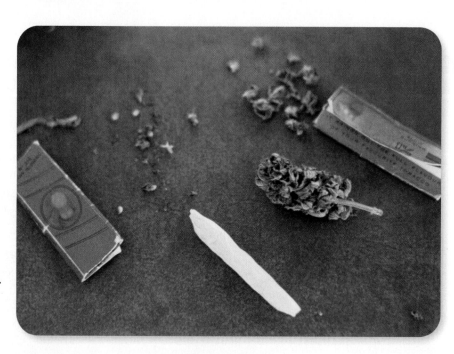

Figure 17 Marijuana is often wrapped in paper and smoked.

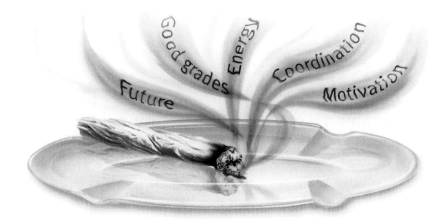

Figure 18 Smoking marijuana makes your health and dreams go up in smoke.

Is Marijuana Harmful?

Marijuana can cause many problems, both physical and psychological. The most common problems are the inability to concentrate and lack of motivation. For this reason, many people who use marijuana perform poorly in school or at work. Marijuana also affects coordination and the ability to react quickly. This effect makes many activities, such as driving and sports, difficult.

People who use marijuana for a long time become psychologically dependent on the drug. People who are psychologically dependent on marijuana are often irritable or unable to sleep if they do not use the drug. Long-term users also need to take more of the drug in order to get the same effect.

Long-term use of marijuana also causes physical damage. Smoking the drug can cause lung problems, including coughing, frequent colds, and lung cancer.

Lesson Review

Using Vocabulary

1. Describe the relationship between marijuana and THC.

Understanding Concepts

2. What are some of marijuana's effects? What can affect a person's reaction to this drug?

3. What physical and psychological problems can happen because of long-term marijuana use?

Critical Thinking

4. **Making Inferences** Some of the harmful effects of marijuana come from smoking the drug. Does that mean eating marijuana is safe? Explain your answer.

5. **Analyzing Ideas** If you could remove all of the THC from marijuana, would it be completely safe? Explain your answer.

Hallucinogens and Inhalants

Cameron's friend talked him into taking a drug called LSD at a party. Before long, Cameron was seeing and hearing things that didn't exist. He became very frightened and had to be taken to the hospital.

What You'll Do

■ **Identify** the dangers of using hallucinogens.

■ **Identify** the dangers of using inhalants.

Terms to Learn

• hallucinogen

• inhalant

Start Off
Write

Why is it dangerous to inhale household products?

LSD, the drug Cameron took, is also called *acid* and belongs to a group of drugs called *hallucinogens*. Hallucinogens (huh LOO si nuh juhns) and another group of drugs called *inhalants* (in HAY luhntz) can produce very strong effects. These effects come with some serious dangers.

Hallucinogens

Drugs that cause a person to sense things that don't actually exist are called **hallucinogens.** Examples of hallucinogens include LSD and magic mushrooms, also called *psilocybin*. Hallucinogens cause the user to experience events in a distorted way or to sense things that don't exist. Hallucinogens also affect the emotions. A person may feel several emotions at once or may swing rapidly from one emotion to another. Being on hallucinogens is often frightening and can cause panic or dangerous actions. Physical reactions to hallucinogens may include nausea, increased heart rate and blood pressure, and sweating.

One long-term effect of hallucinogens is called a flashback. A *flashback* is a sudden reliving of the hallucinogen experience. Flashbacks can happen any time—even months or years after a hallucinogen was last used.

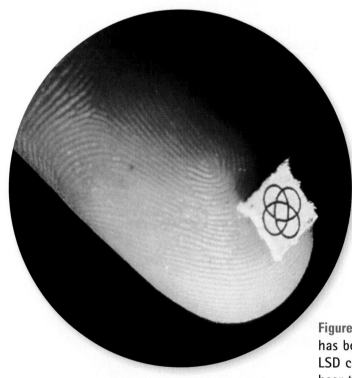

Figure 19 This piece of paper has been soaked in LSD. LSD can make you see or hear things that don't exist.

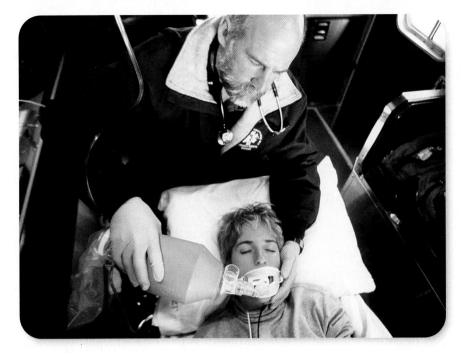

Figure 20 This teen tried inhalants only once, but that was all it took to damage her brain and almost kill her.

Inhalants

A very dangerous group of drugs that is increasing in popularity is called inhalants. **Inhalants** are drugs that are inhaled directly and that enter the bloodstream through the lungs. Inhalants do not include drugs that are smoked. Many products, including common household cleaning supplies, contain chemicals that can be used as inhalants.

When breathed in, inhalants replace the oxygen that goes to the brain. Because they prevent oxygen from reaching your brain, inhalants damage your brain with each use. Some inhalants can cause breathing to stop. Immediate death, coma, or serious brain damage can result from using inhalants just once.

The effects of inhalants are very intense but very short-lived. These effects can include hallucinations, numbness, and the inability to move.

Myth & Fact

Myth: Inhalants stay in your body for only a minute or two, which isn't long enough to do any real damage.

Fact: While the effects of inhalants last only a short while, these chemicals can remain in your body for weeks. Even if they were to remain in your body for only a minute or two, that length of time is more than enough time to kill brain cells, damage your lungs, or even stop your heart.

Lesson Review

Using Vocabulary

1. Define *hallucinogen*.

2. What is an inhalant?

Understanding Concepts

3. What are the main short-term and long-term dangers of using hallucinogens?

4. How do inhalants work on the body?

5. List five dangers of using inhalants.

Critical Thinking

6. **Analyzing Ideas** What kind of dangers could a hallucinogen flashback produce, even if it happened years after the drug was used?

Staying Drug Free

Raoul is a very fast runner. One day, he hopes to make it to the Olympics. Raoul turns down drugs when they are offered to him because he knows that using drugs could make his dream impossible.

What You'll Do

- **List** four reasons to remain drug free.
- **Identify** five ways to refuse drugs.
- **Describe** activities and skills that can help one avoid drugs.

Start Off
Write

How could using drugs negatively affect your plans for the future?

Raoul has a reason to stay drug free. He also knows how to resist the pressure to do drugs. By staying drug free, Raoul has a much better chance of making his dream come true.

Reasons to Be Drug Free

No one else is quite like you. Because you are unique, you will have your own reasons for wanting to stay drug free. Here are some of the best reasons to stay drug free. Perhaps one of these reasons works for you. Or maybe they all do!

- Drugs can damage your health. They can cause permanent effects, such as heart disease, brain damage, or emotional problems. Some drugs can even kill you.

- Drugs can mess up your body and your mind. They can interfere with your ability to succeed in sports and other activities. Drugs can also damage your memory and destroy your desire to accomplish things. As your ability to learn decreases, so will your success in school. A poor school record can limit your choices both now and later in life.

- Drugs can destroy your relationships. They can make you forget about the people who are close to you. You can lose interest in everything except drugs and can behave in ways that are harmful to you and your relationships with your family and friends.

- Drugs are illegal. Even legal drugs, such as nicotine and alcohol, are illegal for someone your age. If you use illegal drugs, you could be arrested. Using drugs can also lead to other illegal behaviors. Going to jail can ruin your future.

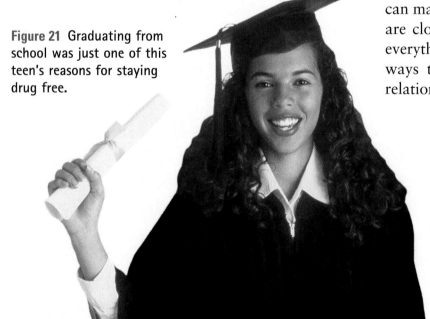

Figure 21 Graduating from school was just one of this teen's reasons for staying drug free.

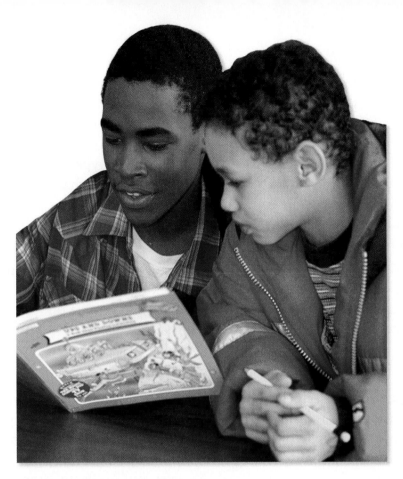

Figure 22 This teen is staying away from drugs by volunteering in his community.

Ways to Stay Drug Free

One of the best ways to protect yourself from drugs is to be involved in activities with others who want to stay drug free. Another way to stay drug free is to stay away from situations where there may be pressure to use drugs. Here are some ways to stay drug free.

- Participate in sports or get involved in school clubs or activities, such as drama or music.

- Develop a hobby, such as doing magic tricks, gardening, or making video movies.

- Get involved in community service by volunteering at a local daycare center or animal shelter.

- Play games with friends, read a book, or write a story.

- Identify students who you think are using drugs, and stay away from them. They may pressure you to do drugs.

- Identify places and situations where drugs are likely to be used, and stay away from these situations.

- Learn ways to handle stress in your life so you won't feel tempted to try to feel better by using drugs.

- Stay connected to a trusted adult, such as a parent, a coach, a relative, or a teacher.

Hands-on ACTIVITY

WHY STAY DRUG FREE?

1. Work in groups of two. Interview 10 people, which consist of both adults and students.
2. Ask each person why he or she wants to stay drug free. Record their answers.

Analysis

1. Categorize your results into four or five areas, such as health, family, education, and other responsibilities.
2. Illustrate your results by making a pie graph. What was the most popular reason for staying drug free?

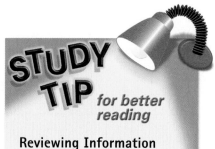

STUDY TIP for better reading

Reviewing Information
As you read the different ways to refuse drugs in the table on the next page, make a chart of your own. Draw a line down the middle of a sheet of paper. On one side, write down the ways to refuse drugs. On the other side, write a personal example of each way.

Refusing Drugs

At some point, people you know may pressure you to use drugs. If so, you are not alone. Even adults have this problem. Often, the people who pressure you are your friends, which can make it even more difficult to say no. When this type of situation arises, it is important to remember the reasons that you have decided to stay drug free. Think about all of the things that you could be giving up if you use drugs. Remember that it is up to you to protect your dreams and your future.

Knowing how to refuse drugs and get out of a pressure situation is also very important. You never know when you might be offered drugs, so it is best to be prepared. The table on the next page shows several different ways to refuse drugs.

Saying No Is OK

Once you've decided to refuse drugs, you can take pride in your decision. By refusing to take drugs, you are saying that you refuse to damage your mind, your relationships, and your future. You will discover that you are not alone in your decision. Not everyone is using drugs. In fact, most young people are NOT using drugs.

If someone stops being your friend just because you refuse to take drugs, that person was not a true friend to begin with. Remember that friendship is based on respect. Anyone who would force you to do something that could hurt you doesn't respect you.

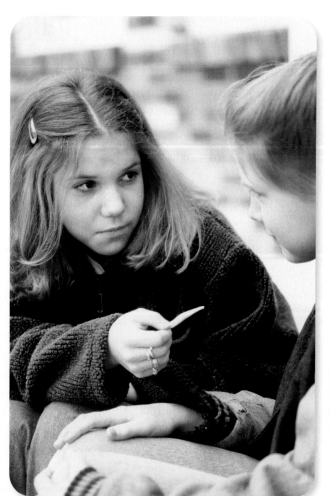

Figure 23 Knowing how to refuse drugs is important, especially when your friends pressure you to use drugs.

TABLE 2 Different Ways to Refuse Drugs

Refusal skill	How it works
Say, "No, thank you."	Very clearly explain to the person who is offering you drugs that you don't want to take them. This is the clearest and easiest way to refuse drugs.
Give a reason.	Explain to the person why you can't take the drugs or why you don't want to take them. Say something like, "I have a big test tomorrow," or "I'm on the track team, and that stuff will just slow me down."
State the consequences.	Describe some of the consequences that may occur if you used the drug offered to you. Say something like, "I would be grounded for a month if I did drugs," or "That stuff could mess up my mind or even kill me!" This might make the person offering the drugs think twice about using the drugs.
Suggest another activity.	Come up with an idea for something that you could do that doesn't involve taking drugs. You could suggest going to a movie, playing a game, going shopping, going to get something to eat, or going for a walk in the park. Try to suggest something fun so that the temptation to use drugs will be less.
Walk away.	If all of your other strategies fail, just walk away from the situation. Nobody can pressure you to do drugs if you aren't there.

Health Journal

Describe a time when you had to say no to a friend. What did you say to convince your friend that you meant no?

Lesson Review

Understanding Concepts

1. How can using drugs affect a person's future?

2. What are four different actions you can take to help keep yourself drug free?

3. List five ways to refuse drugs.

4. What is one reason that you want to stay drug free? Use a reason that is not listed in the text.

Critical Thinking

5. **Analyzing Ideas** Describe an out-of-school activity that you might be interested in. Describe how this activity could make you less likely to use drugs.

6. **Using Refusal Skills** Suppose a friend of yours is trying to get you to smoke marijuana, and he won't take no for an answer. Describe how you would handle this situation.

Chapter Summary

■ A drug is any substance other than food that changes a person's physical or psychological state. ■ Drugs can enter your body in several different ways. ■ Some medicines require a prescription from a doctor, while others do not. ■ Carefully follow all instructions when taking any medicine. ■ Drug abuse is misusing a legal drug on purpose or using any illegal drug. ■ Drug abuse can lead to drug addiction. ■ Drug addiction can cause problems with relationships, money, health, and the law. ■ There are many good reasons to stay drug free, and everyone's reasons will be different. ■ Knowing how to avoid drugs and how to refuse drugs will help you stay drug free.

Using Vocabulary

For each pair of terms, describe how the meanings of the terms differ.

1 drug/medicine

2 prescription medicine/over-the-counter medicine

3 drug misuse/drug abuse

4 physical dependence/psychological dependence

For each sentence, fill in the blank with the proper word from the word bank provided below.

hallucinogen	stimulant
medicine	marijuana
drug addiction	withdrawal

5 A drug that is used to treat disease, injury, or pain is a(n) ___.

6 A drug that speeds up the activity in your body is a(n) ___.

7 A(n) ___ is a drug that can make a person sense things that don't exist.

8 The dried leaves and flowers of the *Cannabis* plant are better known as ___.

Understanding Concepts

9 List the five ways that drugs enter the body, and briefly describe each way.

10 What four rules should you follow when taking medicine?

11 What is drug addiction, and how is it related to dependence?

12 What is withdrawal?

13 What dangers are involved in using marijuana?

14 In your own words, compare the effects of stimulants with the effects of depressants.

15 Explain how inhalants work and how this process presents dangers.

16 What are four reasons to stay drug free?

17 How can certain activities help keep you drug free?

18 Describe five ways to refuse drugs, and give an example of each.

19 What are the most common problems experienced by marijuana users?

Analyzing Ideas

20 Some medicines are sold in over-the-counter and prescription forms. What differences would you expect between these two forms of a medicine?

21 Pilar has been taking a prescription asthma medicine for a few days. She knows that she is supposed to use the medicine only twice a day, but she uses it four times a day because it really helps her asthma. Is Pilar misusing or abusing this drug? What should she do?

22 People who have used hallucinogens in the past may have a flashback at any time. What kind of dangers could an unexpected flashback cause?

23 Tyler is the captain of his school's academic team. Recently, Tyler's friends have started asking him to smoke marijuana with them. How could smoking marijuana affect Tyler's position on the team? Explain your answer.

Making Good Decisions

24 Imagine that a friend of yours has a prescription for a headache medicine. One day, you are having a bad headache, and you complain about it to your friend. He says that you should take some of his medicine because it works very well. He also says that it's safe for you to take the medicine because he has a prescription for it from a doctor. Is your friend right? Should you take his medicine? Explain your answer.

25 Alice has a prescription for a certain medicine. When she took the medicine to school, the label on the medicine fell off and she lost it. Alice is pretty sure that she remembers all of the instructions, but she isn't positive. Should she keep taking the medicine anyway? Explain.

26 Use what you have learned in this chapter to set a personal goal. Write your goal, and make an action plan by using the Health Behavior Contract for drugs. You can find the Health Behavior Contract at go.hrw.com. Just type in the keyword HD4HBC15.

Name _____ Class _____ Date _____

(Health Behavior Contract)
Teens and Drugs

My Goals: I, _____, will accomplish one or more of the following goals:
I will use medicines properly.
I will avoid situations in which I might be pressured to use drugs.
I will refuse drugs if they are offered to me.
Other: _____

My Reasons: By using medicines properly, I will avoid many health problems, such as drug abuse and addiction. By avoiding situations in which I may be pressured to use drugs and by refusing drugs if they are offered to me, I can protect myself from the problems that are caused by drug use.
Other: _____

My Values: Personal values that will help me meet my goals are
_____
_____

My Plan: The actions I will take to meet my goals are
_____
_____
_____
_____

Evaluation: I will use my Health Journal to keep a log of actions I took to fulfill this contract. After 1 month, I will evaluate my goals. I will adjust my plan if my goals are not being met. If my goals are being met, I will consider setting additional goals.
Signed _____
Date _____

Reading Checkup

Take a minute to review your answers to the Health IQ questions at the beginning of this chapter. How has reading this chapter improved your Health IQ?

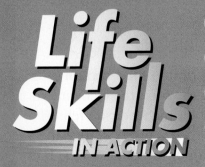

Life Skills IN ACTION

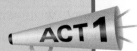

Coping

At times, everyone faces setbacks, disappointments, or other troubles. To deal with these problems, you have to learn how to cope. Coping is dealing with problems and emotions in an effective way. Complete the following activity to develop your coping skills.

The Drug Problem

Setting the Scene

Sasha's older sister Michelle is addicted to drugs. Their parents know about the problem and have been working with Michelle to break her habit. Michelle is having a hard time quitting, and she is often very moody. Michelle yells at Sasha a lot and sometimes refuses to talk to her. Sasha is unhappy about the situation with Michelle. She used to look up to Michelle, and they used to be good friends.

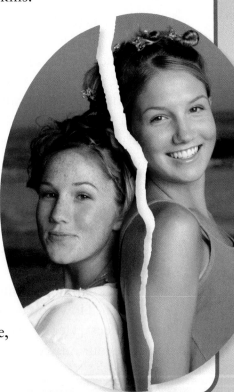

The **5** Steps of Coping

1. Identify the problem.
2. Identify your emotions.
3. Use positive self-talk.
4. Find ways to resolve the problem.
5. Talk to others to receive support.

Guided Practice

Practice with a Friend

Form a group of three. Have one person play the role of Sasha and another person play the role of one of Sasha's parents. Have the third person be an observer. Walking through each of the five steps of coping, role-play Sasha dealing with Michelle's drug addiction. When you reach step 5, Sasha should talk to one of her parents. The observer will take notes, which will include observations about what the person playing Sasha did well and suggestions of ways to improve. Stop after each step to evaluate the process.

Check Yourself

After you have completed the guided practice, go through Act 1 again without stopping at each step. Answer the questions below to review what you did.

1. What are some emotions that Sasha may have?

2. What could Sasha say to herself when using positive self-talk?

3. What are some ways that Sasha could solve her problem?

4. Why is it important for Sasha to talk to someone to receive support for her problem?

ACT 2

On Your Own

Sasha's family has been planning to take a long vacation at the beach. A week before they are scheduled to leave, Sasha's father tells her that they will not be going after all. Michelle is still receiving treatment for her drug problem, and her counselor thinks it would be best for Michelle if the entire family stays home. Sasha is very disappointed and wishes that Michelle wasn't her sister anymore. Write a short story that describes how Sasha uses the five steps of coping to deal with the cancelled vacation plans.

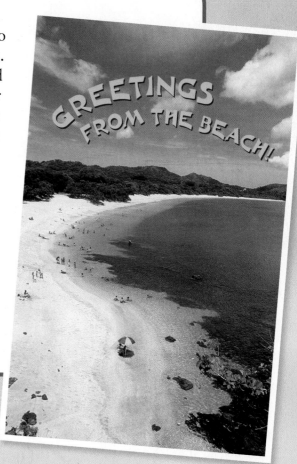

GREETINGS FROM THE BEACH!

CHAPTER 14

Infectious Diseases

Check out **Current Health** articles related to this chapter by visiting **go.hrw.com**. Just type in the keyword **HD4CH29**.

> " Last year, I got a **flu shot** and was one of the only kids in my class who didn't get **sick** and miss several days of **school**. This year, I wasn't so **lucky**. "

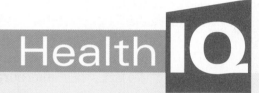

PRE-READING

Answer the following true/false questions to find out what you already know about infectious diseases. When you've finished this chapter, you'll have the opportunity to change your answers based on what you've learned.

1. The term *infectious diseases* refers to diseases that can be passed from person to person.

2. All infectious diseases are caused by tiny organisms called *bacteria*.

3. Antibiotics are drugs that are used to kill bacteria.

4. A common cold is actually an illness that is caused by many different viruses.

5. There is no way to prevent catching viral diseases.

6. *Abstinence* means "being very careful about who you have sex with."

7. HIV infection from blood transfusions is rare now, thanks to testing of donor blood.

8. HIV and AIDS exist only in America and Africa.

9. Frequent hand washing is a very useful tool against catching an infectious disease.

10. If you have a contagious disease, you should avoid public places, such as school.

11. Strep throat is caused by a virus.

12. There is no cure for AIDS at this time.

13. Tuberculosis is a disease of the past and is rarely seen today.

ANSWERS: 1. false; 2. false; 3. true; 4. true; 5. false; 6. false; 7. true; 8. false; 9. true; 10. true; 11. false; 12. false; 13. false

What Is an Infectious Disease?

What You'll Do

- **Describe** the difference between infectious diseases and contagious diseases.
- **List** four common ways that contagious diseases spread.

Terms to Learn

- infectious disease

Start Off *Write*

How does a cold or flu spread from one person to another?

Daryl went to visit his friend Hector, who had been sick for several days. Daryl stayed and talked to Hector for only a few minutes. A few days later, Daryl had the same illness that Hector had. Why did Daryl get sick?

Daryl became ill because the tiny organisms that were making his friend sick infected Daryl's body, too.

Infectious Diseases

Daryl caught an infectious disease. An **infectious disease** (in FEK shuhs dih ZEEZ) is an illness that is caused by microorganisms. *Microorganisms* (MY kroh AWR guhn iz uhmz) are very small things that are found everywhere. Most microorganisms do not cause disease. In fact, there are millions of microorganisms in your body all of the time. Many of these microorganisms help your body function normally.

However, certain microorganisms do cause infectious diseases. Infectious diseases that can spread directly or indirectly from one person to another are called *contagious* diseases. Contagious diseases include sexually transmitted diseases (STDs) and many common infections, such as colds and influenza. However, not all infectious diseases are contagious.

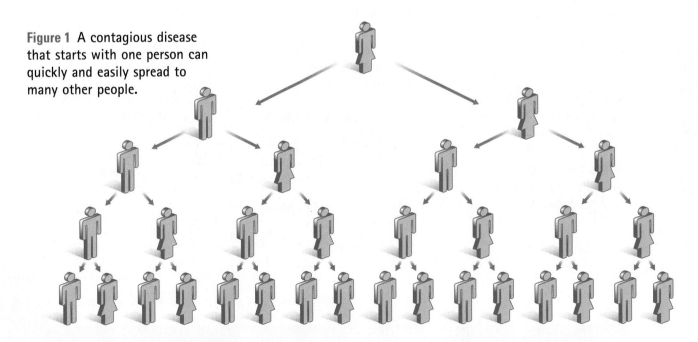

Figure 1 A contagious disease that starts with one person can quickly and easily spread to many other people.

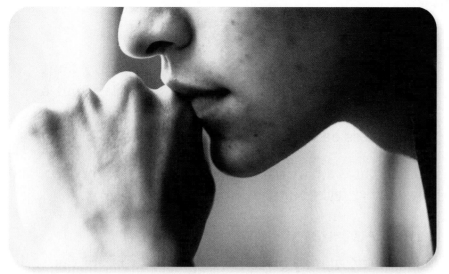

Figure 2 Touching your face passes germs from your hands to your mouth, nose, or eyes.

How Diseases Spread

Infections can come from another person, an animal, or an object. Once you have an infection, you can spread it in many ways. Here are a few of the most common ways that infections are spread.

- **Touching** Your hands are often covered in germs. Germs can be easily passed to people or objects by touching.

- **Coughing or Sneezing** Coughing or sneezing releases many germs into the air. Nearby people can inhale these germs.

- **Sharing** Sharing is usually a good thing, but sharing an infection is not. You can easily catch or spread an infection by sharing objects or food and drink with another person.

- **Sexual Contact** Certain infections are spread through sexual contact.

Hands-on ACTIVITY

INFECTIOUS HANDSHAKE

1. Your teacher will secretly select a member of your class to be a "disease carrier." This person will give a special handshake.
2. Everybody will shake hands. If you receive the secret handshake, you must give this handshake to anyone else whose hand you shake.
3. After everyone has shaken hands with five people, the people who received the secret hand-shake will raise their hands.

Analysis

1. Figure out the percentage of students who caught the "disease."

Lesson Review

Using Vocabulary

1. List three infectious diseases that can be passed from person to person.

2. What is a *contagious* disease?

Understanding Concepts

3. List four ways that contagious diseases can be spread. Give three examples of contagious diseases.

Critical Thinking

4. **Identifying Relationships** Not all infectious diseases are contagious. Are all contagious diseases infectious? Explain your answer.

5. **Making Inferences** Steven caught an infectious disease from eating a piece of meat that had gone bad. Is this type of disease contagious? Explain your answer.

What You'll Do

- **Identify** three common bacterial infections and their symptoms.
- **List** five ways to avoid bacterial infections.
- **Describe** one way to treat bacterial infections.

Terms to Learn

- bacteria
- antibiotic

Start Off
Write

How are bacterial infections treated?

Bacterial Infections

Tina's throat started hurting so badly that Tina could barely swallow. She also had a fever. Her doctor told her that she had an illness called strep throat.

Strep throat is a bacterial infection. But what are bacteria, and how do they make a person ill?

What Are Bacteria?

Some of the most common infectious diseases are caused by bacteria. **Bacteria** (bak TIR ee uh) are very simple single-celled microorganisms that are found everywhere. Bacteria reproduce very quickly by dividing in half. One bacterium can divide into two identical bacteria in as little as 20 minutes. Because they can reproduce so rapidly, a few bacteria can often cause a serious infection very quickly. Bacteria invade a host, such as a human, animal, or plant. Once inside the host, the bacteria get nutrients from the host's cells. In the process, the bacteria may cause damage to the host. If left untreated, bacterial infections can be very serious or deadly.

Figure 3 A single bacterium can double once every 20 minutes. At this rate, a single bacterium may become 4,096 bacteria in only 4 hours.

1 Bacterium
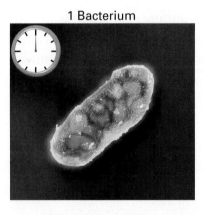

8 Bacteria
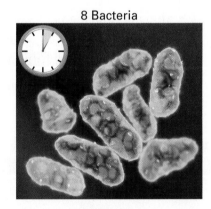

64 Bacteria
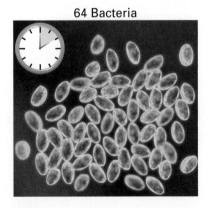

512 Bacteria
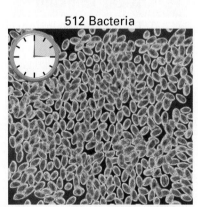

4096 Bacteria
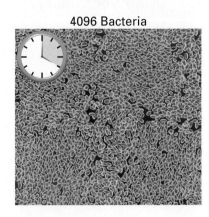

Strep Throat

Strep throat is caused by a type of bacterium called *streptococcus* (STREP tuh CAHK uhs). Although strep throat infections most commonly cause pain in the throat, these infections can also cause body aches elsewhere. The main symptom of strep throat is pain when you try to swallow. Most people also have a fever with strep throat.

If your doctor thinks you might have strep throat, he or she may take a throat culture. A *throat culture* is a test in which a doctor uses a cotton swab to wipe the back of the throat. The material on the swab is then tested for strep bacteria. If the throat culture shows that you have strep throat, the doctor will give you medicine to fight the bacteria. Take all of the medicine even if you feel better in a few days. You must take all of the medicine to make sure that all infectious bacteria have been killed. If strep throat infections are not treated properly, they can cause a condition called *rheumatic fever*. This disease can affect your heart valves and large joints. It can make you sick long after the sore throat is gone.

Figure 4 The throat in the picture on the bottom is healthy. The throat in the top picture is infected with bacteria that cause strep throat.

Sinus Infections

The *sinuses* (SIEN uhs uhz) are spaces located within the front of the skull. There are several pairs of sinuses located in the front of the head, above the mouth. Most, but not all, of the sinuses have a small tube that drains fluid down into the nose or throat. If this tube gets blocked by something, the sinus can become clogged. Clogging of the sinuses can cause the sinuses to become inflamed, which means that they swell and begin to hurt. This inflammation of a sinus is called *sinusitis* (SIEN uhs IET is).

Sinusitis is often caused by bacterial infections. These infections can be caused by many different types of bacteria. Bacterial sinus infections are rarely transmitted from person to person. In other words, bacterial sinus infections are usually not contagious. Often, sinusitis may be confused with colds or flu. The symptoms of sinusitis include congestion, a runny nose, a fever, or a headache. If you have bacterial sinusitis, your doctor will give you medicine to kill the bacteria.

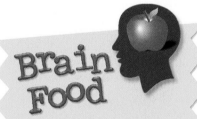

Brain Food

Most bacteria are completely harmless. In fact, there are millions of bacteria in your body right now. Some of these bacteria are necessary for your body to work correctly. For example, bacteria in your intestines play an important role in digestion of your food.

Tuberculosis

Tuberculosis is a serious disease caused by a slow-growing bacterium. This bacterium is in the family of long, thin bacteria called *mycobacteria*. People who have tuberculosis may feel very tired and may have a fever, night sweats, and a cough. Tuberculosis is usually spread through a very contagious cough. However some people with tuberculosis have few or no symptoms. Their tuberculosis is said to be inactive. A person who has inactive tuberculosis cannot pass the disease to others. Your doctor can find out if you have been exposed to tuberculosis by doing a simple test. During this test, your doctor injects a small amount of a special fluid under your skin. If you have been exposed to tuberculosis, your skin will have a reaction to this fluid. Tuberculosis kills about 3 million people a year worldwide. Because tuberculosis is so contagious, all cases must be reported to the health department.

Avoiding Bacterial Infections

There are many ways to reduce your chances of getting a bacterial infection. The best ways are listed below.

- Limit your contact with people who have a bacterial infection.
- Avoid sharing food or drink with others, especially if they have an infection.
- Wash your hands frequently and carefully with soap and warm water.
- Take warm showers frequently.
- Be sure to eat properly and get enough sleep. Then your body will be stronger and more able to fight infections.

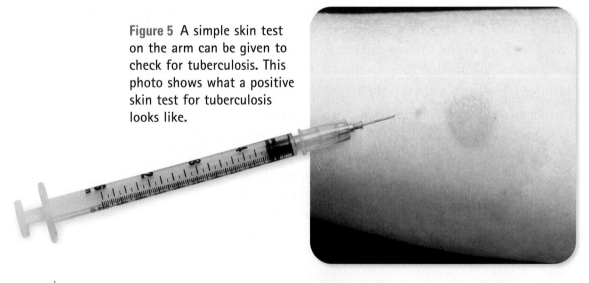

Figure 5 A simple skin test on the arm can be given to check for tuberculosis. This photo shows what a positive skin test for tuberculosis looks like.

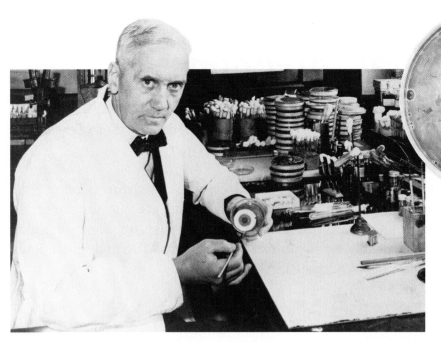

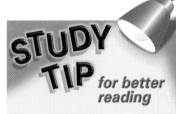

Figure 6 Alexander Fleming discovered penicillin when he noticed that bacteria in a dish were dying around a spot where a mold was growing.

Antibiotics

Fortunately for the millions of people who develop bacterial infections each year, doctors can treat these infections with antibiotics. An **antibiotic** is a drug that can kill bacteria or slow the growth of bacteria. Antibiotics are made naturally by many different organisms, such as other bacteria and molds. Humans have used these substances to fight dangerous bacteria. Penicillin, the first antibiotic, was discovered by accident in 1928. This discovery happened when a scientist named Alexander Fleming noticed that bacteria in a Petri dish were dying where a mold was growing. But it wasn't until the 1940's that antibiotics became available to many people. If you take an antibiotic, you should follow the doctor's instructions carefully. Complete all of the antibiotics. This will ensure that you get rid of all of the bacteria that are making you sick.

Lesson Review

Using Vocabulary

1. What are bacteria?

2. What is an antibiotic?

Understanding Concepts

3. Identify three common bacterial infections, and describe their symptoms.

4. What are five things you can do to keep from catching or spreading a bacterial infection?

Critical Thinking

5. Making Inferences Look at the figure on the first page of this lesson. Why were so many more bacteria produced in the fourth hour than were produced in the first hour?

internet connect

www.scilinks.org/health
Topic: Bacteria

HealthLinks code: HD4012

HEALTH LINKS. Maintained by the National Science Teachers Association

Viral Infections

Have you ever had a cold? Probably; most people are sick with a cold about twice a year. But what causes colds?

The common cold is caused by a virus. A **virus** is one of the smallest and simplest disease-causing agents. Viruses are everywhere. They are responsible for many diseases, some of which can be deadly. For example, viruses cause AIDS and severe acute respiratory syndrome (SARS).

Are Viruses Alive?

Most scientists do not consider viruses to be living things. Like living things, viruses contain proteins and genetic material. *Genetic material* is chemical information that is passed on during reproduction. However, unlike living things, a virus cannot reproduce on its own. A virus must reproduce by invading a living thing, such as an animal or person. The virus then uses the organism's cells to produce more viruses. When viruses invade your cells and use them to produce more viruses, a viral infection occurs. Viruses can be passed by touching living or nonliving objects, coughing, sneezing, insect bites, blood, or sexual contact.

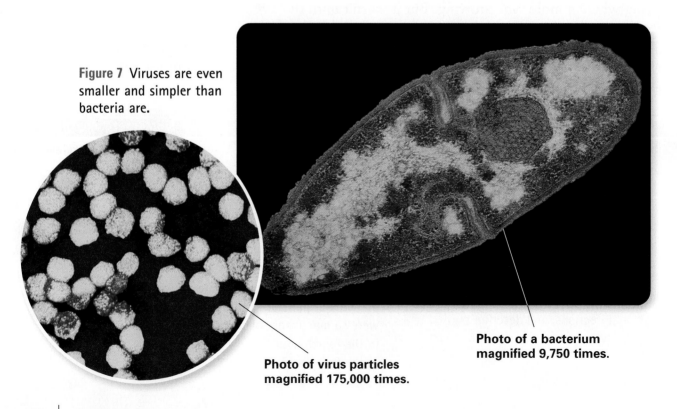

Figure 7 Viruses are even smaller and simpler than bacteria are.

Photo of virus particles magnified 175,000 times.

Photo of a bacterium magnified 9,750 times.

TABLE 1 The Symptoms of Common Infections	
Infections	**Symptoms**
A common cold	congestion, runny nose, sore throat, sneezing, and coughing
Influenza	body aches, headaches, high fever, chills, congestion, cough, and sore throat
Viral sinus infection	congestion, runny nose with thick mucus, high fever, and headache

The Common Cold

The most common viral infection is the cold. The common cold is actually caused by many different kinds of viruses. On average, each person gets about two colds a year. Colds are spread from person to person by coughing, sneezing, or touching. The symptoms of a cold include congestion, a runny nose, a sore throat, sneezing, and coughing. There are many medicines that can treat the symptoms of a cold. If you have a cold, you should drink a lot of fluid and get plenty of rest. Because colds are very contagious, you should also stay away from school or other public places if you have a cold.

Influenza

Influenza, or the "flu," is a viral infection that is very common in the winter months. There are three types of influenza, each of which has many different *strains,* or variations. Like the common cold, the flu is spread by touching, coughing, or sneezing. The symptoms of the flu include body aches, headaches, a high fever, chills, congestion, cough, and a sore throat. When you have the flu, you may have any or all of these symptoms. Many of these symptoms are similar to cold symptoms. A high fever is the main difference between the two viral infections. If you think that you might have the flu, you should talk to your doctor right away.

It is hard to predict when an influenza outbreak will happen. The number of flu cases varies from year to year. One way to avoid the flu is to be given a vaccine. A **vaccine** is a substance that helps the body build a resistance to a certain disease. Vaccines cannot completely stop the spread of a virus. In fact, a new flu vaccine must be developed every year because new strains of the flu develop every year. Receiving the flu vaccine one year may not protect you against the flu the next year.

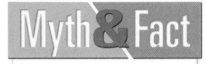

Myth: You catch a cold when you are out in cold or wet weather.

Fact: Colds are caused by viruses, not by the weather.

Health Journal

Have you ever received a flu vaccine? How did you feel after you received the shot? Did you get the flu that season? Write about the experience in your Health Journal.

Mononucleosis

Mononucleosis (MAHN oh NOO klee OH sis), also known as *mono* or the *kissing disease,* is caused by a virus called the *Epstein-Barr virus,* or EBV. In the United States, mono is most common in older teens and young adults. EBV is spread from person to person by coughing, sneezing, kissing, or sharing food and drink. Mononucleosis can make you tired for weeks. It can also give you a bad sore throat, a fever, a swollen spleen, and swollen lymph nodes. *Lymph nodes* are small oval structures located throughout the body that help remove harmful substances from the fluids surrounding your cells. About three-fourths of the people who get infected with mononucleosis have no symptoms at all. People who have mononucleosis but have no symptoms can still pass the disease to others.

Fighting Viral Infections

Most viral infections will make you uncomfortable but will do little harm. However, some viral infections can cause more serious problems, especially for babies, older people, and people who get sick easily. Your body has many defenses and natural chemicals that successfully fight off viral infections. For example, your saliva contains chemicals that help kill some viruses. The mucus in your nose also traps viruses and keeps them from getting into your body. Antiviral drugs are now available to treat a few viral infections. Most viral infections run their course while you take care of your body with extra rest.

Science ACTIVITY

The Epstein-Barr virus has been linked to diseases other than mono. Research this virus, and describe two other diseases (or syndromes) associated with EBV.

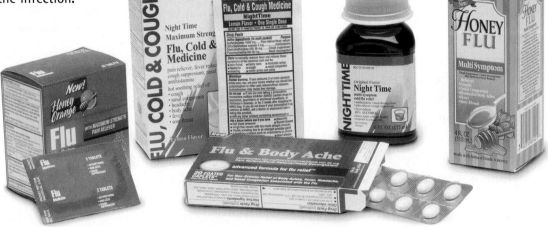

Figure 8 Most flu "remedies" do not cure the flu. Rather, they treat only the symptoms of the infection.

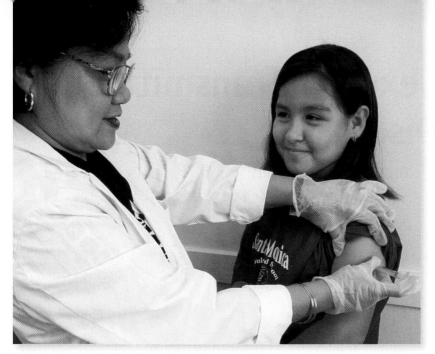

LIFE SKILLS ACTIVITY

PRACTICING WELLNESS

Talk to your parents or guardians about which vaccinations you have had recently. Find out when you were vaccinated and when you are supposed to receive additional vaccinations. Make a chart for yourself that contains all of this information.

Getting Your Shots

The best tools available to prevent viral diseases are vaccines. Today, vaccines are used all over the world to prevent many serious diseases. A vaccine contains viruses or parts of viruses that have been specially treated so that they don't make you sick. Instead of infecting you with a virus, vaccines fool your body into thinking it has been infected. This causes your body to produce chemicals to fight the infection. These chemicals then give you protection from the real virus. Although common vaccines can sometimes—though very rarely—cause harm, their benefits far outweigh their risks. Students are often legally required to get vaccines before they are allowed to go to school. Some vaccines require only one or two doses, but others, like the flu vaccine, should be received every year. Your doctor can tell you if you have had all of the shots that you need.

Lesson Review

Using Vocabulary

1. What is a virus?

2. What is a vaccine?

Understanding Concepts

3. How do viruses reproduce?

4. Identify three common viral infections, and describe the symptoms of each one.

5. How do the symptoms of influenza differ from the symptoms of a common cold?

Critical Thinking

6. **Making Good Decisions** Your mom has made an appointment for you to get a flu shot at the clinic. But you just had one last year. Will last year's shot prevent the flu this year? Explain your answer.

🖷 internet connect

www.scilinks.org/health
Topic: Viruses
HealthLinks code: HD4104

HEALTH LINKS Maintained by the National Science Teachers Association

Sexually Transmitted Diseases

One in every four people newly infected with a sexually transmitted disease is a teenager!

Every year there are millions of new cases of diseases that are spread through sexual contact. Many of these diseases not only are painful, but several of them also have no cure.

What Are STDs?

Herpes is just one of the incurable diseases that can be sexually transmitted. A **sexually transmitted disease** (STD) is any disease that can be passed from person to person by any form of sexual contact. STDs can be caused by bacteria, viruses, fungi, or parasites.

The symptoms of STDs vary. Some STDs cause very serious and painful symptoms. Other STDs cause no symptoms at all in some people. This means that a person with an STD can sometimes not know that he or she has the infection. This person can then unknowingly spread the disease to others. If untreated, some STDs can cause lasting pain and *infertility,* or the inability to produce children. Other STDs can cause brain damage, paralysis, and death. The only sure way to protect yourself from these diseases is to practice sexual abstinence. **Sexual abstinence** is the refusal to take part in sexual activity.

What You'll Do

- **Explain** what a sexually transmitted disease is.
- **Identify** seven common sexually transmitted diseases.
- **Explain** the difference between HIV and AIDS.
- **Identify** four ways that HIV can be passed from person to person.

Terms to Learn

- sexually transmitted disease (STD)
- sexual abstinence
- AIDS
- HIV

Start Off Write

How many STDs have you heard of? List them.

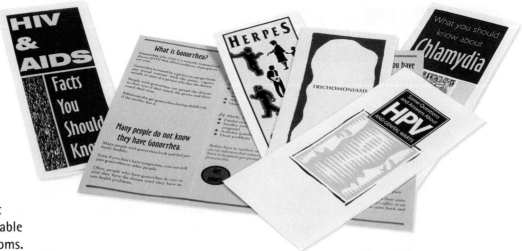

Figure 10 There is a great deal of information available on STDs and their symptoms.

Common STDs

You might think that STDs are dangerous but rare. Nothing could be farther from the truth. STDs are very common. In fact, statistics show that one out of every five people in the United States has an STD. Because STDs are so common, practicing sexual abstinence is very important. Sexual abstinence is the only way to stay completely safe from STDs. Table 2 gives information on the most common STDs and what they do to your body.

TABLE 2 Common Sexually Transmitted Diseases

Disease	Symptoms	Treatment or cure	Long-term consequences
Chlamydia (kluh MID ee uh)	Some people show no symptoms, especially women; others have a discharge from the genitals, painful urination and severe abdominal pain.	Chlamydia can be cured with antibiotics taken by mouth.	If left untreated, chlamydia can cause sterility; damage to the prostate gland, seminal vesicles, and testicles; and complications during pregnancy.
Human papilloma-virus (HPV) (HYOO muhn PAP i LOH muh vie ruhs)	Some people show no symptoms, others have warts on the genital area, and women have an abnormal Pap-smear test.	HPV can be treated, but not cured; sometimes, warts can be removed; Pap-smear tests help to identify precancerous conditions.	HPV can cause cervical cancer in women.
Genital herpes (JEN i tuhl HUHR PEEZ)	Symptoms include outbreaks of painful blisters or sores around the genital area that recur, swelling in the genital area, and burning during urination.	Genital herpes cannot be cured. Treatment with antiviral medicines can decrease the length and frequency of outbreaks, and can decrease the spread of herpes.	Herpes may cause cervical cancer in women; can cause deformities in unborn babies.
Gonorrhea (GAHN uh REE uh)	Some people show no symptoms; others have a discharge from the genitals, painful urination, and severe abdominal pain.	Gonorrhea can be cured with antibiotics, although a new strain of this bacteria has shown resistance to antibiotics.	If left untreated, gonorrhea can cause sterility, can cause liver disease, and can spread to the blood and joints.
Syphilis (SIF uh lis)	Symptoms, if present, may include sores, fever, body rash, and swollen lymph nodes.	Syphilis can be cured with antibiotics.	If left untreated, syphilis can cause mental illness, heart and kidney damage, and death.
Trichomoniasis (TRIK oh moh NIE uh sis)	Symptoms include itching, discharge from the genitals, and painful urination.	Trichomoniasis can be cured with medication.	Trichomoniasis has been linked to an increased risk of infection by HIV.

HIV and AIDS

Even though many STDs are painful and often incurable, they are not usually fatal diseases. However, unlike most STDs, AIDS is a deadly disease. **AIDS,** or acquired immune deficiency syndrome (uh KWIERD im MYOON dee FISH uhn see SIN DROHM), is a disease that is caused by HIV (human immunodeficiency virus), an infectious virus. **HIV** is a virus that attacks the immune system, which is the group of cells and tissues that defends your body against disease. As HIV infects a person, it slowly destroys the person's ability to fight disease. Once a person is infected with HIV, the infection does not go away. Eventually, the patient starts to develop the symptoms of AIDS. The symptoms of AIDS vary widely and can include such things as fever, weight loss, and sores covering the body. Once a person develops AIDS, he or she becomes gradually more and more ill. Eventually, he or she dies. People who die from AIDS actually die from secondary infections, such as pneumonia, that AIDS has left their body unable to fight. There are now combinations of drugs to treat HIV and AIDS as well as the related infections. Although very unpleasant and expensive, these treatments have extended the lives of many patients. However, as of the writing of this book, there is no cure for HIV or AIDS.

How HIV Is Spread

You can protect yourself from AIDS by avoiding exposure to HIV. HIV is spread in several of the following ways:

- **Sexual Contact** HIV is most often spread through exchange of bodily fluids during sexual intercourse.

- **Mother to Child** A mother can spread HIV to her unborn child while she is pregnant or to her child while she is breast-feeding.

- **Drug Use** Many people are infected by sharing hypodermic needles while using illegal drugs.

- **Blood Transfusion** Some people are infected through blood transfusions at hospitals. This type of infection is now extremely rare, because all blood in this country is tested for diseases before it is used.

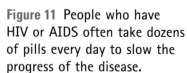

Myth: You can get HIV by using a toilet after somebody who has HIV.

Fact: HIV can only be passed in certain ways. You cannot get HIV by using a toilet after anybody.

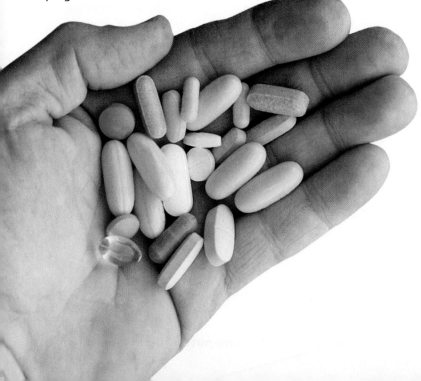

Figure 11 People who have HIV or AIDS often take dozens of pills every day to slow the progress of the disease.

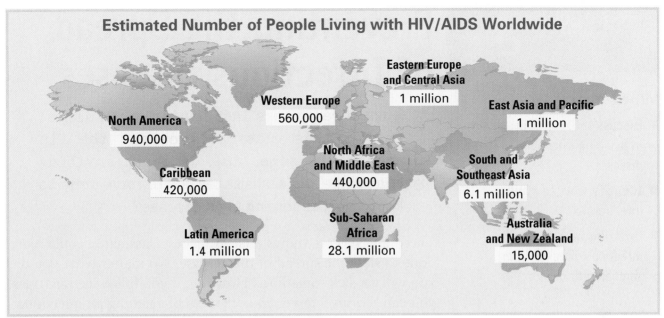

Estimated Number of People Living with HIV/AIDS Worldwide

North America
940,000

Western Europe
560,000

Eastern Europe
and Central Asia
1 million

East Asia and Pacific
1 million

Caribbean
420,000

North Africa
and Middle East
440,000

South and
Southeast Asia
6.1 million

Latin America
1.4 million

Sub-Saharan
Africa
28.1 million

Australia
and New Zealand
15,000

Source: Joint United Nations Program on HIV/AIDS.

Figure 12 Since the HIV/AIDS epidemic started, the disease has spread to every continent and has claimed tens of millions of victims.

The HIV/AIDS Problem

Since the first AIDS cases were reported in 1981, the disease has spread worldwide. Cases are now reported from virtually every country in the world. Africa has been hit very hard, but the number of cases is rising everywhere. HIV infection is increasing most quickly in poorer countries, where education and healthcare are lacking.

If you think you might have been exposed to HIV, you should be tested for the virus. There are several very simple tests to detect HIV infection. HIV is not transmitted by casual contact. So do not be afraid to show your love to people who are infected with this deadly disease.

Lesson Review

Using Vocabulary

1. What is a sexually transmitted disease?

2. Define *sexual abstinence* in your own words.

Understanding Concepts

3. What are some symptoms common among the STDs listed in the table on the second page of this lesson?

4. What is the difference between HIV and AIDS?

5. Describe four ways that HIV can spread from person to person.

Critical Thinking

6. Making Inferences HIV is spreading more quickly now than it was in the early 1980s. Why might HIV spread to more people per year now than it did in the 1980s?

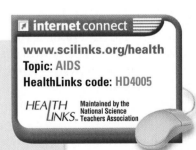

internet connect

www.scilinks.org/health

Topic: AIDS

HealthLinks code: HD4005

HEALTH
LINKS

Maintained by the
National Science
Teachers Association

Preventing the Spread of Infectious Diseases

What You'll Do

- **Discuss** the role of hygiene in avoiding infectious diseases.

- **Identify** ways to avoid infection.

- **Describe** ways to prevent infectious diseases from spreading to others.

Start Off Write

What can you do to prevent the spread of a disease?

Angelo remembers last winter, when almost half of his classmates caught the flu around the same time. Is there anything that Angelo's classmates could have done to keep from catching this disease?

There are several things that Angelo's classmates could have done to slow the spread of this disease. No matter what you do, you will get sick sometimes. However, if you follow certain rules, you can seriously lower your chances of catching an infection.

Keeping Clean

The first step you can take to prevent the spread of a disease is to practice good hygiene. Remember that contagious infections are spread more often by touch than by any other method. Wash your hands before you eat. Germs that collect on your hands can infect you when you touch your mouth, eyes, or nose or when you eat. Every time you use the bathroom, wash your hands with soap and warm water. If your hands get dirty, wash them as soon as you can. Also be sure to take warm showers regularly. Showering with soap washes off many of the germs that are on your body, lowering your risk of infection.

Figure 13 Washing your hands regularly with soap and warm water lowers your risk of infection.

▶ Always use soap because washing your hands with water alone does not kill germs.

▶ Use warm water.

▶ Scrub your hands with soap for at least 20 seconds. Pay attention to your fingernails, where germs may be trapped.

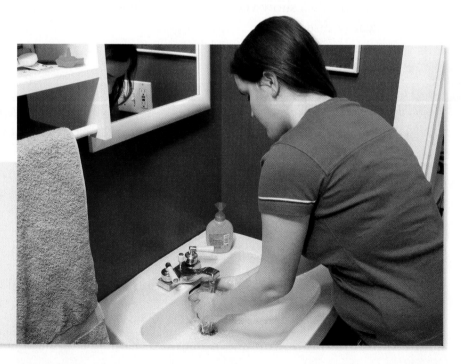

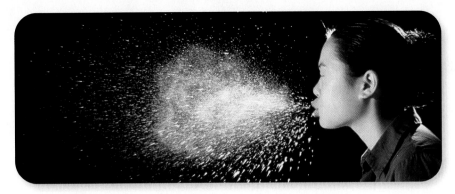

Figure 14 When a person sneezes, he or she can release millions of germs into the air.

Avoiding Infection

The only sure way to avoid an infectious disease is to stay away from the source of the infection. However, this is not always possible. If you must be around somebody who has a contagious infection, do the following things to protect yourself:

- Keep distance so that you don't get infected by a cough or sneeze.

- Avoid sharing food or drink with the infected person.

- If you touch the infected person or objects that he or she has touched, wash your hands with soap and warm water.

Protecting Others

When you have a contagious illness, you should do certain things to keep from infecting others. First, if you feel ill, you should stay away from school or other public places until you start to feel better. By going to school, you could spread the infection to many of your classmates. If you do have to be around other people, remember not to touch others or share food and drink with them. Also, remember to cover your mouth when you cough or sneeze.

Myth & Fact

Myth: You should cover your mouth and nose with your hand when coughing or sneezing.

Fact: You should cover your mouth or nose with the inner part of your elbow or with a tissue. This keeps the germs from getting on your hands, where they could be easily passed to others.

Lesson Review

Understanding Concepts

1. How does washing your hands lower your risk of catching an infectious disease?

2. How should you protect yourself if somebody around you has a contagious infection?

3. What are three things you can do to protect others from infection?

Critical Thinking

4. **Making Good Decisions** Imagine that you are on the soccer team. You have a big game coming up. You need to go to practice, but you are sick. You don't feel that bad, though. And you don't have a fever. Should you go to practice anyway? Explain.

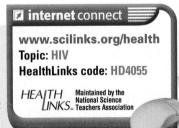

internet connect

www.scilinks.org/health
Topic: HIV
HealthLinks code: HD4055

HEALTH LINKS. Maintained by the National Science Teachers Association

Chapter Summary

■ Infectious diseases are caused by microorganisms and viruses. ■ Some infectious diseases are contagious, which means that they can be passed from person to person. ■ Many common infections are caused by bacteria, which are single-celled organisms that can reproduce quickly. ■ Antibiotics are drugs that kill bacteria or slow the growth of bacteria. ■ Many common infections are caused by viruses, which are extremely small disease-causing agents. ■ Some infections are passed from person to person through sexual contact. ■ AIDS is a deadly disease that is caused by HIV, a virus. ■ You cannot avoid all infections, but certain behaviors can lower your risk of infection. ■ If you have a contagious infection, you should try to avoid passing it to others.

Using Vocabulary

For each pair of terms, describe how the meanings of the terms differ.

1 infectious disease/contagious disease

2 bacteria/virus

3 AIDS/HIV

For each sentence, fill in the blank with the proper term from the word bank provided below.

HIV	antibiotic
infertility	EBV
throat culture	chlamydia
influenza	sexual abstinence

4 ___ is the virus that causes mononucleosis.

5 A drug that kills bacteria or slows the growth of bacteria is called a(n) ___.

6 Avoiding all sexual contact is called ___.

7 If a doctor thinks that you might have strep throat, he or she will give you a test called a(n) ___.

8 If untreated, some STDs can cause ___, or the inability to have children.

Understanding Concepts

9 What causes infectious diseases?

10 How can coughing or sneezing pass contagious infections?

11 Describe the symptoms of strep throat.

12 What are the sinuses, and how can they become infected?

13 Why are viruses not considered living things?

14 How do the symptoms of influenza differ from the symptoms of the common cold?

15 Do all people who have an STD get sick? Explain.

16 Describe the relationship between HIV and AIDS.

17 What is the most common way that HIV is passed from person to person?

18 How does a vaccine work?

19 How does washing your hands and taking warm showers lower your risk of catching an infectious disease?

20 Compare and contrast bacterial infections and viral infections.

Applying Concepts

21 If you vaccinated every living thing that a certain virus could infect, could you be sure that the virus would be eliminated? Explain your answer.

22 Does everybody that has HIV also have AIDS? Explain your answer.

23 Imagine that one morning in January, you wake up feeling sick. Your head hurts, you have a sore throat, your muscles ache, and you have a very high fever. What disease do you most likely have? Explain your answer.

Making Good Decisions

24 A man speaks to your school about HIV. During his speech, he tells everybody that he is HIV positive, meaning that he is infected with HIV. After the speech, you want to shake the man's hand, but you are afraid of catching HIV. Should you shake the man's hand or not? Explain your answer.

25 Your doctor prescribes an antibiotic for your strep throat. You take the medicine for a few days, and you start feeling better. The instructions for the medicine say that you should keep taking it until it is gone. During the last few days, the medicine has been giving you stomachaches. What should you do in this situation? Explain your answer.

26 If you were in charge of lowering the rate of HIV infection in your city, what three things would you do? Explain your answer.

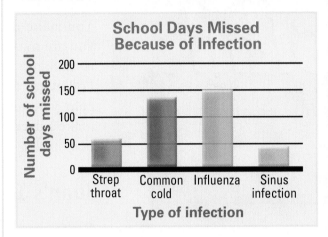

The graph above shows the number of missed days that were caused by each different infection. Use this graph to answer questions 27–31.

27 How many days of school were missed because of bacterial infections?

28 How many days of school were missed because of viral infections?

29 Which infection caused the most missed school days?

30 Fewer students at the school caught influenza than common colds, yet the cold caused less total missed days. What would explain this?

31 About how many more days of school were missed because of strep throat infections than were missed because of sinus infections?

Reading Checkup

Take a minute to review your answers to the Health IQ questions at the beginning of this chapter. How has reading this chapter improved your Health IQ?

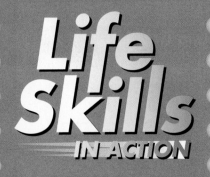

Making Good Decisions

You make decisions every day. But how do you know if you are making good decisions? Making good decisions is making choices that are healthy and responsible. Following the six steps of making good decisions will help you make the best possible choice whenever you make a decision. Complete the following activity to practice the six steps of making good decisions.

Juan's Illness

ACT 1

Setting the Scene

Juan does not feel very well this morning. His body aches, and he thinks he has a fever. Juan's mother suggests that he stay home from school because he might have the flu. But Juan tells her that he wants to go to school because the school band is having solo tryouts. He has been practicing on his trumpet for weeks, and he doesn't want to miss his chance to audition.

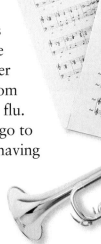

The 6 Steps of Making Good Decisions

1. Identify the problem.
2. Consider your values.
3. List the options.
4. Weigh the consequences.
5. Decide, and act.
6. Evaluate your choice.

Guided Practice

Practice with a Friend

Form a group of three. Have one person play the role of Juan and another person play the role of Juan's mother. Have the third person be an observer. Walking through each of the six steps of making good decisions, role-play Juan deciding whether or not to go to school. Juan's mother can help him brainstorm options and weigh the consequences of each option. The observer will take notes, which will include observations about what the person playing Juan did well and suggestions of ways to improve. Stop after each step to evaluate the process.

Independent Practice

Check Yourself

After you have completed the guided practice, go through Act 1 again without stopping at each step. Answer the questions below to review what you did.

1. What values should Juan consider while making his decision?

2. What options does Juan have?

3. What are the possible consequences of Juan's options?

4. Think about a time when you went to school while you were ill. What were the consequences of your decision? Would you make the same decision again?

ACT 2

On Your Own

One day during band practice, Juan drops his trumpet. When he picks it up, he discovers that it is badly dented. Juan starts to worry about what will happen when he tells his parents. Then, his friend Mark tells Juan that he thinks he can fix the trumpet in the school's metal shop. Make an outline that shows how Juan could use the six steps of making good decisions to decide what to do about his trumpet.

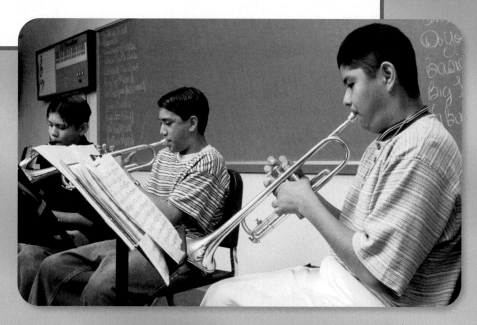

Noninfectious Diseases and Disorders

Lessons

Check out
Current Health
articles related to this chapter by
visiting go.hrw.com. Just type in
the keyword **HD4CH30**.

> " Usually, my grandmother is pretty **healthy.** She did **break** her left **hip** last year.
>
> It's OK now. She's never had a **medical emergency** or anything like that.
>
> I remember she had a really bad allergy attack once. The medicine she took made her feel a whole lot better. Now she's fine. "

Health IQ

PRE-READING

Answer the following multiple-choice questions to find out what you already know about noninfectious diseases. When you've finished this chapter, you'll have the opportunity to change your answers based on what you've learned.

1. A body system is a group of ___ that work together.
   a. cells
   b. tissues
   c. organs
   d. hormones

2. Your heart is a muscular pump with ___ chambers
   a. two
   b. four
   c. six
   d. eight

3. ___ is a respiratory disease that causes parts of the lung to narrow.
   a. Appendicitis
   b. Cystic fibrosis
   c. Type 2 diabetes
   d. Asthma

4. The ___ is the main organ of the nervous system.
   a. brain
   b. spinal cord
   c. central nervous system
   d. peripheral nervous system

5. ___ is a disease in which the body produces no insulin.
   a. Type 2 diabetes
   b. Heart failure
   c. Hyperthyroidism
   d. Type 1 diabetes

6. Digestion of food begins in the
   a. large intestine.
   b. small intestine.
   c. stomach.
   d. mouth.

7. Most kidney disease results from diabetes and
   a. high blood pressure.
   b. cancer.
   c. drinking too little water.
   d. cataracts.

ANSWERS: 1. c; 2. b; 3. d; 4. a; 5. d; 6. d; 7. a

Noninfectious Diseases and Body Systems

What You'll Do

■ **Identify** three noninfectious causes of diseases.

Terms to Learn

- organ
- body system
- noninfectious disease

Start Off
Write

What is a noninfectious disease?

In 1996, Lance Armstrong was told that he had a type of cancer. His cancer was treated, and in 1999, he won his first Tour de France, the world's toughest bicycle race.

Cancer is a serious disease that can attack any part of the body. But with proper support, the body has an amazing ability to fight diseases, such as cancer, and to heal.

Body Systems and Noninfectious Diseases

Your body is made up of cells, tissues, and organs. *Cells* are the simplest units of living organisms. A *tissue* is a group of similar cells that perform a single function. An **organ** is two or more tissues working together. Your heart, stomach, and brain are organs. A **body system** is a group of organs that work together. Different body systems work together to keep you healthy.

But sometimes, a disease can cause an organ or system not to work properly. A *disease* is any harmful change in your body's normal activities. A **noninfectious disease** is a disease that is not caused by a virus or living organism. Common noninfectious diseases include many kinds of cancer, most types of heart disease, and inherited disorders.

TABLE 1 Noninfectious Causes of Diseases		
Cause of disease	**Example**	**Organ or system affected**
Congenital (present at birth)	cleft lip	mouth
Hereditary	cystic fibrosis	respiratory and digestive systems
Accident	brain injury	brain
Nutritional defect	iron deficiency (anemia)	blood and all systems
Metabolic disorder	diabetes	endocrine
Cancer	leukemia breast, lung, and stomach cancer	blood any organ or tissue
Immune defect (allergy)	asthma	respiratory system, eyes, and skin
Multiple causes	high blood pressure	heart and circulatory system

TABLE 2 Body Organs and Systems

Body organ or system	Importance to your body
Heart (organ)	pumps blood to every cell in the body; part of circulatory system
Circulatory system	carries blood and nutrients to every cell in the body; includes the heart, arteries, capillaries, and veins
Lungs	are used for breathing; part of the respiratory system
Respiratory system	takes oxygen into the body and releases carbon dioxide into the atmosphere; system includes the nose, trachea, bronchi, and lungs
Brain (organ)	controls and coordinates all mental and physical activity; part of the nervous system
Nervous system	controls the body's actions and reactions and the body's adjustments to the environment
Endocrine system	produces chemical messengers called *hormones;* includes the pituitary gland, thyroid gland, parathyroid glands, adrenal gland, pancreas, ovaries, and testes
Digestive system	provides the body with nutrients by acting on food and excretes digestive waste products; includes the mouth; esophagus, stomach, intestines, and anus
Urinary system	excretes urine, which is mostly water and waste products from cells; includes kidneys, ureters, urinary bladder, and urethra
Skin (organ)	encloses the body, protects the body from pathogens, insulates the body, and helps the body get rid of wastes
Skeletal system	provides structure and support for the body; protects organs such as the brain and the lungs
Muscular system	provides movement inside and outside of the body
Eyes	organs of sight
Ears	organs of hearing

Lesson Review

Using Vocabulary

1. Explain the difference between an organ and a body system.

Understanding Concepts

2. Give three noninfectious causes of diseases.

3. Explain how noninfectious diseases are different from infectious diseases.

Critical Thinking

4. **Analyzing Ideas** How may severe brain injuries be similar to a non-infectious disease?

5. **Making Inferences** Your body's immune system destroys most disease-causing organisms. Explain how being born with a disease of the immune system may affect a person's life.

internet connect

www.scilinks.org/health

Topic: Inherited Diseases
HealthLinks code: HD4062

Topic: Noninfectious Diseases
HealthLinks code: HD4070

HEALTH LINKS Maintained by the National Science Teachers Association

Circulatory System

What You'll Do

- **Identify** the parts of the circulatory system.
- **Identify** two noninfectious diseases of the circulatory system.

Terms to Learn

- heart attack
- congenital disorder
- hypertension
- leukemia

Start Off
Write

What is a heart attack?

Tony had a physical exam when he tried out for the track team. His doctor found a heart murmur. Tony wants to know if he will be able to run track.

Tony learned that there are many kinds of heart murmurs. Tony's doctor told him that his heart murmur is not unusual. The murmur is not dangerous, so Tony will be able to join the track team.

Your Heart

Your *circulatory system* is made up of your heart and blood vessels, through which blood circulates. The heart is a muscular pump that has four chambers. The two upper chambers hold the blood and are called the *atria* (singular, *atrium* [AY tree uhm]). The two lower chambers pump the blood and are called the *ventricles* (VEN tri kuhlz). Blood enters the right atrium from all parts of the body. This blood is low in oxygen. Blood goes into the right ventricle and is then pumped into the lungs. Between the atrium and the ventricle are valves that prevent blood from flowing backwards. In the lungs, blood picks up oxygen. The high-oxygen blood then returns to the left atrium and goes to the left ventricle. The left ventricle pumps the high-oxygen blood to the rest of the body, including to the heart itself. Like all muscles, the heart needs a constant supply of oxygen to keep beating.

Figure 2 Diagram of a Healthy Heart

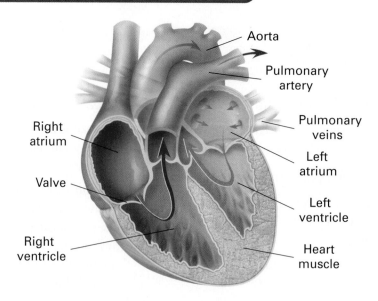

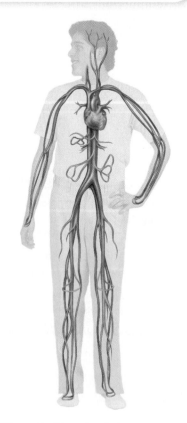

Figure 1 The circulatory system

Heart Disease

Heart disease is any condition that affects the heart's ability to pump blood. There are many kinds of heart disease. For example, sometimes arteries are blocked and do not deliver enough blood to the heart. A **heart attack** happens when part of the heart does not receive enough blood and the heart does not pump well. In a heart attack, part of the heart muscle dies.

Heart failure is a condition that slowly develops as the heart muscle gets weaker. Having heart failure does not mean that your heart stops. During heart failure, the heart cannot pump enough blood to keep the body going. This condition may be caused by high blood pressure, a heart attack, or a congenital disorder. A **congenital disorder** is any disease, abnormality, or defect that is present at birth but is not inherited.

There are more than thirty kinds of congenital heart disease. For example, some babies are born with a hole between the two ventricles in their heart. This defect can be fixed with surgery. Tony's heart murmur is caused by a congenital defect that affects his heart valves. Some congenital defects are detected at birth, but some defects are not discovered for years.

Fighting Heart Disease

The best way to fight heart failure and heart attacks is to prevent them from happening at all. Good health habits can be started in middle school. These health habits are important for preventing heart disease later in life. Eating a nutritious diet, getting plenty of exercise, not being overweight, and not smoking can prevent most heart attacks. Some heart disease may be controlled with medicine, but some heart disease requires surgery. Surgery can also correct many congenital heart defects. But the best medicine for fighting heart disease is to make good health choices from the start.

Your Blood Vessels

There are three major types of blood vessels—arteries, veins, and capillaries. *Arteries* carry blood away from the heart to various organs. *Veins* carry blood from various parts of the body back to the heart. *Capillaries* (KAP uh LER eez) are very small tubes that connect arteries and veins. Some capillaries are so small that you need a microscope to see them.

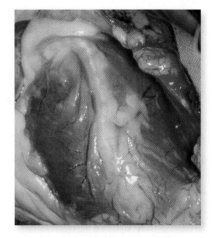

Figure 3 This heart has suffered a heart attack and part of the heart muscle was damaged.

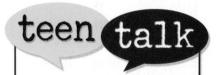

Teen: "I didn't know teens can have heart attacks. How would I know if I was having one?"

Expert: "Usually, a heart attack has warning signs such as the following:

- A sudden pressure, squeezing, or pain in the chest, possibly spreading to the arms, shoulders, neck, or jaw

- Sickness, nausea, or weakness

- Rapid, weak, or irregular pulse

- Sweating, fainting, shortness of breath, lightheadedness, or fear

- Pale or blue skin

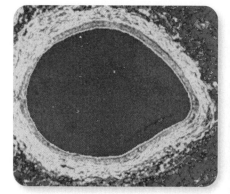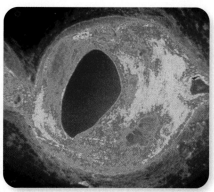

Figure 4 Healthy arteries, such as the one on the left, let blood flow freely to all parts of the body. Blood flow is reduced in a blocked or damaged artery, such as the one on the right.

Hands-on ACTIVITY

HEARTBEATS

1. Feel your pulse by placing two fingers at the pulse point on your neck or wrist.

2. Using a clock or stopwatch, count the number of beats you feel in 15 seconds.

3. Multiply this number by 4 to get the number of times your heart beats each minute. Record this number.

Analysis

1. Organize the data in step 3 into a data table.

2. Draw a bar graph to show what the range of heart rates for the class is and how often each rate happens.

Your Blood

Your heart pumps blood to the cells in your body. Blood has a liquid part, called *plasma*, and a solid part. Plasma is mostly water, but also includes other chemicals and nutrients.

The solid part of your blood is made up of two types of blood cells—red blood cells and white blood cells. *Red blood cells* carry oxygen to the cells of your body. Every cell in your body needs oxygen in order to keep working. *White blood cells* help fight infections. When you are sick, your white blood cell count may increase to help you fight the infection. Your blood also contains *platelets* (PLAYT lits) which are not true cells. Platelets help stop bleeding by plugging leaks in your arteries, veins, and capillaries.

When the heart tries to pump blood through a blocked artery, the result may be hypertension (HIE puhr TEN shuhn). **Hypertension** is a condition in which the pressure inside your large arteries is too high. Therefore, hypertension is also called *high blood pressure*. This disease can damage your arteries, heart, kidneys, and brain. High blood pressure can also be fatal.

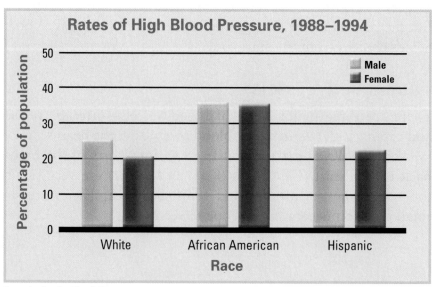

Rates of High Blood Pressure, 1988–1994

Source: American Heart Association.

Figure 5 High blood pressure can affect anyone. Some groups have higher rates of hypertension than others, but scientists do not know why.

Fighting Blood Diseases

Blood diseases may affect red blood cells, white blood cells, and platelets. *Anemia* (uh NEE mee uh) is a disease in which your body does not have enough red blood cells. Without these blood cells, your body cells cannot get enough oxygen. Anemia has several causes. For example, your body may not produce enough red blood cells because of a disease. Sometimes, severe blood loss from an accident or an injury can cause anemia. You may lose blood faster than your body can replace it, so you become anemic. You may also become anemic if your diet does not have enough iron. Eating foods high in iron, such as fish, lean meat, and green, leafy vegetables will help prevent anemia. Some diseases, such as sickle cell anemia, cause the body to make defective red blood cells. These defective blood cells cannot carry enough oxygen to the body cells.

White blood cells can be affected, too. For example, some medicines may affect your body's production of white blood cells and make your white cell count too low. And some diseases, such as leukemia (loo KEE mee uh), increase the number of white blood cells. **Leukemia** is cancer of the blood. It causes defective white cells to form in very large numbers.

Platelet diseases happen when there are too few or too many platelets. With too few platelets, you may bruise easily or bleed too much. With too many platelets, your blood may clot too easily. Blood clots can be dangerous if they travel to your heart, lungs, or brain and stop the flow of blood to these vital organs. In some diseases, platelets do not form clots as they should.

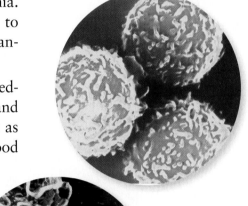

Figure 6 The top photo shows normal white blood cells. The bottom photo shows hairy cell leukemia white blood cells.

Lesson Review

Using Vocabulary

1. Define *congenital disorder*.

Understanding Concepts

2. Identify the parts of the circulatory system.

3. Describe the flow of blood after it enters the right atrium. Draw a diagram if necessary.

4. Describe two noninfectious diseases of the circulatory system.

Critical Thinking

5. Making Inferences Aspirin reduces the clumping or clotting ability of platelets. Doctors sometimes tell patients who have had a heart attack caused by blood clots to take aspirin. Before the patient takes aspirin, what other problem should the doctor warn them about?

Lesson 3

Respiratory System

Estebán's lungs sometimes fill with mucous and he feels as if he cannot breathe. Estebán loves soccer, but playing even part of a game makes him exhausted and weak.

Estebán has a disease called *cystic fibrosis* (SIS tik fie BROH sis), or CF. Cystic fibrosis impairs a person's breathing, or *respiration*. Respiration is the process by which a body takes in and uses oxygen and gets rid of carbon dioxide and water.

What You'll Do

■ **Describe** how the respiratory system works.

■ **Identify** two noninfectious diseases of the respiratory system.

Terms to Learn

- asthma
- emphysema

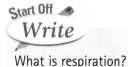

Start Off Write

What is respiration?

Your Respiratory System

Respiration is made possible by the respiratory system. The respiratory system consists of the nose, mouth, throat, voice box, trachea (TRAY kee uh), and lungs. Air enters the body through the nose and mouth and then enters the trachea. The trachea splits into two tubes called the *bronchi* (BRAHNG kie). Each of the bronchi attaches to a lung. In the lungs, the bronchi divide several times into very small tubes called *bronchioles*. Bronchioles end in small, thin air sacs called *alveoli* (al VEE uh LIE). In the alveoli, oxygen from the air enters your blood and carbon dioxide and water from your blood go into the air.

Respiration is controlled by the brain. You don't even have to think about it. Muscles in the chest and between the chest and the abdomen move your chest and help you breathe. Some noninfectious diseases, such as CF, interfere with the airflow in the lungs. Other diseases affect the muscles that help you breathe.

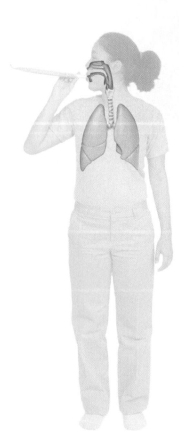

Figure 7 The respiratory system

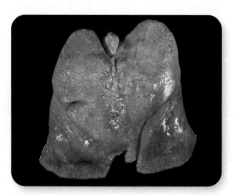

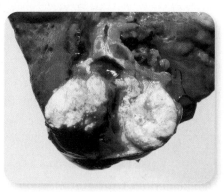

Figure 8 Healthy lungs, shown at left, provide oxygen to your body. A diseased lung, below, cannot provide the oxygen your body needs.

Respiratory Diseases

Estebán's CF is a respiratory disease. In CF, mucus in the lungs is thick and sticky, and it clogs the lungs. People with CF sometimes feel like they cannot breathe.

A common respiratory disease is asthma. **Asthma** causes the small bronchioles in the lung to narrow. Asthma causes shortness of breath, wheezing, or coughing. Allergies to smoke, dust, pollen, or other things in the environment may cause asthma attacks. Cold air, exercise, and respiratory infections may also trigger asthma attacks.

Emphysema is a respiratory disease that causes the alveoli to become thin and stretched. Oxygen and carbon dioxide cannot move through the damaged alveoli. As a result, a person with emphysema has difficulty breathing. Emphysema is strongly tied to cigarette smoking and is a disease mainly of adults.

Fighting Respiratory Diseases

Most noninfectious respiratory diseases cannot be cured, but they can be treated. For some respiratory diseases, such as CF and asthma, people take medicine to make breathing easier. People who have these diseases can often lead fairly normal lives. Emphysema, which is one of the worst respiratory diseases, cannot be cured or even treated very well. But emphysema can be almost completely prevented by not smoking cigarettes.

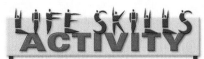

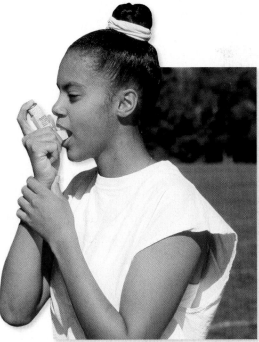

LIFE SKILLS ACTIVITY

MAKING GOOD DECISIONS

Suppose that a friend wants you to start smoking. What would you do? Use the steps for making decisions to show what you would decide. Explain why you would or would not choose to smoke.

Figure 9 Some respiratory diseases, such as asthma, can be controlled with medication.

Lesson Review

Using Vocabulary

1. What is the difference between asthma and emphysema?

Understanding Concepts

2. Describe how the respiratory system works.

Critical Thinking

3. **Identifying Relationships** Air contains about 21 percent oxygen gas. If a person has trouble breathing because of an asthma attack or emphysema, what could a doctor do to help the person get more oxygen?

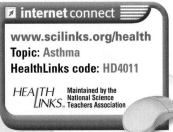

internet connect

www.scilinks.org/health
Topic: Asthma
HealthLinks code: HD4011

HEALTH LINKS Maintained by the National Science Teachers Association

Nervous System

Gwen's aunt has Alzheimer's disease. Gwen has offered to help take care of her aunt as the disease worsens.

What You'll Do

■ **Identify** parts of the nervous system.

■ **Identify** two noninfectious diseases of the nervous system.

Terms to Learn

• Alzheimer's disease

• central nervous system

• peripheral nervous system

Start Off
Write

What happens if messages from your brain can't get through to your body?

Gwen learned that **Alzheimer's disease** (AHLTS HIE muhrz di ZEEZ) is a disease of the brain that affects thinking, memory, and behavior. Eventually, her aunt will need almost constant care.

Your Brain and Nervous System

The *nervous system* is the command and control system for the body. It consists of several parts that connect to each other and that work together. The two main parts of the nervous system are the central nervous system (CNS) and the peripheral nervous system (PNS).

The **central nervous system** is made up of the *brain* and the *spinal cord*. The brain, located inside the skull, is the main organ of the nervous system. The *spinal cord* is the bundle of nerves that runs down the back, inside the backbone. The spinal cord is the main pathway for messages between the brain and the peripheral nervous system. The **peripheral nervous system** is made of all of the nerves outside the brain and the spinal cord. The PNS has two main parts, the *somatic* (so MAT ik) *nervous system* and the *autonomic* (ot uh NOM ik) *nervous system*. The somatic nervous system contains the nerves that send information between the CNS and bones, muscles, and skin. The autonomic nervous system controls body functions, such as digestion, breathing, blood pressure, and heart rate, which you do not usually control.

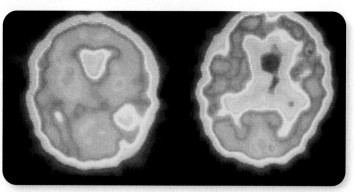

Normal   **Alzheimer's disease**

Figure 11 These photos show brain activity. The yellow and blue colors represent areas of reduced activity.

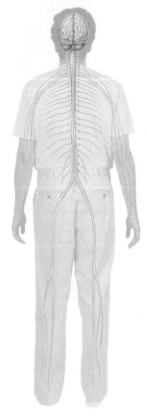

Figure 10 The nervous system

TABLE 3 Examples of Nervous System Diseases

Disease	Description	Treatment or cure
Alzheimer's Disease	a degenerative disease of the brain that often causes loss of memory and changes in behavior	no known cure
Brain tumors	abnormal tissue growth in the brain; Brain tumors may be cancerous or noncancerous.	surgery, chemotherapy, radiation therapy, and medicine
Parkinson's disease	a degenerative disease of the nervous system that is usually associated with trembling of the arms, legs, and face, stiffness of the limbs, and slow movement	no known cure; Medicines may slow the progress of the disease.
Guillain-Barré syndrome	a disorder in which the body's immune system attacks part of the peripheral nervous system; first causes muscle weakness and a tingling sensation in the legs but then may cause paralysis and breathing difficulty	no known cure; The symptoms can be treated, and physical therapy may be used to keep the muscles flexible.

Noninfectious Nervous System Diseases

Some nervous system diseases, such as Alzheimer's disease and brain tumors, affect the brain. Other diseases, such as Guillain-Barré (ge LAN bah RAY) syndrome, affect nerves, or parts of nerves, outside the brain. Many diseases of the nervous system have no known cure, but the symptoms and effects of the diseases can be controlled and treated.

Injuries are another source of nervous system diseases. Head injuries may damage the brain and can affect your ability to think, move, remember, or speak. Spinal cord injuries can stop messages from traveling between your body and your brain. People who have spinal cord injuries may not be able to walk or use their hands. But many brain and spinal cord injuries can be prevented by wearing proper safety equipment and by being careful.

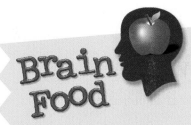

Brain Food

Young adults, in the 16- to 30-year-old age group, account for 55 percent of spinal cord injuries. The average age at injury is about 22.

Lesson Review

Using Vocabulary

1. Name the parts of the central nervous system.

Understanding Concepts

2. Describe two noninfectious diseases of the nervous system.

Critical Thinking

3. Making Inferences How might a disease affecting the spinal cord affect a musician or a dancer?

4. Applying Concepts Why are the symptoms of a serious brain injury likely to be similar to the symptoms of a serious brain disease?

Lesson 5

Endocrine System

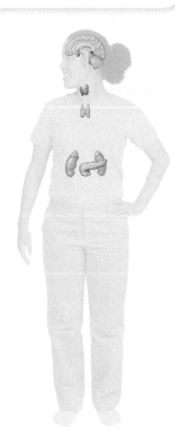

Figure 12 The endocrine system

What You'll Do

- **Describe** the function of the endocrine system.
- **Identify** three noninfectious diseases of the endocrine system.

Terms to Learn

- endocrine gland
- hormones
- type 1 diabetes
- type 2 diabetes

Start Off
Write

What do hormones do?

Anthony's friend Sandra asked him to get ice cream with her. Anthony has diabetes and has to watch what he eats. But because he knows that his diabetes is under control, Anthony decides to go.

Diabetes is a disease that affects the body's ability to use sugar for energy. Anthony controls his diabetes by giving himself insulin shots every day. The insulin controls the level of sugar in Anthony's blood. By being careful, Anthony can eat a normal diet, including some ice cream occasionally.

Your Endocrine System

Diabetes is a disease of the endocrine system (EN doh krin SIS tuhm). The *endocrine system* is a network of glands throughout the body that produce chemicals that control many body functions. An **endocrine gland** is a group of cells or an organ that produces hormones. **Hormones** are the chemicals released directly into your blood by the endocrine system to regulate body functions.

Some hormones regulate your growth, and some help with digestion. Other hormones cause your body to change from being a child to being an adult. In fact, hormones affect nearly every body function, including your body's metabolism. *Metabolism* (muh TAB uh LIZ uhm) includes all the processes by which your body breaks down food and converts the energy in food into energy your body can use for growth and repair.

TABLE 4 Glands of the Endocrine System	
Pituitary gland	growth hormone
Thyroid gland	thyroid hormone (necessary for growth and metabolism)
Parathyroid gland	parathyroid hormone (necessary for calcium metabolism)
Pancreas	insulin (necessary for sugar metabolism)
Adrenal gland	sex hormones and hormones for salt metabolism
Testes	male sexual-development hormones
Ovaries	female sexual-development hormones

Endocrine System Diseases

There are two types of diabetes. Both types of diabetes may cause serious health problems, including blindness, heart disease, circulatory problems, stroke, and kidney disease. In **type 1 diabetes,** the body produces little or no insulin. *Insulin* is a hormone produced in the pancreas that helps your body store glucose, or sugar. Insulin also enables cells to use glucose for energy. Anthony controls his type 1 diabetes with daily insulin shots. In **type 2 diabetes,** the body makes insulin but cannot use it properly. Type 2 diabetes usually strikes people over age 40. Type 2 diabetes is linked to obesity and lack of exercise. A healthy diet and plenty of exercise help prevent or control type 2 diabetes.

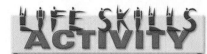

BEING A WISE CONSUMER

One of the main ingredients in fruit juices and regular soft drinks is sugar. Explain why these beverages may not be the best choice for someone with type 1 diabetes.

Another endocrine system disease is hyperthyroidism (HIE puhr THIE royd IZ uhm). Hyperthyroidism causes the thyroid gland to produce too much thyroid hormone. Excess thyroid hormone speeds up metabolism and may cause weight loss and makes a person feel warm, sweaty, and nervous. At the end of the day, a person who has hyperthyroidism may feel very tired but may have trouble sleeping. Hyperthyroidism can usually be treated with medication.

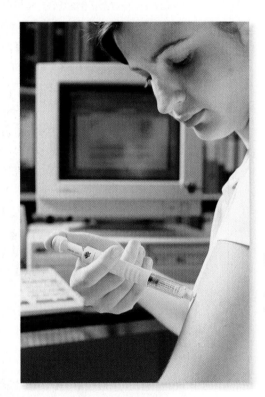

Figure 13 People who have type 1 diabetes can control their disease by taking insulin.

Lesson Review

Using Vocabulary

1. What is the endocrine system?

2. Write a sentence that correctly uses the terms *endocrine gland* and *hormone*.

Understanding Concepts

3. What are three noninfectious diseases of the endocrine system?

Critical Thinking

4. **Making Predictions** If someone takes too much insulin, what happens to the sugar level in his or her blood?

5. **Analyzing Ideas** Type 2 diabetes may be becoming more common among young children and teens. Explain why type 2 diabetes may be increasing in these age groups.

Digestive System

Jasmine often has stomach cramps. She feels sick and is losing weight. Jasmine wants to know why she is sick.

Jasmine's doctor ran a series of tests. The results show that Jasmine has a digestive system disease that keeps her body from absorbing nutrients from food.

Your Digestive System

Your *digestive system* is the body system that breaks down food so that it can be used by your body. Digestion of food begins in the mouth. Food passes from your mouth down your esophagus (i SAHF uh guhs) to the stomach. Your stomach holds food and partially digests it. From your stomach, food passes into the small intestine. In the small intestine, digestion of food is completed and nutrients from food are absorbed. The small intestine connects to the large intestine, where water from food is absorbed. The large intestine, or colon, ends at the rectum. Finally, the rectum ends at the anus. Solid waste—undigested and unabsorbed food—leaves the body through the anus.

Digestive enzymes are special proteins that help digestion. They are produced in the mouth, stomach, and small intestine. These enzymes break down food and make it usable. Your pancreas and liver are also involved in the digestive process. The liver produces *bile*, which helps digest fats. The pancreas produces a mixture of enzymes that help break down fats, proteins, and carbohydrates.

What You'll Do

- **Identify** the parts of your digestive system.
- **Identify** two noninfectious disorders of the digestive system.

Terms to Learn

- celiac disease

Start Off
Write

What happens if your intestines cannot absorb nutrients?

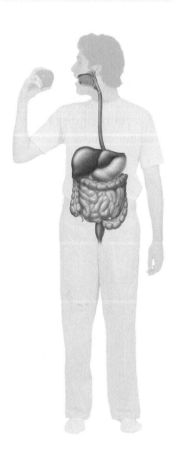

Figure 14 The digestive system

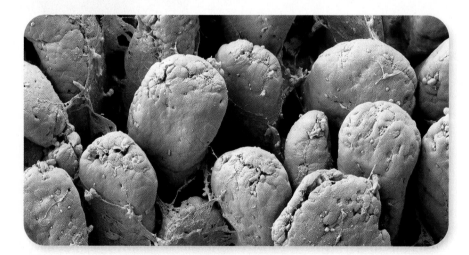

Figure 15 The small and large intestines are lined with villi, shown above. Villi absorb nutrients from food.

Noninfectious Digestive System Diseases

Jasmine has celiac disease (SEE lee AK di ZEEZ). **Celiac disease** is a disease that makes the body allergic to a protein called *gluten* (GLOOT n). Gluten is found in grains, such as wheat, rye, and barley. When someone who has celiac disease eats food with gluten, his or her immune system reacts by damaging the lining of the small intestine. This damage stops the person's intestine from absorbing the nutrients in his or her food. A person with celiac disease can live a normal life if he or she avoids food containing gluten.

Other digestive diseases include Crohn's disease, which attacks the lining of the intestines and causes diarrhea, cramps, and fever. Ulcerative colitis (UHL suhr AY tiv koh LIET is) is a similar disease that attacks the colon. These two diseases are often grouped together as inflammatory bowel disease (IBD). With proper medication and a healthy diet, people with IBD can usually live relatively normal lives.

Stomach cancer is another noninfectious disease of the digestive system. Stomach cancer has no known cause. Factors that may be related to stomach cancer include

- alcohol abuse
- tobacco abuse
- a diet that is high in smoked food and salted fish or meat
- a diet low in fiber and high in starch

Stomach cancer can be treated by surgery, radiation therapy, and chemotherapy. But it is better to avoid stomach cancer entirely. You can reduce your chances of getting stomach cancer by avoiding tobacco and alcohol and by eating a nutritious diet.

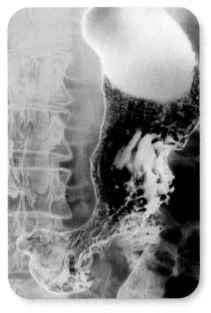

Figure 16 This colored x ray shows a stomach being destroyed by cancer. The pink area (upper right) is healthy stomach wall. The dark purple mass extending downward is the cancer that has attacked part of the stomach.

Lesson Review

Using Vocabulary

1. What is celiac disease?

Understanding Concepts

2. Describe two noninfectious diseases of the digestive system.

3. What are the parts of your digestive system?

Critical Thinking

4. Identifying Relationships Why would diseases such as celiac disease or Crohn's disease affect the health of the entire body even though they are diseases of the digestive system?

Urinary System

Jackson's father has high blood pressure. His father's doctor said that high blood pressure can damage the kidneys.

Jackson is worried because he knows that kidney damage is serious. Jackson's father takes medicine to control his blood pressure. A doctor checks his father's kidneys every few months to make sure that they are healthy and are working properly.

Your Urinary System

Kidneys are organs that remove wastes and water from blood. Wastes removed by the kidneys are products of metabolism inside the cells. These wastes are not the same as digestive wastes. Kidneys are also important in maintaining the level of salt and fluid in the body. Maintaining this level helps control blood pressure.

Kidneys are part of the urinary system. The *urinary system* includes the two kidneys, two ureters (yoo REET uhrz), the urinary bladder, and the urethra (yoo REE thruh). As blood travels through your body, it collects the waste products from your cells. Your kidneys constantly clean your blood through more than a million tiny filters called *nephrons* (NEF RAHNZ). Nephrons collect waste products and water from the blood. Together, the waste products and water form *urine*. Urine leaves the kidneys through the *ureters*. It is transported by the ureters to the urinary bladder, where it is stored. Eventually, urine leaves the body through the *urethra*. The process of releasing urine from the body is called *urination*.

What You'll Do

- **Describe** the urinary system.
- **Identify** three noninfectious diseases that affect the urinary system.

Terms to Learn

- kidneys

Start Off
Write

What do your kidneys do?

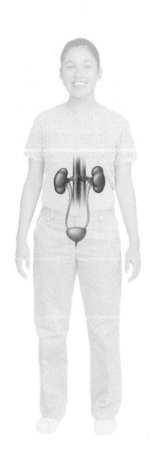

Figure 17 The urinary system

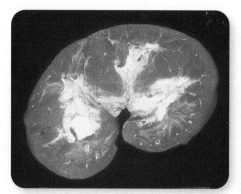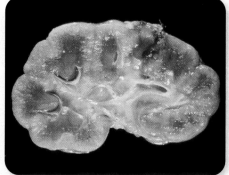

Figure 18 A healthy kidney is shown on the left. A kidney damaged by disease, such as the one shown on the right, cannot remove wastes from the body.

Noninfectious Urinary Diseases

Diabetes and hypertension cause most kidney disease. In diabetes, the body cannot use the sugar in the blood. This unused sugar damages small blood vessels and nephrons in the kidneys. In hypertension, the nephrons are damaged by the stress caused by high blood pressure. When nephrons are damaged, they are unable to filter blood and remove wastes.

In both diabetes and hypertension, wastes can build up in blood and organs and cause a variety of health problems, including complete kidney failure. If untreated, kidney disease can lead to death. Kidney disease can sometimes be treated with diet and medication. In other cases, dialysis is necessary.

Some kidney diseases are inherited. For example, polycystic (PAHL ee SIS tik) kidney disease (PKD) is hereditary. In PKD, hard growths, called *cysts* (SISTS) form in the kidneys. These cysts slowly replace large portions of the nephrons. PKD cannot be cured, but it can be treated with medication and a proper diet.

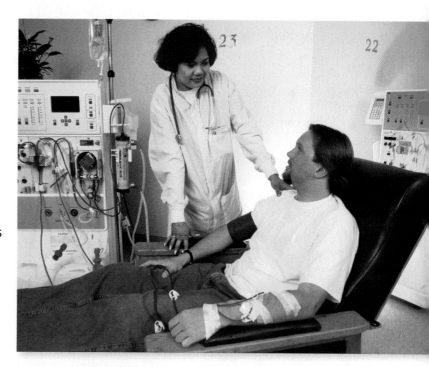

Figure 19 When a person's kidneys are severely diseased, a process called dialysis is used to filter wastes from the person's blood.

Lesson Review

Using Vocabulary

1. What are your kidneys?

Understanding Concepts

2. Draw a diagram showing the parts of the urinary system and the ways in which this system removes waste from the blood.

3. An older man has blockages in both his ureters. Will he be able to urinate?

4. What are three noninfectious diseases that affect the urinary system?

Critical Thinking

5. **Making Inferences** Some desert-dwelling animals, such as gerbils and some lizards, add little or no water to their cellular waste products. What advantage(s) may this system have for animals that use it?

Skin, Bones, and Muscles

Mohandas was hiking across a field when he stepped in a hole and fell. He broke his wrist while trying to break his fall. Now he has to wear a cast for 6 weeks!

Bones are made of connective tissue cells and minerals. Some people think that bones are lifeless. But bones, just like your brain or stomach, are living organs made of several different tissues.

Your Connective Tissues

You are made of more than just skin and bones. Your body has four basic kinds of tissue—epithelial tissue (EP i THEE lee uhl TISH oo), nervous tissue, muscle tissue, and connective tissue. Your skin and your stomach lining are made of epithelial tissue. Nervous tissue is found in your nerves, brain, and spinal cord. Your muscles are made of muscle tissue. And your bones, ligaments, and tendons are all made of connective tissue.

Your *skin* is a protective covering for your body. It receives signals from the environment, such as touch or pain. These signals travel to the brain along nervous tissue. *Bones* are solid structures made of proteins, minerals, and connective tissue. Blood vessels inside your bones deliver nutrients to the living bone cells. Your bones give you stability. They also protect important organs, such as the brain and the spinal cord. Bone marrow, located in the center of the bone, is where blood cells are formed. Your *muscles* are tissue that make it possible for your body to move. Your muscles are controlled by your nerves and your brain.

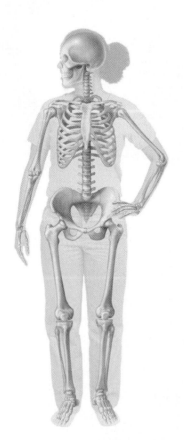

Figure 20 The skeletal system

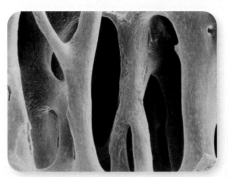

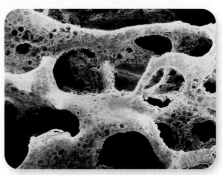

Figure 21 Healthy bone tissue is shown on the left. Bone tissue with osteoporosis, shown below, is weaker and more fragile than healthy bone tissue.

Hands-on ACTIVITY

HOW MUCH SKIN DO YOU HAVE?

1. Use a cloth measuring tape or a piece of string to measure the average circumference and the length of each of the following body parts: head, torso, upper arm, lower arm, upper leg, and lower leg.

2. Multiply the average circumference by the length to get the amount of skin for each part.

3. Add together the amount of skin for each part to get your total amount of skin.

Analysis

1. Record the height, age, and total amount of skin for everyone in the class. Make graphs that show whether the amount of skin depends on height or age.

2. Does the amount of skin a person has depend on how old the person is? how tall the person is? Explain your answer.

Noninfectious Connective Tissue Diseases

There are many skin, bone, and muscle diseases. Some skin diseases, such as skin cancers, are caused by exposure to sunlight. Other skin diseases, such as eczema and psoriasis, have no known cause. Skin is your first line of defense against infection, so skin diseases and breaks in the skin should be treated quickly.

Osteoporosis is a bone disease that causes loss of bone density, so bones become brittle. Osteoporosis usually strikes older adults, especially women. It can be treated with calcium, vitamin D, and sometimes hormones. Another bone disease called *rickets* strikes young children. Rickets results from a lack of vitamin D, and can be treated with a proper diet.

Muscular dystrophy (MD) is a group of several inherited muscle diseases that cause muscles gradually to become weak and disabled. There are no cures for MD, but treatment and therapy can support people who have MD.

Myth & Fact

Myth: Cracking your knuckles makes your knuckles get bigger and will give you arthritis.

Fact: There is actually little scientific data available on this topic. One study concluded that there is no relation between knuckle cracking and damage to the finger joints.

Lesson Review

Using Vocabulary

1. What is osteoporosis?

Understanding Concepts

2. Why are bones, muscles, and skin important?

3. Identify a noninfectious bone disease.

Critical Thinking

4. Making Inferences Cancer is the uncontrolled growth of live cells. Can cancer attack bone tissue? Explain your answer.

5. Making Inferences Why is rickets rarely seen in this country?

Eyes and Ears

> Krishna sits at the front of the class. He still cannot see the board very clearly. He doesn't want to say anything because he is afraid that he will have to wear glasses.

What You'll Do

- **Describe** the function of eyes and ears.
- **Describe** three noninfectious diseases of the eyes and ears.

Terms to Learn

- cataract
- glaucoma
- deafness

Start Off Write

How do your eyes and ears give you information about your world?

Krishna may be right. He may have to get lenses to correct his vision. His vision is blurry, and he is missing important work on the board. But he thinks that glasses will make him look ugly.

Your Eyes and Ears

You are using your eyes to read this sentence. Your eyes are sensory organs that send information from the world around you to your brain. Light passes through the cornea, the pupil, and the lens of your eye. The lens focuses light on the retina. The *retina* is a layer of cells at the back of the eye. The cells of the retina send electrical impulses along the optic nerve to your brain. Your brain changes these electrical impulses into images. Usually, the parts of your eyes work together to make sure that you get this information. The images Krishna sees are blurred because his lenses don't focus light exactly on the retina.

Your ears are sensory organs used for hearing. They send information about sound to your brain. Each ear is divided into three parts—the outer, middle, and inner ears. Sound waves that reach the outer ear are funneled toward the eardrum and make the eardrum vibrate. These vibrations travel through the three small bones of the middle ear—the hammer, the anvil, and the stirrup—to the inner ear. The inner ear converts the vibrations into electrical impulses, which go to the brain. The inner ear also has a second function—maintaining your balance. People with a disease of the middle ear may feel dizzy and nauseated because the inner ear is sending incorrect messages to their brain.

Figure 22 Your eyes and ears are sensory organs.

Retina · Cornea · Light · Pupil · Iris · Lens · Optic nerve

Hammer · Anvil · Stirrup · Cochlea · Eardrum · Ear canal

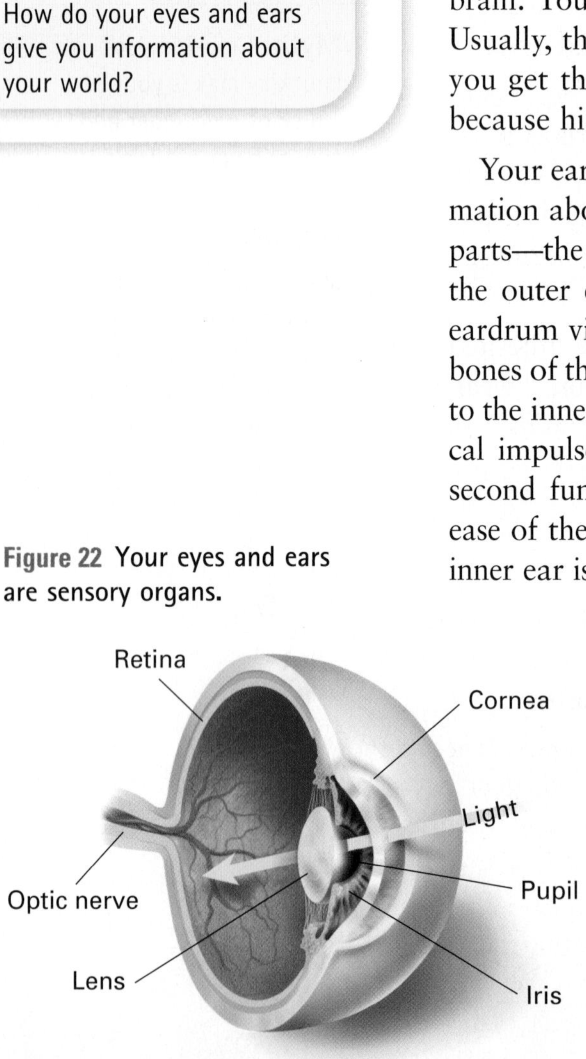

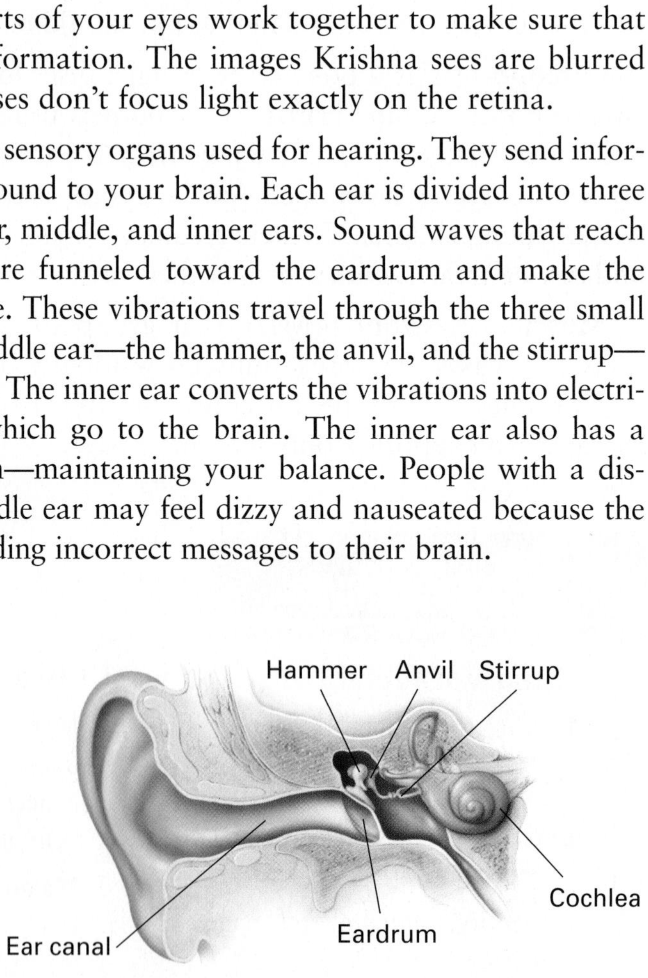

Noninfectious Diseases of the Eyes and Ears

Noninfectious eye diseases include cataracts and glaucoma (glaw KOH muh). A **cataract** is a clouding of the natural lens of the eye. Fortunately, the cloudy lens can be replaced with a plastic lens similar to a contact lens. **Glaucoma** is a disease that causes high pressure in the fluid inside the eye. This high pressure damages the optic nerve and causes a permanent loss of vision. Most cases of glaucoma cannot be cured, but glaucoma can be treated and vision can be saved. With regular eye exams, both cataracts and glaucoma can be detected early, and can be stopped or treated with medicine or surgery.

The most common hearing problem is deafness. **Deafness** is the partial or total loss of the ability to hear. There are many levels of hearing loss, from mild loss to total deafness. Deafness may be hereditary or may happen during the birth process. Infectious diseases, such as meningitis, may cause deafness. Noninfectious diseases, such as diabetes and leukemia, may also cause deafness. In teens, the most common cause of deafness is exposure to loud noise. Loud noise can cause damage to the inner ear, which may leave you unable to hear some sounds. You may be unable to hear parts of normal conversation. How can you tell if the noise is too loud? If you have to shout to be heard over the music, the music may be damaging your hearing.

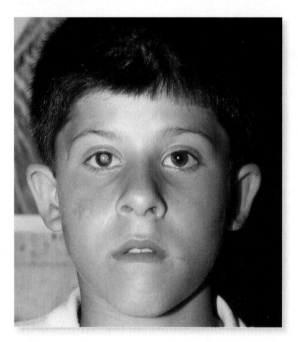

Figure 23 Cataracts, such as the one in this boy's right eye, are a noninfectious eye disease.

Health Journal

Needing glasses to correct vision problems usually does not mean that you have an eye disease. Nevertheless, getting glasses is often very stressful for teens. What would you say to a friend to help relieve his or her stress about getting glasses?

Lesson Review

Using Vocabulary

1. Define *deafness*.

Understanding Concepts

2. What is the function of your eyes and ears?

3. Describe three noninfectious diseases of the eyes and ears.

Critical Thinking

4. **Making Inferences** Your friend is suffering from a severe head cold. He also feels dizzy and sick. Is it possible that there is any connection between his cold and his dizziness? Explain your answer.

Chapter Summary

■ A noninfectious disease is a disease that is not caused by a virus or living organism. ■ Noninfectious diseases can strike any organ or system in the body. ■ Heart failure and heart attacks are two noninfectious diseases of the circulatory system. ■ Asthma is a respiratory disease that makes breathing difficult. ■ The nervous system has two main parts—the central nervous system and the peripheral nervous system. ■ People with brain or spinal cord injuries may not be able to walk or use their hands. ■ A person with diabetes cannot use glucose properly. ■ The digestive system breaks down food so that it can by used by the body. ■ Kidney disease damages the body's ability to remove waste products from the blood. ■ Noninfectious diseases, such as cancer, can strike the skin, bones, and muscles.

Using Vocabulary

For each sentence, fill in the blank with the proper word from the word bank provided below.

organ
osteoporosis
noninfectious disease
cataract

type 1 diabetes
type 2 diabetes
body system
glaucoma

❶ A(n) ___ is a group of organs that work together.

❷ The heart is a(n) ___ that pumps blood throughout the body.

❸ A(n) ___ is not caused by a virus or living organism.

❹ ___ is a bone disease that causes bones to lose density.

❺ ___ is a disease in which the body produces insulin but cannot use it properly.

❻ A(n) ___ is clouding of the natural lens of the eye.

❼ ___ is a disease that causes high fluid pressure inside the eye.

For each pair of terms, describe how the meanings of the terms differ.

❽ central nervous system/peripheral nervous system

❾ noninfectious disease/congenital disease

❿ hypertension/heart attack

⓫ asthma/emphysema

Understanding Concepts

⓬ What is the relationship between kidneys and nephrons?

⓭ If a disease or injury seriously damaged the spinal cord, how might the body be affected?

⓮ What happens to the body if the thyroid gland produces too much hormone?

⓯ Describe the path of food through the digestive system, and explain why enzymes are important to digestion.

⓰ Explain why some airport workers wear protective headphones.

⓱ Why is it so important to avoid high blood pressure?

Critical Thinking

Identifying Relationships

18 Why is it important to know whether a disease is infectious or noninfectious?

19 Type 2 diabetes usually strikes people in their 40s or 50s. But some studies show that type 2 diabetes is becoming more common in young children and teens. Why is it important for teens to develop good eating habits and get plenty of exercise?

20 Why is it important for the small intestine to be working properly?

21 Why is it important not to smoke cigarettes?

22 Describe how your nervous system is working with your skin, muscles, bones, eyes, and ears as you answer this question.

Making Good Decisions

23 Imagine that you have a family history of skin cancer. This type of cancer usually strikes people in their 20s or 30s. You have been offered a summer job working outside at a local swimming pool. Describe the steps you would take in deciding whether to accept the job.

24 Imagine that someone has discovered a drug that will make you 20 percent smarter than you are. Unfortunately, the drug has a side effect. The drug damages bone marrow. Would you take this new "smart pill" or not? Explain your answer.

Interpreting Graphics

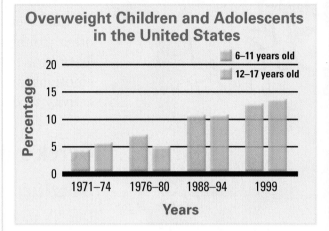

Overweight Children and Adolescents in the United States

Use the graph above to answer questions 25–28.

25 Between which two time periods did the prevalence of overweight adolescents from 12 to 17 years old show the greatest increase?

26 What general statement can you make about the percentage of overweight children in the years from 1988–1994 to 1999?

27 For 1999, what percentage of children ages 6 to 11 are overweight?

28 Being overweight is sometimes related to type 2 diabetes. Looking at the graph, what prediction would you make for the number of type 2 diabetes cases in the years after 2028?

Reading Checkup

Take a minute to review your answers to the Health IQ questions at the beginning of this chapter. How has reading this chapter improved your Health IQ?

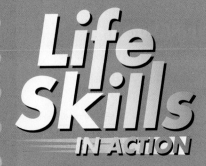

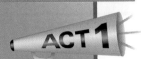

Coping

At times, everyone faces setbacks, disappointments, or other troubles. To deal with these problems, you have to learn how to cope. Coping is dealing with problems and emotions in an effective way. Complete the following activity to develop your coping skills.

Derek's Depression

Setting the Scene

Derek's mother has cancer. She has been receiving treatment for a year now. Sometimes, she seems to get better, but other times she seems to be very sick. Derek's mother remains hopeful that she will be cured and tries to keep Derek and his brother cheerful. But Derek is very worried about her. He has trouble sleeping at night and struggles with many different emotions.

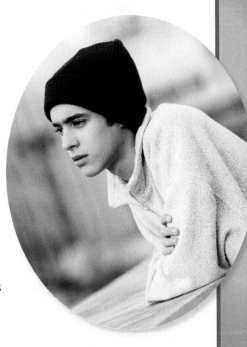

The 5 Steps of Coping

1. Identify the problem.
2. Identify your emotions.
3. Use positive self-talk.
4. Find ways to resolve the problem.
5. Talk to others to receive support.

Guided Practice

Practice with a Friend

Form a group of three. Have one person play the role of Derek and another person play the role of Derek's brother. Have the third person be an observer. Walking through each of the five steps of coping, role-play Derek dealing with his mother's illness. Derek can talk to his brother to receive support. The observer will take notes, which will include observations about what the person playing Derek did well and suggestions of ways to improve. Stop after each step to evaluate the process.

Independent Practice

Check Yourself

After you have completed the guided practice, go through Act 1 again without stopping at each step. Answer the questions below to review what you did.

1. What are some emotions that Derek may be feeling?

2. How can positive self-talk help Derek cope with his problem?

3. Other than Derek's family members, who can Derek speak with to receive support?

4. Think about a time when you faced a difficult problem. How did you cope with the problem?

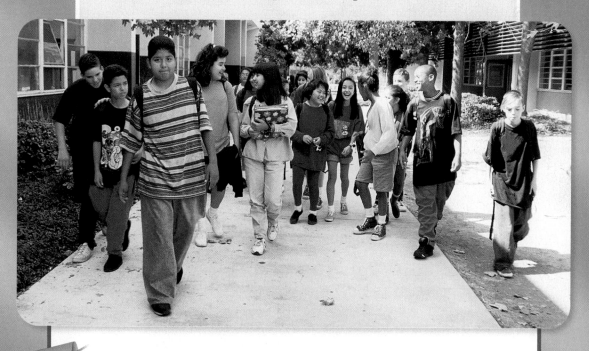

ACT 2 · On Your Own

Derek's mother's health is getting worse. She needs to go to a cancer treatment center in another city, so the family moves there temporarily. Derek and his brother start attending school in the other city. Derek is having trouble fitting in at the new school. No one talks to him, and he is struggling with his schoolwork. Make a poster that shows how Derek could use the five steps of coping to cope with attending a new school.

Check out
Current Health
articles related to this chapter by
visiting go.hrw.com. Just type in
the keyword **HD4CH31**.

> " So much has **changed** since last year. I look **different,** all of my classes are different, and I'm in a **new school.** I also have a lot of new responsibilities. This year, we get to join school sports teams. I'm really excited about joining the track team. "

Health IQ

PRE-READING

Answer the following multiple-choice questions to find out what you already know about reproduction and development. When you've finished this chapter, you'll have the opportunity to change your answers based on what you've learned.

1. **You may look like your brother or sister because**
   a. you live in the same house.
   b. you share some of the same genes.
   c. you have the same last name.
   d. All of the above

2. **How long does a human pregnancy last?**
   a. 9 weeks
   b. 20 weeks
   c. 31 weeks
   d. 40 weeks

3. **Which of the following substances can be harmful to the fetus if the mother uses the substance while she is pregnant?**
   a. alcohol
   b. tobacco
   c. illegal drugs
   d. all of the above

4. **Puberty is part of**
   a. early childhood.
   b. adolescence.
   c. the menstrual cycle.
   d. adulthood.

5. **Which of the following is a condition associated with aging?**
   a. Alzheimer's disease
   b. endometriosis
   c. inguinal hernia
   d. all of the above

6. **Which of the following is NOT a stage of grief?**
   a. denial
   b. acceptance
   c. fear
   d. bargaining

7. **Which of the following body systems helps control growth and development?**
   a. skeletal system
   b. respiratory system
   c. endocrine system
   d. circulatory system

ANSWERS: 1. b; 2. d; 3. d; 4. b; 5. a; 6. c; 7. c

What Makes You You

Jenny is going to the same school that her older brother, Sam, went to. The teachers always say things like "You must be Sam's sister" or "You look just like your brother Sam."

What You'll Do

- **Explain** where your genes come from.
- **Describe** how your growth and development are affected by both heredity and environment.

Terms to Learn

- genes
- heredity
- sex cell
- environment

Start Off Write

How does your environment affect how you look?

Have you ever wondered why some people look like a parent or a brother or a sister and why some people don't? What caused Sam and Jenny to look alike? The answer is in their genes (JEENZ).

From Two to You

The cells of every person carry a set of instructions called **genes** that describe how that person will look and grow. These instructions are passed from parents to children. The passing of traits from parents to children is called **heredity** (huh RED i tee). Each parent donates one-half of a set of instructions to the child through sexual reproduction. In sexual reproduction, a sex cell from the mother and a sex cell from the father join to form a new cell that has a full set of instructions for forming a new person. Over 9 months, this cell will develop into a baby. A **sex cell** is a cell that contains half of the genes of the parent. Because each parent's cell has one-half of the complete set of genes, a child will have some genes from the father and some genes from the mother. You may look like your parents or like your brother or sister because you share some of the same genes.

Your physical appearance isn't all you get from your parents. You also may have inherited some personality traits and some mental characteristics. But you are not only a sum of your genes. Other factors affect your development, too.

Figure 1 Your father's genes + your mother's genes = you

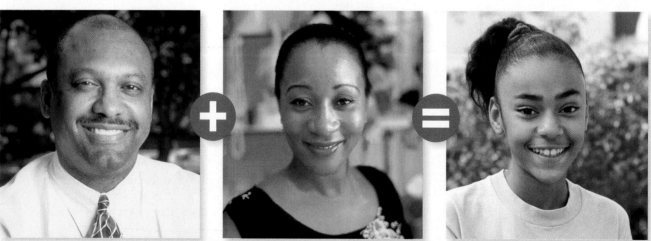

Why You Are Unique

Your growth and development are also influenced by your environment. Your **environment** is your surroundings, including people and places. Many factors affect your environment, including where you live and what your parents do. Your habits and personality are influenced by both people and opportunities. Education, nutritious foods, and a safe place to live all affect how you grow, think, and act. For example, if you live in a colder climate, you will probably dress differently than someone who lives in a warmer climate does. You may also enjoy activities associated with cold weather, such as hockey or ice skating.

No one knows exactly how much your heredity determines who you are and how much your environment does. But you are not a product of only one influence. By making good decisions, planning well, and working both smart and hard, you can have a happy and healthy life.

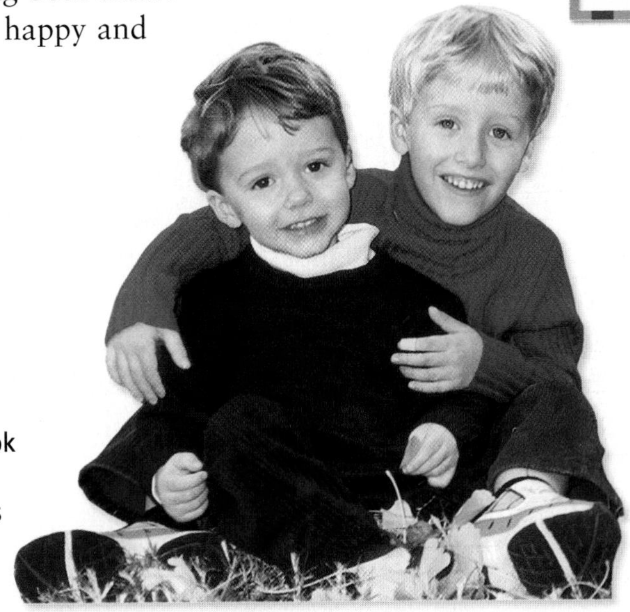

Figure 2 You and your brother or sister may look different because you inherited different genes from the same parents.

Hands-on ACTIVITY

THE EYES HAVE IT

1. Create a "family tree" of your immediate family and as much of your extended family as you can. Show the eye color of each family member.
2. Trace the trait of eye color from one generation to the next.

Analysis

1. What patterns do you see?

Lesson Review

Using Vocabulary

1. What are sex cells?
2. What is the difference between genes and heredity?

Understanding Concepts

3. Is your appearance determined by heredity, or is it determined by your environment?

Critical Thinking

4. **Identifying Relationships** How might nutrition affect your physical appearance?
5. **Analyzing Ideas** Which influence—heredity or environment—do you think is more important in shaping a person's appearance? in shaping a person's personality? Explain your answer.

The Male Reproductive System

The father provides a sex cell that contains half the blueprint for forming a new person. Where in the man's body does this cell form?

In sexual reproduction, the man provides the sex cell called a **sperm.** Sperm is made in organs called **testes** (TES TEEZ). The testes (singular, *testis*), also called *testicles*, also make most of the man's primary sex hormone, *testosterone* (tes TAHS tuhr OHN).

The Male Anatomy

Figure 3 shows the organs of the male reproductive system. Some of these organs are outside the body, and some are inside the body. The outside organs are the penis and scrotum. The scrotum is a sack of skin that holds the two testes and the two epididymises. The reproductive organs inside a man's body are the vas deferens, the prostate gland, the seminal vesicles, the Cowper's glands, and the urethra.

What You'll Do

- **Identify** the parts of the male reproductive system.
- **Describe** how sperm are made.
- **List** seven problems of the male reproductive system.
- **Explain** four ways to protect your reproductive system.

Terms to Learn

- sperm
- testes

Start Off *Write*

Describe one way that males can protect their reproductive health.

Figure 3 The Male Reproductive System

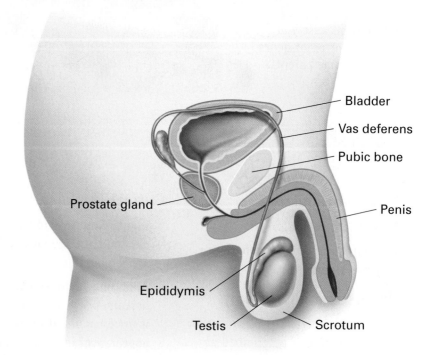

Bladder

Vas deferens

Pubic bone

Prostate gland

Penis

Epididymis

Testis

Scrotum

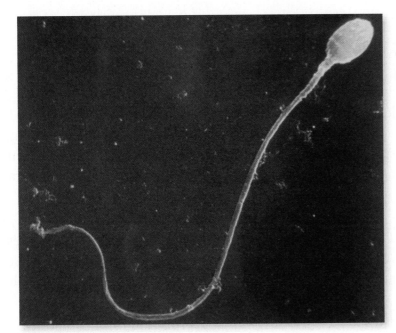

Figure 4 Sperm have a head and a tail. The head carries the genes of the father. The tail's swimming motion propels the sperm.

The Production of Sperm

Sperm are made in tightly coiled tubes inside the testes. The cells in these tubes make copies of their genes and then divide to make more cells. The new cells that form have one-half of the original number of genes. The sperm cells will carry the genes of the father into the mother's body, where the mother's sex cell, called an *egg*, can join with the sperm. But when they leave the testes, the sperm are immature and are not able to combine with a female egg. After about 70 days in the testes, the sperm pass to the epididymis.

Each testis continually releases immature sperm cells into an epididymis. In each epididymis, sperm mature and grow the tails that allow them to swim. Sperm's ability to swim is necessary for them to be able to reach an egg. When the sperm are fully grown, they move into the tubes called the *vas deferens*, each of which is attached to an epididymis. The vas deferens run from each epididymis out of the scrotum. Then, they widen to form a storage area for sperm located just above the prostate gland. Sperm pass through the prostate gland and past the Cowper's glands on their way from the storage area to the urethra. Those glands make a fluid that mixes with the sperm to form a fluid called *semen*. The semen passes to the outside of the body through the urethra, which is a tube that runs through the penis. After 2 weeks in the man's body, the sperm are broken down and reabsorbed by the body.

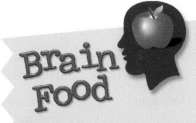

Brain Food

Sperm are kept 4°F (1°C to 2°C) cooler than the rest of the body. The temperature of the testes is controlled by a muscle that moves the scrotum closer to or farther from the body.

Problems of the Male Reproductive System

Most men may not think about the possibility that something could go wrong with their reproductive system. As a result, boys and men often do not think of having checkups by a doctor unless they must do so for school or sports. But regular medical checkups can protect men's health in many ways. For example, during regular medical checkups, a doctor can identify potential problems and treat the problems before they get worse or cause permanent damage.

Some problems with the male reproductive system may produce a bump, a sore, or pain or discomfort in the testes or scrotum. Any bumps, pain, or uncomfortable rashes or sores require immediate medical attention. Other problems may have no visible symptoms. Table 1 describes some problems of the male reproductive system.

TABLE 1 Problems of the Male Reproductive System

Problem	Description	Treatment or prevention
Jock itch	an infection of the skin by a fungus; often happens when scrotum and groin skin stays hot and moist; symptoms are red, itchy, irritated skin	treated with medicated creams or ointments; prevented by keeping the area clean and dry
Sexually transmitted diseases (STDs)	diseases passed by sexual contact that involves the sex organs, the mouth, or the rectum; symptoms may include sores or discharge, but many STDs have no symptoms	medical treatment required; prevented by abstaining from sexual activity
Inguinal (ING gwi nuhl) hernia	a weakness in the lower abdominal wall that allows a small loop of the intestines to bulge through; causes a soft bulging area on the lower abdomen, just above where the legs join the body; may or may not be painful	medical treatment required; often surgery is required to repair a hernia
Trauma (injury)	injury to the scrotum or testicles; usually happens during athletic events, accidents, or falling on an object	treated by resting and by applying ice packs; requires medical care if swelling is massive or pain persists; prevented by wearing a protective cup
Urinary tract infections (UTIs)	infections in the urethra and bladder that cause frequency of and burning during urination, may cause urine to be bloody; relatively rare for men	medical care required; treated with antibiotics
Testicular cancer	uncontrolled growth of cells of the testes; usually does not cause pain; usually found as an enlargement of the testis or as a pea-sized lump on the testis	medical care, including surgery and chemotherapy, required; easily treatable when found early; detected by regular testicular exams
Testicular torsion	twisting of the testis around on the nerves and blood vessels attached to it; usually happens during athletic activity; produces swelling and pain	immediate medical care required

Staying Healthy

Some medical problems can damage your body for the rest of your life. Some tips for staying healthy are listed below.

- Bathe every day. Don't wear damp or tight clothing longer than you have to.

- Always wear protective gear when playing sports.

- Do regular testicular self-exams. Ask your doctor how to do these exams. See a doctor about any unusual pain, swelling, or tenderness or any unusual lumps or growths.

- To prevent STDs, abstain from sexual activity.

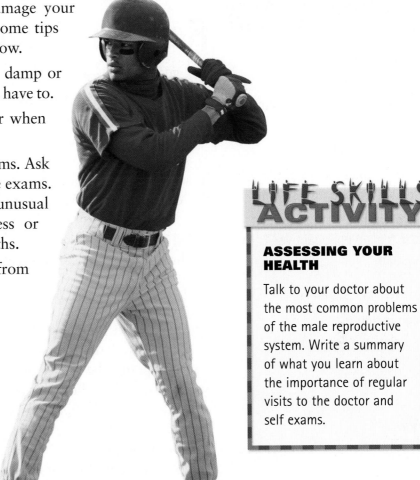

Figure 5 Wearing protective gear, such as a cup, when playing sports can help protect your reproductive system.

LIFE SKILLS ACTIVITY

ASSESSING YOUR HEALTH

Talk to your doctor about the most common problems of the male reproductive system. Write a summary of what you learn about the importance of regular visits to the doctor and self exams.

Lesson Review

Using Vocabulary

1. Name the male sex cell. Briefly describe how the cell is made.

Understanding Concepts

2. Which organs of the male reproductive system are outside the body? Which are inside the body?

3. List three problems of the male reproductive system, and describe how to prevent them.

Critical Thinking

4. Identifying Relationships How does wearing protective gear when playing sports help protect the male reproductive system?

5. Analyzing Ideas Why is it important that sperm cells contain only one-half of the man's genes?

The Female Reproductive System

The father supplies the sex cell known as sperm. Which sex cell does the mother provide? Where in the woman's body does this cell form?

What You'll Do

■ **Identify** the parts of the female reproductive system.

■ **Describe** the typical menstrual cycle.

■ **List** seven problems of the female reproductive system.

■ **Explain** five ways to protect the female reproductive system.

Terms to Learn

● egg (ovum)
● ovulation
● menstruation

Start Off
Write

What is the menstrual cycle?

In sexual reproduction, the woman provides the sex cell called the **egg,** or **ovum.** Women are born with all the eggs they will ever have; they do not make more. The eggs are stored in organs called *ovaries.* The ovaries make most of the woman's primary sex hormone, *estrogen* (ES truh juhn).

The Female Anatomy

Figure 6 shows the female reproductive system. A fallopian (fuh LOH pee uhn) tube runs between each ovary and the uterus. The fallopian tube does not actually connect to the ovary. The egg is drawn into the fallopian tube by sweeping movements of the ends of the fallopian tubes. The egg then travels through the tube to the uterus. The uterus is a muscular organ that holds a fetus during pregnancy. The uterus meets the vagina at the cervix. The vagina is the muscular organ that connects the outside of the body with the uterus. A woman's breasts are also a part of her reproductive system.

Figure 6 The Female Reproductive System

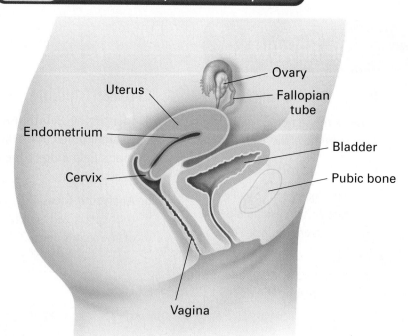

Figure 7 The Menstrual Cycle

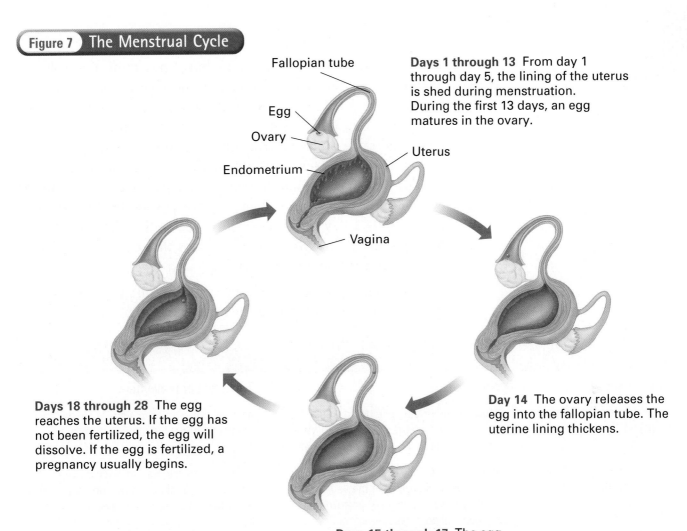

Days 1 through 13 From day 1 through day 5, the lining of the uterus is shed during menstruation. During the first 13 days, an egg matures in the ovary.

Fallopian tube

Egg

Ovary

Endometrium

Uterus

Vagina

Day 14 The ovary releases the egg into the fallopian tube. The uterine lining thickens.

Days 18 through 28 The egg reaches the uterus. If the egg has not been fertilized, the egg will dissolve. If the egg is fertilized, a pregnancy usually begins.

Days 15 through 17 The egg travels through the fallopian tube, toward the uterus.

The Menstrual Cycle

Every month, one of the ovaries releases a mature egg in a process called **ovulation** (AHV yoo LAY shuhn). During this time, the lining of the uterus thickens to prepare for a possible pregnancy. The uterine lining is called the *endometrium* (EN doh MEE tree uhm). If the egg is fertilized by a sperm cell in the fallopian tube, the fertilized egg will attach to the wall of the uterus and a pregnancy will begin. If the egg is not fertilized, the lining of the uterus will be shed. When the lining is shed, blood and tissue leave the body through the vagina. The monthly breakdown and shedding of the endometrium is called **menstruation** (MEN STRAY shuhn), or the menstrual period.

Ovulation and menstruation usually happen in a cycle, called the *menstrual cycle*, that lasts roughly 28 days. The typical menstrual cycle is shown in Figure 7. Girls often have their first menstrual period between the ages of 9 and 16.

Myth & Fact

Myth: Women always ovulate on the 14th day of the menstrual cycle.

Fact: The timing of ovulation can be irregular for every woman. Ovulation can happen at unusual times without a woman knowing it. However, ovulation generally happens toward the middle of the cycle.

Problems of the Female Reproductive System

Most healthy young women do not have any significant problems with their reproductive system. But the changes in the female reproductive system can cause young women a great deal of stress. Many of the health concerns of young women are related to the menstrual cycle and menstruation. Girls normally have irregular periods for the first few years after starting menstruation. Irregular periods vary in length and heaviness. Periods can come as often as every 3 weeks or as infrequently as every 6 weeks. Bleeding can last for only 1 day or for as long as 8 days. Both light and heavy bleeding are normal. Abdominal cramps that come with periods are also normal, unless the cramping is extremely severe.

Some female reproductive health problems are listed in Table 2. All of the problems listed in the table require medical care.

TABLE 2 Female Reproductive Problems

Problem	Description	Treatment or prevention
Urinary tract infections (UTIs)	infection of the urinary bladder, urethra, or kidneys that causes frequency of and burning during urination; may cause bloody urine	medical care required; usually treated with antibiotics and plenty of fluids
Vaginitis (VAJ uh NIET is)	infection of the vagina that causes itching, odor, and/or discharge from the vagina; caused by bacteria, fungi, or protozoans; sometimes called a *yeast infection*	medical care required; usually can be treated with antibiotics; may be prevented by keeping the area clean and dry and by not wearing damp clothes longer than is necessary
Endometriosis (EN doh MEE tree OH sis)	growth of tissue like that of the endometrium outside the uterus and inside a woman's body; during the menstrual period, bleeding inside the woman's body causes pain; may lead to infertility	medical care for severe cramps with periods may be required; treated with hormones and/or surgery
Sexually transmitted diseases (STDs)	diseases passed by sexual contact that involves the sex organs, the mouth, or the rectum; symptoms may include sores or discharge, but many STDs have no symptoms	medical treatment required; prevented by abstaining from sexual activity
Toxic shock syndrome	an infection by bacteria; most common in women who use tampons during menstruation; causes fever, chills, weakness, a rash, and many other symptoms	emergency medical care required; treated with hospitalization and antibiotics; may be prevented by changing tampons every 4 to 6 hours
Cervical, uterine, or ovarian cancer	uncontrolled growth of cells of the cervix, uterus, or ovaries; usually does not cause pain; is usually found by doctors during annual Pap smear tests and physical examinations	detected by annual pelvic exams and Pap-smear tests by a doctor; may be prevented by avoiding sexual activity to avoid contracting STDs that may increase the chance of cancer
Breast cancer	uncontrolled growth of cells of the breast; usually does not cause pain	can be detected during monthly self-examinations; your doctor can explain how to do these exams

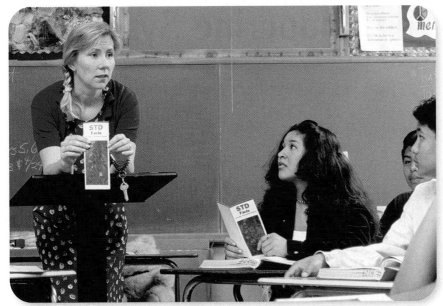

Figure 8 Learning about your reproductive health can help you make good decisions.

teen talk

Teen: I hear a lot about doing breast self-examinations and getting tested for cancer. How often should these tests be done?

Expert: Being tested regularly for different cancers of your reproductive system is very important. You can do breast self-examinations once a month. Once you reach age 18, you should start getting annual pelvic examinations and Pap tests. Ask your doctor for more information about these exams.

Staying Healthy

Some medical problems can damage your body for the rest of your life. Some tips for staying healthy are listed below.

- Bathe every day. Do not wear damp or tight clothing longer than is necessary.

- If you have questions about your health, talk to a parent or another trusted adult. See a doctor if necessary.

- Start going to a doctor for annual exams at age 18.

- Maintain good hygiene during menstrual periods. Bathe every day, and change sanitary pads or tampons every 4 to 6 hours.

- To protect yourself from STDs, do not have sex before marriage.

Lesson Review

Using Vocabulary

1. What is the female sex cell?

2. Describe the menstrual cycle.

Understanding Concepts

3. List the parts of the female reproductive system.

4. List six problems of the female reproductive system.

5. Describe five ways a woman can protect her reproductive health.

Critical Thinking

6. Analyzing Ideas Why do you think the endometrium is shed every month if a pregnancy does not begin?

The Endocrine System

Keeshawn grew 6 inches last year. His body is changing so quickly that his mom teases him about having to buy new clothes every month.

What You'll Do

- **Summarize** the role of hormones in growth and development.

Terms to Learn

- endocrine system
- gland
- hormone

Start Off
Write

How does the endocrine system affect growth and development?

Keeshawn is growing so quickly because of his endocrine (EN doh KRIN) system. The **endocrine system** is a group of glands that release special chemicals that control much of how your body functions. A **gland** is a group of cells that make these chemicals for your body. The endocrine system is shown in Figure 9.

What Are Hormones?

Each gland produces its own specific type of hormone. **Hormones** are chemicals produced by the endocrine glands that travel through the bloodstream and cause changes in different parts of the body. Hormones regulate the growth and activity of the organs of your body. Hormones are responsible for how your body grows and changes. How you react to stress is also related to the release of hormones. The actions of hormones in the body are amazing: hormones are produced in tiny amounts but have a huge impact on the body's functions.

Figure 9 The Endocrine System

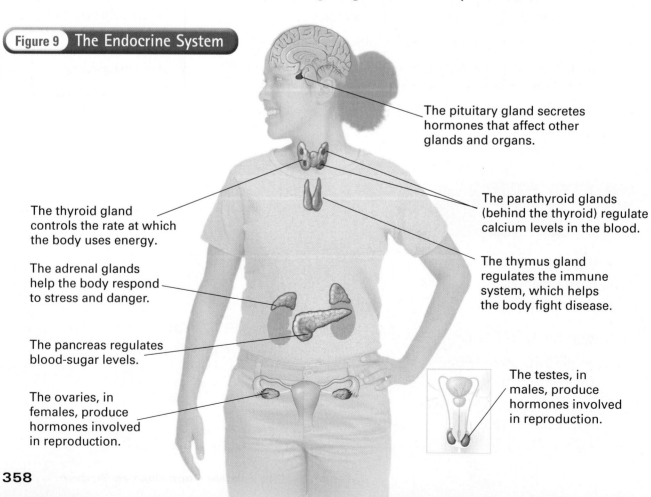

The pituitary gland secretes hormones that affect other glands and organs.

The parathyroid glands (behind the thyroid) regulate calcium levels in the blood.

The thymus gland regulates the immune system, which helps the body fight disease.

The thyroid gland controls the rate at which the body uses energy.

The adrenal glands help the body respond to stress and danger.

The pancreas regulates blood-sugar levels.

The ovaries, in females, produce hormones involved in reproduction.

The testes, in males, produce hormones involved in reproduction.

TABLE 3 Human Endocrine Glands and Their Hormones

Gland	Hormone	Function
Ovary	estrogen, the primary female sex hormone	causes physical changes during puberty; essential for menstruation
	progesterone	prepares the lining of the uterus for pregnancy
Testis	testosterone, the primary male sex hormone	causes physical changes during puberty; essential for sperm production
Thyroid	thyroid hormones	regulate how the body stores and uses energy
Pituitary	human growth hormone	stimulates body growth

How Hormones Work

You may wonder how hormones affect some parts of your body and not others. Your body's organs and tissues chemically respond only to certain hormones. Hormones target certain organs and cause only the targeted organs to respond. When a hormone reaches the target organ, that organ responds to the hormone by reacting in a certain way. Although the amount of each hormone is very small, it must be precisely the right amount to cause the organ to respond correctly. For example, if you have too much of a given hormone, you will grow too much. If you have too little of that hormone, you will not grow enough. Table 3 describes how some hormones affect your body.

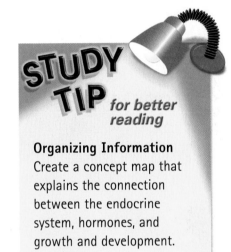

STUDY TIP *for better reading*

Organizing Information
Create a concept map that explains the connection between the endocrine system, hormones, and growth and development.

Lesson Review

Using Vocabulary

1. What is a gland?
2. Define *hormone*. List two functions of hormones.

Understanding Concepts

3. How do hormones work in the body?

4. Why do hormones affect some parts of your body and not others?

Critical Thinking

5. **Making Inferences** Why might males and females have different primary sex hormones?
6. **Analyzing Ideas** Why is it important that hormones be released directly into the blood?

internet connect

www.scilinks.org/health
Topic: Growth and Development
HealthLinks code: HD4048

HEALTH LINKS. Maintained by the National Science Teachers Association

Growing Up

When the two separate sex cells combine, a new human cell is created. During pregnancy, this new cell grows into a baby.

What You'll Do

- **Describe** the development of a fetus.
- **Summarize** the stages of childhood.

Terms to Learn

- pregnancy
- embryo
- fetus

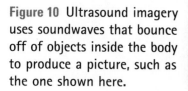

Start Off
Write

Describe what happens during birth.

The time when a woman is carrying a developing baby in her uterus is called **pregnancy.** Pregnancy begins with fertilization (FUHR t'l uh ZAY shuhn). Fertilization is the process by which the egg and sperm join and the genes of the mother and father combine. The new cell that forms during fertilization begins to grow based on the instructions from the parents' genes.

Pregnancy

From fertilization until the end of the eighth week of pregnancy, the developing cells are called an **embryo.** From the start of the ninth week until birth, the developing cells are called a **fetus.** The distinction between an embryo and a fetus is made because by the ninth week, all major organs have started to form. For the mother, the pregnancy is divided into three specific time periods called *trimesters.* Each trimester is about 3 months, or 13 weeks, long. Development during pregnancy is described in Figure 11.

While a fetus is inside its mother, it receives nutrition and oxygen through its umbilical cord. The umbilical cord is attached to what becomes the baby's "bellybutton." The other end of the umbilical cord is attached to the placenta. The *placenta* is a temporary organ attached to the inside wall of the mother's uterus during pregnancy. Nutrients and oxygen pass through the placenta from the mother's blood to the fetus. Waste products flow from the fetus's blood across the placenta to the mother.

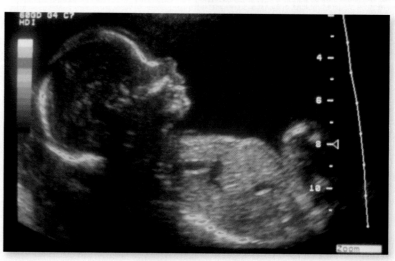

Figure 10 Ultrasound imagery uses soundwaves that bounce off of objects inside the body to produce a picture, such as the one shown here.

Figure 11 Pregnancy Timeline

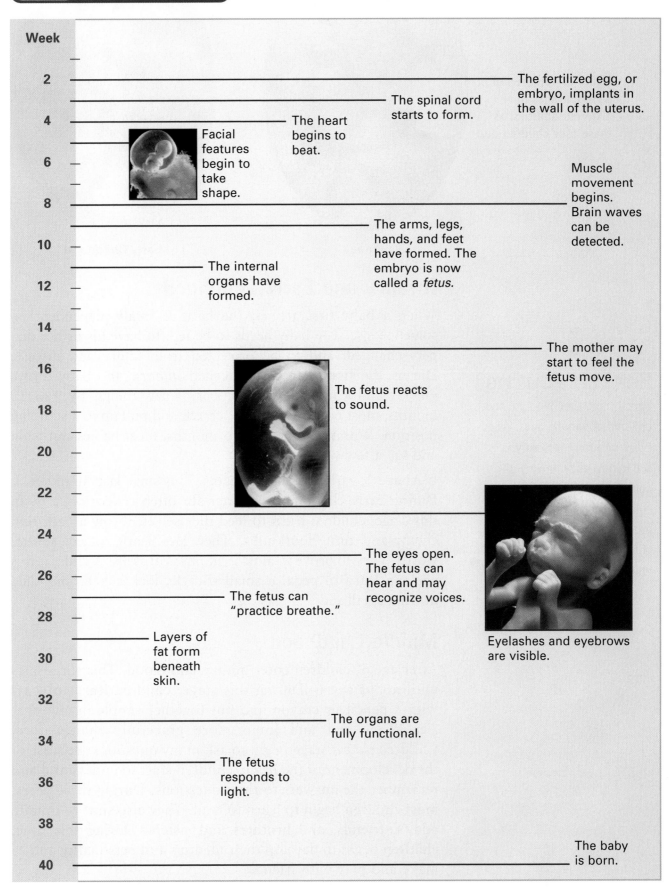

Week

2 — The fertilized egg, or embryo, implants in the wall of the uterus.

The spinal cord starts to form.

4 — The heart begins to beat.

Facial features begin to take shape.

6 —

Muscle movement begins. Brain waves can be detected.

8 —

The arms, legs, hands, and feet have formed. The embryo is now called a *fetus*.

10 —

The internal organs have formed.

12 —

14 —

The mother may start to feel the fetus move.

16 —

The fetus reacts to sound.

18 —

20 —

22 —

24 —

The eyes open. The fetus can hear and may recognize voices.

26 —

The fetus can "practice breathe."

28 —

Layers of fat form beneath skin.

30 —

Eyelashes and eyebrows are visible.

32 —

The organs are fully functional.

34 —

The fetus responds to light.

36 —

38 —

The baby is born.

40 —

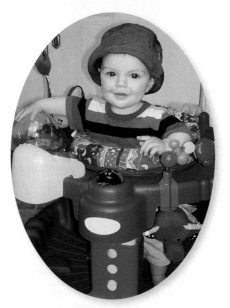
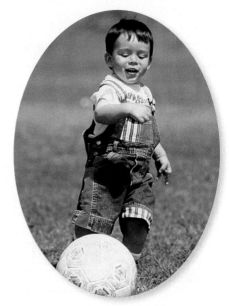

Infancy   **Early Childhood**

Figure 12 Children of different ages have different abilities, as these four children do.

Health Journal

Spend some time with younger children of varying ages. What types of differences do you see in how they move and communicate? How do they communicate with others around them? How does communication change as children get older?

Infancy and Early Childhood

When a baby first arrives, the baby is totally dependent on someone else. The baby needs to be fed, to have his or her diapers changed, and to be protected from injury and disease. During the first year of life, called *infancy*, the baby grows quickly and learns to do a number of new things. By 9 or 10 months, most babies can sit up, crawl, and pull up to a standing position. Within another 3 to 6 months, most babies can walk and say a few words.

At age 1, early childhood begins. This stage lasts until age 3. During early childhood, children are often called *toddlers*. In this stage, children learn to feed themselves, throw a ball, run, climb, and turn doorknobs. They also learn to say several words. They improve in almost all physical skills. A child at this age can learn to pedal a small tricycle, kick a ball, and slide down a small slide.

Middle Childhood

After age 3, children enter middle childhood. This stage lasts until about age 6. During this stage, children learn to draw with a pencil or crayon and put together simple jigsaw puzzles. They run and jump more gracefully than before. Children in this stage begin to ask many questions. Because of the development of the brain, children start to understand and remember the answers to their questions. During these years, most children begin to learn to read. They also start to imitate adults, friends, and brothers and sisters. During this time, children begin to develop their identity and personality and to make and play with friends.

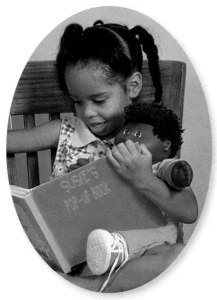

Middle Childhood

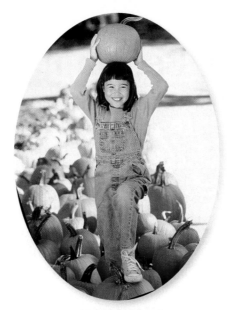

Late Childhood

Late Childhood

Late childhood lasts from age 6 until about age 11. During these years, physical ability dramatically improves, and physical size increases. Growth during this time takes place in spurts. These rapid physical changes sometimes make children feel awkward and self-conscious.

Children in this stage need to be active physically, mentally, and socially. Participating in physical activity can help children stay strong and healthy. Exploring skills and interests helps older children develop mentally. Late childhood is also a time of increased social development. Forming friendships with others of the same age becomes important and allows children to develop new social skills. At the end of late childhood, children are prepared to enter adolescence.

LANGUAGE ARTS ACTIVITY

Write a short story about a child who is in one of the stages between infancy and late childhood. Write the story in the first person. The language in the story should reflect the age of the child who is telling the story.

Lesson Review

internet connect

www.scilinks.org/health
Topic: Pregnancy
HealthLinks code: HD4077

HEALTH LINKS. Maintained by the National Science Teachers Association

Using Vocabulary

1. Define *pregnancy*.

2. What is the difference between an embryo and a fetus?

Understanding Concepts

3. Summarize the development of a fetus.

4. Summarize the development of children between birth and age 11.

Critical Thinking

5. Making Inferences Why is it important for infants and toddlers to receive a lot of physical and emotional care?

6. Analyzing Ideas The mother passes nutrients to the fetus through the placenta. Why is it important for the mother to avoid alcohol, tobacco, and other drugs?

Becoming an Adult

Hassan noticed that he looked different in the mirror. He was getting taller, and the shape of his body was changing. His shoulders were getting wider, and hair was starting to grow on his face.

Your body changes as you get older. The changes Hassan is seeing are only the beginning of the changes he will go through as he becomes an adult.

Adolescence

The time in life when a person matures from a child to an adult is called **adolescence.** Adolescence begins with puberty and lasts until the person is physically mature. **Puberty** is the stage of development when the reproductive organs mature and the person becomes able to reproduce. Puberty begins at different times for different people. In general, puberty starts earlier for girls than it does for boys. This growth from childhood to maturity involves mental, emotional, physical, and social growth.

The physical changes of adolescence are caused by increased amounts of hormones in the body. High levels of hormones cause girls to have a menstrual cycle and to develop breasts. Different hormones cause boys to start making sperm. Both boys and girls have growth spurts and begin to grow body hair.

Both boys and girls go through mental, social, and emotional changes, too. These changes prepare them for adulthood. Adolescents must learn how to interact with others and how to perform tasks of adults, such as taking care of a family and holding a steady job.

What You'll Do

- **Explain** how the physical, mental, social, and emotional changes of adolescence prepare you for adulthood.
- **Describe** what happens to the body during aging.
- **List** the five stages of grief.

Terms to Learn

- adolescence
- puberty
- adulthood
- grief

Start Off
Write

What does *being an adult* mean?

Figure 13 All of these boys are normal. Growth spurts during adolescence happen at different times for different people.

Preparing for Adult Roles

During adolescence, you grow mentally as your brain matures. You learn to understand more-complex concepts. You learn the importance of making good decisions and accepting the consequences of your decisions and actions. These mental changes prepare you for adult tasks, such as getting a job.

The sex hormones your body produces may make you interested in romantic relationships with others. Friendships and dating relationships help you prepare for adult relationships. Learning to be more independent and more responsible prepares you for having a job or a family.

All of the changes of adolescence can be confusing and even scary. Sometimes, adolescents are tempted to engage in risky behaviors as a way of dealing with these changes. Parents and other trusted adults can help you deal with the changes you are experiencing and can help you prepare to take on adult roles.

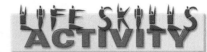

LIFE SKILLS ACTIVITY

MAKING GOOD DECISIONS

Form a group discussion in which the topic of debate is how intensely teens should begin planning for future goals while they are still in middle school and high school.

Adulthood

An adult is a person who is fully grown physically and mentally. **Adulthood** is the stage of life that follows adolescence and lasts until the end of life. During adulthood, many people fulfill personal and vocational goals. Adulthood is the time in life when people establish careers. Many adults get married and have children. Many adults find fulfillment in participating in community events and in continuing to learn.

Adults must be responsible for their own health and safety. They must pay their bills and provide food, shelter, and clothing for themselves and, if they have a family, for their spouse and children. These responsibilities can be stressful for adults.

Adults who have developed physically, mentally, emotionally, and socially are best able to cope with the demands of adulthood. Emotional and mental development during adolescence helps adults maintain stable home and work lives. This stability allows them to work well with others and provide for the needs of their families.

Figure 14 Many adults achieve personal and vocational goals through their careers.

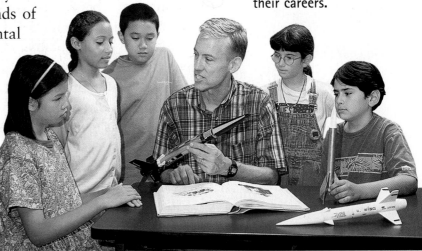

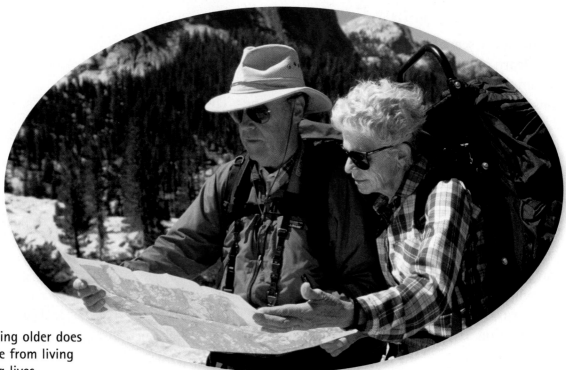

Figure 15 Growing older does not keep people from living happy, fulfilling lives.

Health Journal

Interview someone whom you consider a role model. This person can be anyone you admire. In what ways can you be like that person? In what ways do you not want to be like that person? Explain your answers.

Aging

Part of adulthood is growing older, or *aging*. Even during adulthood, our bodies continue to change. Over time, our bodies begin to wear down, and eventually they work less efficiently. One way to stay as healthy as possible for as long as possible is to take good care of yourself now. Taking good care of yourself includes eating nutritious foods and exercising regularly. It also means avoiding many risky behaviors, such as using tobacco, alcohol, and other drugs, and avoiding unnecessary physical risks, such as not wearing protective gear and seat belts.

As people age, health problems such as arthritis, Alzheimer's disease, heart disease, and cancer may arise. While each condition can be treated, many have no cure. Some of these conditions can be prevented by maintaining good health habits for an entire lifetime. Other conditions are related to heredity or environmental factors that are beyond your control. Many conditions can be managed because of advances in medical technology. These advances have improved the quality of life for many people and have increased the length of time that people live.

Even as they get older, most adults find ways to be fulfilled. Many older adults retire and begin to spend more time with their families and friends. They have more time to travel and work on their hobbies. Most adults stay healthy and active for most of their lives.

Death

Life expectancy for both men and women in the United States is the highest it has ever been. *Life expectancy* is the average number of years that people are expected to live. People are living longer because medical advances are keeping people healthy longer. Everyone eventually dies. *Death* is the end of life. At death, all of the body functions that are necessary for life stop.

Dealing with death will always be difficult. When someone you love dies, you will probably feel grief. **Grief** is a deep sadness about a loss. Many people go through five stages when dealing with death: denial, anger, bargaining, despair, and acceptance. Going through these stages helps people come to terms with their loss and prepare to live their lives without the person who has died.

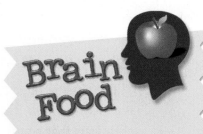

Brain Food

The average life expectancy in the United States for a man is 74 years. The average life expectancy for a woman in the United States is 80 years.

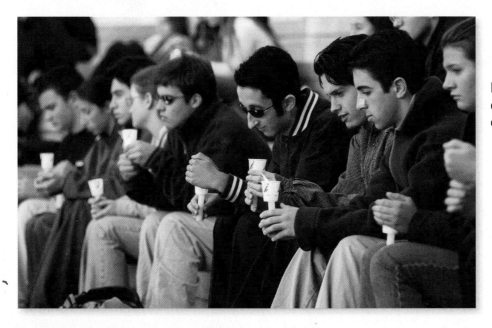

Figure 16 Many people rely on their family or friends for comfort when they grieve.

Lesson Review

Using Vocabulary

1. What is the difference between adolescence and puberty?

Understanding Concepts

2. How do changes during adolescence prepare you for adult roles?

3. Describe what happens to the body during aging.

4. List the five stages of grief.

Critical Thinking

5. **Making Inferences** Why might your health habits as a young person influence your health as you grow older? Give two examples of health habits that can have negative effects on your long-term health. Explain your answer.

Chapter Summary

■ The passing of genes from parent to child is called *heredity*. ■ The male sex cell is called *sperm*. ■ The female sex cell is called the *egg*, or *ovum*. ■ Hormones are chemicals that control the growth and activity of the body. ■ When egg and sperm combine, a new human cell forms and develops into a fetus. ■ Pregnancy is divided into three trimesters; each trimester is about 3 months long. ■ During infancy and childhood, people grow rapidly both physically and mentally. ■ Adolescence is the stage of development from the start of puberty to adulthood. ■ An adult is a person who is fully developed physically and mentally. ■ Aging is a natural part of life. ■ Death is the end of life. People experience grief when someone dies.

Using Vocabulary

For each sentence, fill in the blank with the proper word from the word bank provided below.

testes uterus
penis ovaries
heredity environment

1 The passing of characteristics from parent to child is called ___.

2 The ___ are the male reproductive organs that make sperm and testosterone.

3 The organs that release eggs are called the ___.

4 Your surroundings, including your home and your family, are your ___.

5 During pregnancy, the fetus develops inside the mother's ___.

For each pair of terms, describe how the meanings of the terms differ.

6 hormone/gland

7 menstruation/ovulation

8 embryo/fetus

9 adolescence/puberty

Understanding Concepts

10 Briefly describe how sex cells combine to pass on the genes of both mother and father.

11 How are growth and development affected by heredity and environment?

12 What are sperm, and how are they made?

13 List and describe two problems of the male reproductive system and two problems of the female reproductive system.

14 Identify four ways to protect your reproductive system from harm.

15 What role does the endocrine system play in growth and development?

16 Summarize the typical menstrual cycle.

17 Describe what happens to the body during aging.

18 Describe human development from fertilization to birth.

19 Summarize the stages of childhood.

20 Explain how changes that happen during adolescence prepare people for adult roles.

21 What are the five stages of grief?

Critical Thinking

Analyzing Ideas

22 A fetus in the uterus receives all of its nourishment from its mother. Why should expectant mothers avoid using alcohol and other drugs?

23 Having the sexually transmitted disease human papillomavirus, HPV, increases the chances that a woman will get cervical cancer. Explain how abstaining from sexual activity can reduce a woman's chance of getting cervical cancer later in life.

24 Explain how differences in growth and development patterns in adolescents, such as the onset of puberty, may affect personal health.

25 What are some health problems that you could have if your body produced too much or too little of the thyroid hormone that regulates how your body stores fat and uses energy?

Using Refusal Skills

26 Some students on your sports team have been taking hormones called *steroids* to make their muscles grow bigger and faster. One day, they offer you some steroids. What reasons would you give for refusing the steroids?

27 Imagine that you are baby-sitting for an infant. After you have been baby-sitting for about an hour, your friend calls and invites you to go with him to the movies. He says that you'll be gone for only two hours and that the baby will be all right alone for that long. How do you explain to him that you can't leave the baby alone?

Interpreting Graphics

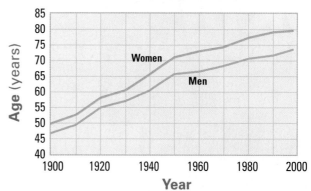

Average Life Expectancy in the United States

Use the figure above to answer questions 28–31.

28 The graph above shows average life expectancy in the United States from 1900 to 1997. What was life expectancy for men in 1940? What was life expectancy for women in 1930?

29 By how many years did life expectancy for men increase between 1900 and 1997? By how many years did life expectancy change for women between 1900 and 1997?

30 What was the difference (in years) between life expectancy for men and life expectancy for women in 1980?

31 What may have caused the increase in life expectancy over the last 100 years?

Reading Checkup

Take a minute to review your answers to the Health IQ questions at the beginning of this chapter. How has reading this chapter improved your Health IQ?

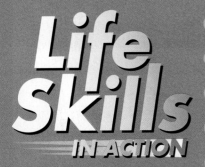

Life Skills IN ACTION

Assessing Your Health

Assessing your health means evaluating each of the four parts of your health and examining your behaviors. By assessing your health regularly, you will know what your strengths and weaknesses are and will be able to take steps to improve your health. Complete the following activity to improve your ability to assess your health.

Puberty Blues

ACT 1

Setting the Scene

Maura is going through puberty, and she doesn't like it. She grew several inches over the last half year and her body seems to change shape daily. None of Maura's clothes fit well any more, and she feels awkward just walking down the hallway at school. Maura used to be a cheerful person, but now her mood changes very often and very rapidly.

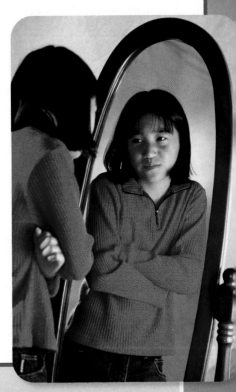

The 4 Steps of Assessing Your Health

1. Choose the part of your health you want to assess.
2. List your strengths and weaknesses.
3. Describe how your behaviors may contribute to your weaknesses.
4. Develop a plan to address your weaknesses.

Guided Practice

Practice with a Friend

Form a group of two. Have one person play the role of Maura, and have the second person be an observer. Walking through each of the four steps of assessing your health, role-play Maura analyzing one of the four parts of her health. The observer will take notes, which will include observations about what the person playing Maura did well and suggestions of ways to improve. Stop after each step to evaluate the process.

Independent Practice

Check Yourself

After you have completed the guided practice, go through Act 1 again without stopping at each step. Answer the questions below to review what you did.

1. Which part of her health did Maura assess? Why did you choose that part?

2. What are Maura's strengths and weaknesses?

3. What plan did Maura develop to address her weaknesses?

4. Name a weakness in one of your health behaviors. What can you do to improve this health behavior?

ACT 2 On Your Own

Over the last few months, Maura has felt like spending more and more time alone. She doesn't hang out with her friends as much as she used to, and she prefers staying in her room when she is home with her family. When Maura is alone, she reads and writes in her journal. Yesterday, Maura's best friend called and asked why Maura didn't like her anymore. Make a flowchart showing how Maura could use the four steps of assessing your health to assess her social health.

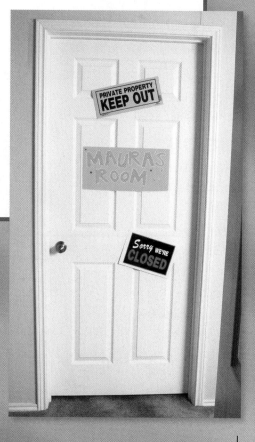

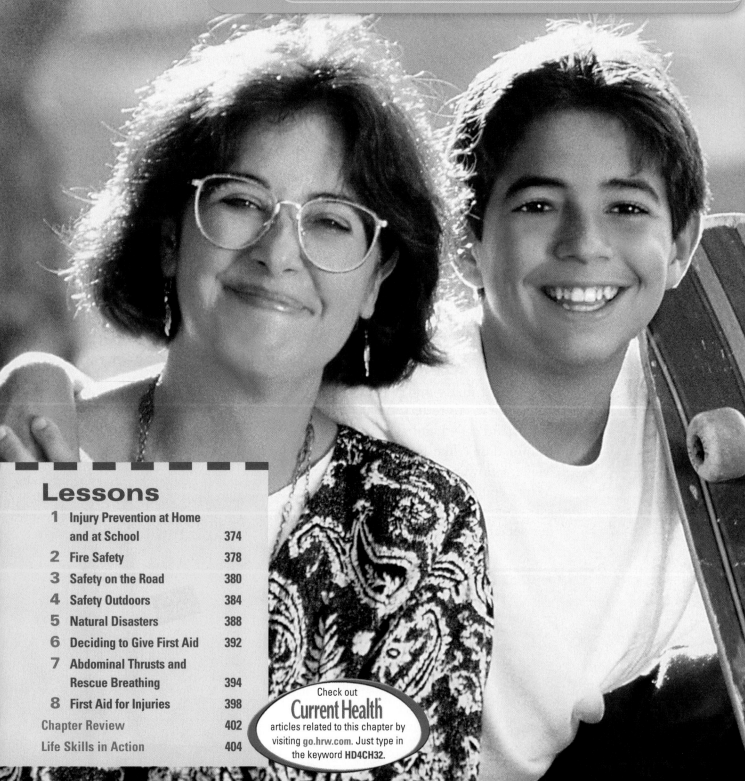

Check out
Current Health®
articles related to this chapter by
visiting go.hrw.com. Just type in
the keyword **HD4CH32**.

> **"** My mom **worries** about me when I go **skateboarding.**
>
> So, I make sure I skateboard **safely.** I always use my helmet, elbow pads, knee pads, and wrist guards. And I always go with a group of my friends. Mom also worries less when I tell her where I'll be. **"**

Health IQ

PRE-READING

Answer the following multiple-choice questions to find out what you already know about safety. When you've finished this chapter, you'll have the opportunity to change your answers based on what you've learned.

1. **What can you do to avoid violence at school?**
   a. walk away
   b. use conflict management skills
   c. tell an adult
   d. all of the above

2. **To give first aid for a cut, you should**
   a. use sterile gloves.
   b. remove soaked gauze.
   c. always elevate the injured limb.
   d. None of the above

3. **Which of the following should NOT be used on a grease fire?**
   a. fire extinguisher
   b. salt
   c. water
   d. baking soda

4. **A second-degree burn**
   a. affects all layers of skin.
   b. forms blisters.
   c. looks dark or dry and white.
   d. affects the top layer of skin.

5. **Which of the following should NOT be done to save a choking infant?**
   a. firm blows to the infant's back with the heel of your hand
   b. thrusts to the breastbone
   c. removing the object from the infant's mouth using your fingers
   d. none of the above

6. **A below-normal body temperature is called**
   a. frostbite.
   b. heat exhaustion.
   c. hypothermia.
   d. heatstroke.

ANSWERS: 1. d; 2. a; 3. c; 4. b; 5. c; 6. c

Injury Prevention at Home and at School

Yuli has a 2-year-old brother. Yuli and his family do a lot to make sure that Yuli's brother doesn't get hurt. They're careful to pick up anything he might choke on and to close cabinet doors.

Yuli and his family are trying to make sure that Yuli's brother doesn't have an accident. An **accident** is an unexpected event that may lead to injury.

Accidents at Home

Many accidents can happen at home. The following are four common types:

- **Falls** The most common accidents are falls. Move objects out of walkways, and wipe up spills to prevent falls.
- **Fires** Burns and smoke inhalation from fires can lead to death. Open flames, unattended stoves, and some chemicals can cause fires.
- **Electrical shock** Bare wires and overloaded outlets can cause electrical shock. Also, using electrical appliances near water can lead to electrical shock.
- **Poisoning** Household chemicals can cause poisoning if they are mistaken for something that is safe to eat or drink. Medicines can poison someone if taken incorrectly.

Figure 1 Home Safety Tips

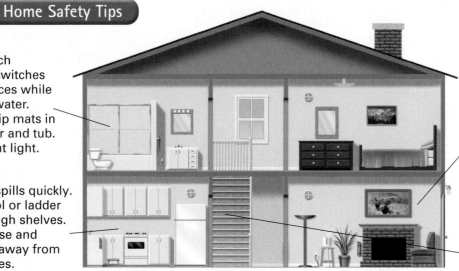

Bathroom
- Never touch electrical switches or appliances while touching water.
- Use nonslip mats in the shower and tub.
- Use a night light.

Kitchen
- Clean up spills quickly.
- Use a stool or ladder to reach high shelves.
- Keep grease and drippings away from open flames.

Living room
- Keep electrical cords out of walkways.
- Do not plug too many electrical devices into one outlet.

Stairs
- Use a railing.
- Never leave objects on stairs.

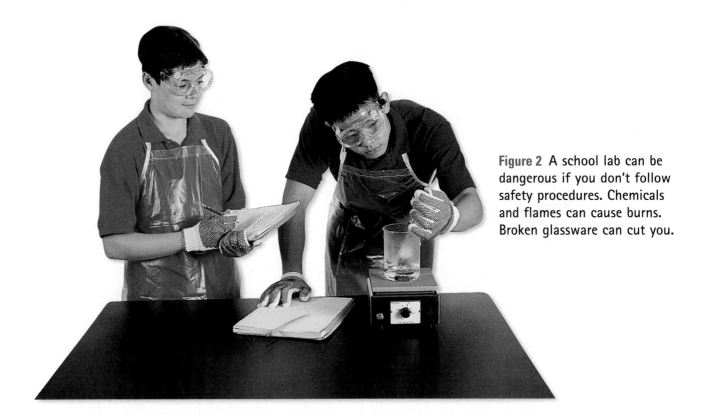

Figure 2 A school lab can be dangerous if you don't follow safety procedures. Chemicals and flames can cause burns. Broken glassware can cut you.

Safety in Class

Many of the injuries that happen at home can also happen at school. But some accidents are more likely to happen only at school. For example, injuries can happen during a lab class or in the wood shop. Glass containers, Bunsen burners, and chemicals can cause injury during a lab class. A shop class has dangerous equipment, such as saws. You should follow your teacher's instructions to avoid injury. You should also wear safety equipment, such as goggles, aprons, and gloves, to avoid injury.

Violence at School

Using physical force to hurt someone or to cause damage is called **violence.** Anger, stress, illegal drugs, prejudice, and peer pressure may make someone act violently. *Gangs* are groups of people who often use violence.

The best way to avoid violence or gangs is to walk away from any situation that could become violent. You can also use your refusal skills and your conflict management skills to avoid violence. Some situations are hard to handle on your own. If you don't think you can avoid violence, talk to your parents or a school counselor. One of the best ways to avoid violence and gangs is to look for positive alternatives. Join the school band or a sports team. Start a new club. Volunteer at the local nursing home or food bank.

Health Journal

Write about a time when you or someone you know got hurt accidentally at home or in class. Describe how the accident could have been avoided.

Gun Safety

Maybe you've seen articles or news reports about school shootings. School shootings don't happen very often. In fact, many gun-related injuries are accidental. Guns are dangerous. But you can do the following to stay safer:

- Avoid guns. If you find a gun, walk away and tell an adult right away. Don't touch the gun.

- Lock up guns in the home. If your parents have a gun, ask them to keep it locked up. Also, ask your parents to keep the gun unloaded.

- Many families hunt or shoot together. Before you go hunting, take a class in gun safety. A shooting range or local organization may offer these classes.

- Always hunt or shoot with an experienced adult. You should never use a gun without supervision.

Guns have no place in school. School shootings are frightening reminders of the harm that guns can do. Maybe you know about a student carrying a gun to school. If so, let an adult know. You should also tell an adult if you hear a student talking about hurting others. The student may just be joking. He or she may not actually want to hurt someone else. But don't take the risk. When you tell an adult, you're not just protecting yourself. You're also protecting other people.

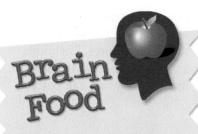

Brain Food

In 1999, about 4 percent of unintentional deaths of 10- to 14-year-olds in the United States were caused by gunshot wounds.

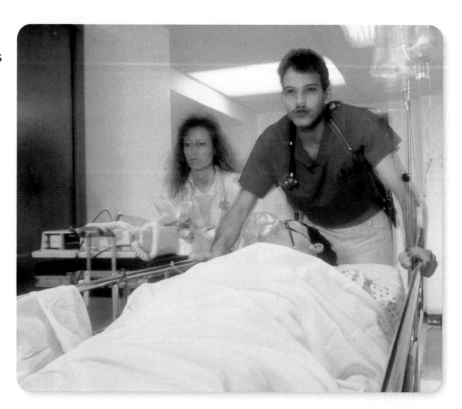

Figure 3 Each year, thousands of people visit the hospital with gunshot wounds.

Seven Ways to Protect Yourself

Many accidents don't cause an injury. But some accidents can be very serious. People have accidents every day, but you can avoid many accidents. The following are seven things you can do to stay safer:

1. **Think before you act.** Think about the consequences of your actions. Don't do something you know is dangerous.

2. **Pay attention.** Be aware of your surroundings. Look out for dangers around you.

3. **Know your limits.** Some things are safe only if you know what you're doing. Don't do something you know you aren't ready to do.

4. **Practice refusal skills.** Learn to say no when something is not safe.

5. **Use safety equipment.** Safety equipment helps keep you from getting hurt.

6. **Change risky behavior.** Change bad habits that put you or anyone else at risk.

7. **Change risky situations.** If you see a risky situation, try to fix it. Or, if you can't fix it, tell an adult about it.

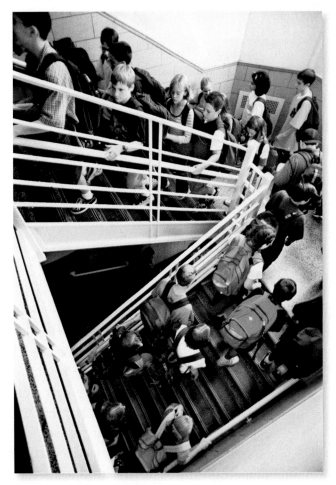

Figure 4 A busy school hallway provides plenty of opportunities for a person to have an accident.

Lesson Review

Using Vocabulary

1. What is an accident?

2. Define *violence*.

Understanding Concepts

3. Describe four common accidents.

4. What are two risky places at school? What could cause injuries in these two places?

5. List seven ways to avoid accidents.

Critical Thinking

6. **Making Good Decisions** Teddy's family goes hunting in the fall. Teddy has taken a gun safety class. If he finds an unlocked gun, what should he do?

7. **Applying Concepts** Identify the possible accidents in the following scenario: Fred's brother left his robe on the bathroom floor and the hairdryer next to the tub. Also, Fred's brother didn't wipe off the floor after he took a shower.

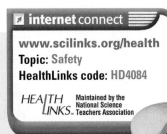

internet connect

www.scilinks.org/health
Topic: Safety
HealthLinks code: HD4084

HEALTH LINKS Maintained by the National Science Teachers Association

Fire Safety

What You'll Do

- **Describe** two devices that protect you from fire.
- **List** four ways to put out small fires.

Terms to Learn

- smoke detector
- fire extinguisher

Start Off Write

How should you put out a grease fire?

Tori and her family sat down one evening and made a family evacuation plan. They drew a map of the house with ways to escape in case of a fire. They even started practicing their evacuation plan once a month.

Many people don't understand how dangerous fire is. Fire can spread quickly and cause a lot of damage.

Fire Prevention and Detection

Many things can cause fires. Open flames, unattended stoves, overloaded circuits, and even a large pile of newspaper can start a fire. Avoiding these situations can help you stay safe.

Not all fires can be avoided. But if you have smoke detectors in your home, you will know about fires when they happen. A **smoke detector** is an alarm that detects smoke from a fire. Ask your parents to install smoke detectors in every major room of your house. Check the smoke detectors monthly to make sure they still work. Replace the batteries once a year or as needed.

What do you do when the smoke detector goes off? You need to get out of the building right away! Your family should make a family evacuation plan and practice it. This plan will help you get out of the building faster during a fire. Never go back into the building once you've left.

Figure 5 A fire evacuation plan can save your life.

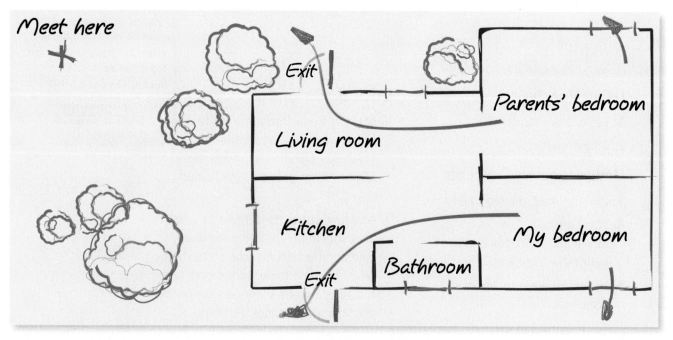

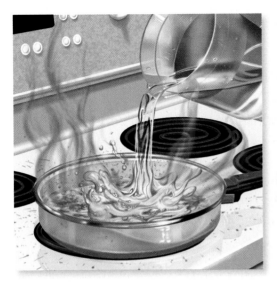
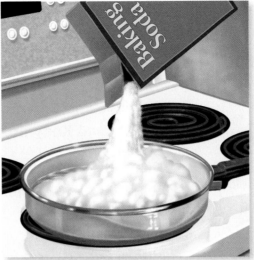

How to Put Out Small Fires

Some fires are small enough to be put out with a fire extinguisher. A **fire extinguisher** is a device that releases chemicals to put out a fire. You should put fire extinguishers in areas where fires are likely to start, such as the kitchen. Read the instructions on the fire extinguisher. Then, you'll know how to use it. Also, have your fire extinguisher checked each year to make sure it still works.

You can use the fire extinguisher to put out a small fire. You can also use water, baking soda, or salt to smother a fire. But don't use water on a grease fire. The figure above discusses how to put out a grease fire.

Putting out a fire can be dangerous. If you have any doubts about whether you can put a fire out, leave the building. Call for help from a neighbor's home. Do not go back into the building.

Figure 6 Grease floats on water. So, if you try to put out a grease fire by using water, the fire will spread. Instead, use baking soda or salt to smother the fire. You can also put the lid over the pan.

Health Journal

Walk through your home. Make a list of some fire hazards that you see. Describe ways you can fix them.

Lesson Review

Using Vocabulary

1. How do a smoke detector and fire extinguisher protect you?

Understanding Concepts

2. List four ways to put out small fires.

3. Why should you have a family evacuation plan?

Critical Thinking

4. Applying Concepts Kira is cooking some bacon when it catches on fire. The fire is not a very big fire. What should Kira do?

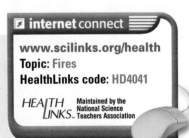

🔲 internet connect

www.scilinks.org/health
Topic: Fires
HealthLinks code: HD4041

HEALTH LINKS™   Maintained by the National Science Teachers Association

Lesson 3

Safety on the Road

Donnie has been teaching his younger sister, Katy, about road safety. He wants to make sure she is safe when she walks to school. He showed Katy how to use the **crosswalk**.

Donnie is teaching Katy how to stay safe near a road. Roadways are some of the most dangerous areas. People can get hurt while walking, riding a bike, skating, or riding in a car.

Safety While Walking

Walking down the street may not seem like a risky activity. But if you don't pay attention, you could get hurt. By paying attention, you'll know when it is safe to cross the street. You'll also be aware of automobile drivers who may not be paying attention to you. Follow these tips to stay safer:

- Use sidewalks when they are available.
- Walk facing the traffic.
- Cross the street only at crosswalks.
  - Always look both ways before crossing the street, even if you're in a crosswalk. Before crossing, look for traffic to the left, to the right, and to the left again.
  - Make sure the driver can see you if you're crossing in front of a vehicle.
  - Try to avoid walking at night. If you must walk somewhere in the dark, wear bright or reflective clothing.
  - Don't wear headphones when you're walking. Headphones may keep you from hearing approaching danger.

What You'll Do

- **Describe** seven ways to protect yourself while walking.
- **Explain** why you should use a helmet while cycling and skating.
- **Describe** how seat belts and air bags protect you.
- **List** four bus safety practices.

Start Off
Write

Why do you think it is important to wear a bicycle helmet every time you ride your bike?

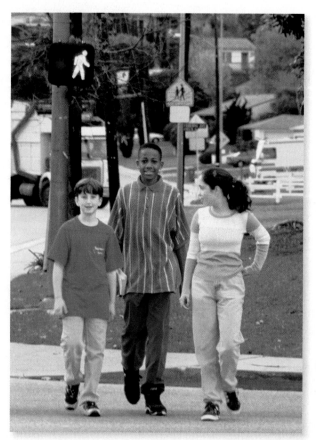

Figure 7 Using the crosswalk reduces your chances of injury.

Safety on Wheels

Cycling and skating are fun ways to exercise. But more than 300,000 people get hurt each year in cycling accidents. People also get hurt when they are in-line skating or skateboarding.

Head injuries are the most serious type of cycling and skating injury. You should wear a helmet every time you ride or skate, even if you're just going down the street. In fact, many states and cities have laws requiring teens to wear helmets while riding their bikes. Helmets aren't the only way to protect yourself. You should also remember the following safety tips:

- Wear your safety equipment. In addition to helmets, you can use knee and elbow pads to prevent injury. Skaters can also use wrist guards to protect their wrists if they fall.

- Pay attention to traffic. Watch out for busy intersections. If you are riding a bike, walk it through the intersection.

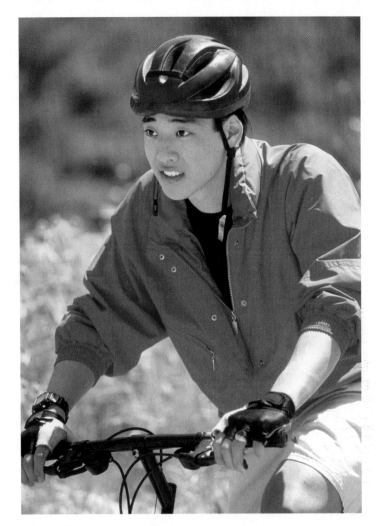

Figure 8 Helmets can keep you from getting seriously hurt if you fall while riding your bike.

- Follow the rules of the road. For example, cyclists should ride with traffic and follow the same rules as cars do.

- Wear the right clothes. Baggy clothes may get caught in bicycle chains. Wear brightly-colored clothes so that you are visible to traffic.

- Ride and skate only in designated areas. Cyclists should stay to the side of the road. Also, many communities have parks and trails set aside for cyclists and skaters to enjoy.

- Always ride and skate with friends. Friends can help you if you have an accident or if you have a problem with your equipment.

- Avoid riding and skating at night. If you have to ride at night, make sure you have a headlight and blinking taillight on your bike. If you're skating, you should also use a light. Wear bright, reflective clothing.

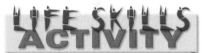

COMMUNICATING EFFECTIVELY

Imagine that you work for a bicycle, in-line skate, or skateboard company. Design an advertisement for your product that promotes the safe use of your product. Show your ad to your classmates. Does your ad inspire them to use your product safely? If not, how could you improve your ad?

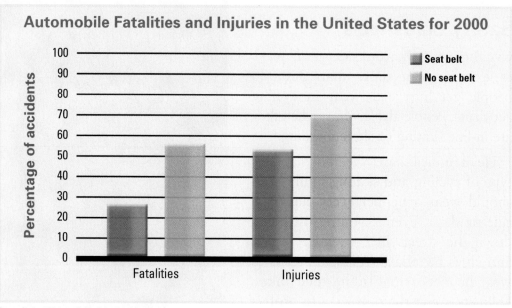

Automobile Fatalities and Injuries in the United States for 2000

Source: National Highway Traffic Safety Administration.

Figure 9 Many people die or get hurt in auto accidents because they are not wearing seat belts.

Vehicle Safety

Did you know that automobile accidents are a leading cause of death for people under age 14? Many of these people weren't wearing their seat belts. Seat belts keep you from being thrown around in a car. They also keep you from being thrown out of the vehicle. You should wear your seat belt every time you ride in a car, truck, or SUV.

Air bags inflate during an accident. Air bags, along with seat belts, keep passengers from hitting the dashboard or windshield. But air bags are made to protect larger people. They may hurt a smaller person. For the best protection, anyone under age 12 should ride in the back seat. Also, infants and smaller children should ride in child safety seats or booster seats until they are big enough to use a seat belt correctly.

Hands-on ACTIVITY

CAR HABITS

1. For 1 week, watch the members of your family when you ride in the car. Write down where each member of your family sits in the car.

2. Write down how often everyone uses a seat belt. Record the length of each trip.

Analysis

1. Did everyone use seat belts? If not, do you think the length of your trip was the reason?

2. Did anyone in your family sit in an unsafe position in the car?

3. How can you promote vehicle safety in your family?

Bus Safety

Many teens travel to and from school on a bus. Follow these tips to stay safer.

- Don't distract the driver. He or she needs to concentrate on the road.
- Sit down while the bus is moving. This way you won't fall if the bus goes over a bump or stops suddenly.
- Make sure the driver can see you when you get off the bus. Don't cross the street behind the bus or bend over while in front of the bus.
- Learn where the emergency exits are located. If there is an emergency, follow the driver's instructions.

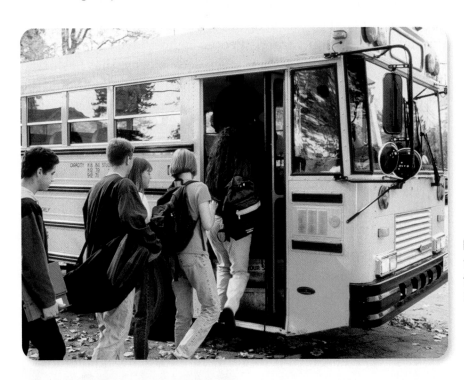

Figure 10 A bus is a convenient way to get to school. By following the safety tips, you can make sure it is a safe trip!

Lesson Review

Understanding Concepts

1. List seven ways to stay safe while walking down the street.

2. Why should you wear a helmet while cycling and skating?

3. How do seat belts and air bags protect you?

4. What are four ways to stay safe when riding the bus?

Critical Thinking

5. **Applying Concepts** Eduardo's parents have a car with air bags. If Eduardo is 11 years old, where in the car should he sit? Eduardo has a 3-year-old sister. Where should she sit?

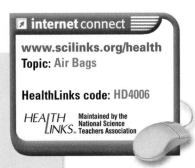

internet connect

www.scilinks.org/health
Topic: Air Bags

HealthLinks code: HD4006

HEALTH LINKS Maintained by the National Science Teachers Association

Lesson 4 · Safety Outdoors

What You'll Do

- **List** two injuries caused by cold weather.
- **Identify** two injuries caused by hot weather.
- **Describe** three ways to protect yourself while doing outdoor activities.

Terms to Learn

- hypothermia
- frostbite
- heat exhaustion
- heatstroke

Start Off *Write*

How can you avoid heat-related injuries when you exercise on a hot day?

> Jenny was watching a special on TV about climbers on Mount Everest. Some of the climbers died because of the extreme cold.

Winter weather may look pretty in pictures, but it can be dangerous. Hot weather can be dangerous, too.

Safety on a Cold Day

You may have noticed that you shiver when you get cold. Shivering helps keep you warm. But people who are cold for a long time or who get wet on a cold day may develop hypothermia (HIE poh THUHR mee uh). **Hypothermia** is a below-normal body temperature. People who have hypothermia shiver uncontrollably. They also feel sleepy, have slurred speech, and seem confused. A hypothermia victim should be kept warm. Remove any wet clothes, and wrap the victim in dry blankets. Call for help.

Cold weather can also cause frostbite. **Frostbite** is damage to skin and other tissues that is caused by extreme cold. Frostbite usually affects the fingers, toes, ears, or nose. Frostbitten skin is pale, stiff, and numb. If someone has frostbite, call for help. Put the affected area in lukewarm water until help arrives.

You can avoid hypothermia and frostbite by dressing in layers on cold days. Also, wear gloves and a hat to protect your hands and ears. Avoid going outside on extremely cold days. Go inside if you start shivering.

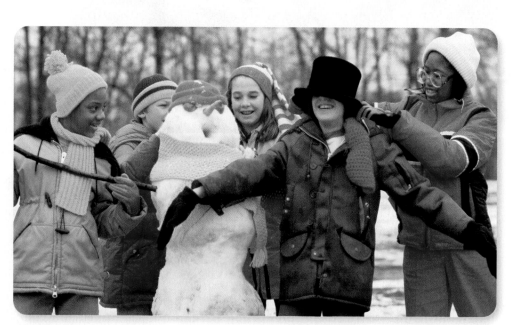

Figure 11 Dressing for the weather can keep you warm on chilly days.

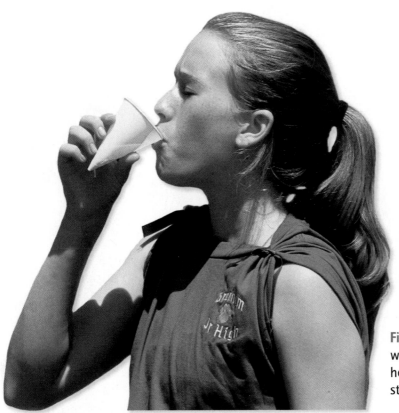

Figure 12 Drinking plenty of water is one way to avoid heat injuries. Also, try to stay in the shade.

Safety on a Hot Day

Summer is a great time to go outside and enjoy exercise. But did you know that summer weather can cause injury? Sometimes, it gets so hot that your body can't keep cool. If you can't stay cool, you can develop heat exhaustion (eg ZAWS chuhn) or heatstroke.

Heat exhaustion is a condition caused by too much water loss through sweating on a hot day. On hot days, your body absorbs heat from the sun and the air. Exercising makes you even warmer. Sweating helps your body cool down. But if you don't drink enough water to replace the water you lose as sweat, you may get heat exhaustion. Signs of heat exhaustion include headache, dizziness, nausea, and clammy skin. The best way to treat heat exhaustion is to stop exercising. Go inside, and drink cool fluids. If the symptoms do not improve, call for help.

Heatstroke is an injury that happens when the body cannot control its temperature. A person who has heatstroke can't sweat. His or her body temperature rises. The signs of heatstroke are high fever and dry skin. Sometimes, a victim may collapse and have convulsions. Someone with heatstroke should be taken to a doctor right away. Heatstroke can be life threatening.

The best way to avoid heat injuries is to drink plenty of water. Take plenty of breaks in the shade. If you're outside for a long time, you may also want to eat. Water and food help your body keep you cool.

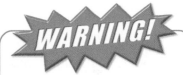

Heatstroke

Adolescents are more likely to get heatstroke than adults are. Your body is still developing, so your body's cooling system is not as advanced as an adult's system is. Because your body doesn't cool as efficiently as an adult's body does, you should be very careful on hot days.

Figure 13 Playing It Safe Outdoors

Hiking and Camping Safety

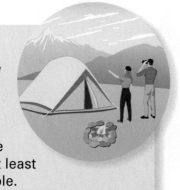

✔ Don't camp or hike by yourself. For more remote areas, go with at least three other people.

✔ Leave a plan of your activities with friends and park headquarters.

✔ Plan for emergencies. Carry emergency signal devices. Know where you can find ranger stations or telephones along your route.

✔ Carry a first-aid kit.

✔ Carry plenty of food and water.

✔ Carry bug repellant and sunscreen.

✔ Become familiar with the area. Carry a map and compass.

✔ Be aware of dangerous wildlife.

✔ Make sure all campfires are properly contained and extinguished.

Water Safety

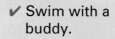
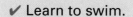

✔ Learn to swim.

✔ Swim with a buddy.

✔ Swim in designated areas. Avoid areas that aren't supervised.

✔ Obey posted warning signs.

✔ Don't run near water.

✔ Don't dive into unfamiliar bodies of water.

✔ Swim parallel to shore instead of away from shore.

✔ When at the beach, check surf conditions before getting in the water.

✔ Watch out for water plants and animals that may be dangerous.

✔ Wear a life jacket when boating.

Playing Safe

Outdoor adventures are exciting and fun. But they can be risky, too. The figure above provides some tips for hiking and camping, water safety, skiing and snowboarding, and mountain biking. Remember the following tips whenever you go outside:

• Drink plenty of water. Drinking water is important in both hot and cold weather. Water helps your body regulate its temperature.

• Use sunscreen, even on cold or cloudy days. This will prevent sunburn. Sunscreen can also prevent skin cancer. Wear a hat and sunglasses to protect your head and eyes.

• Watch the weather. Be ready for weather changes. Dress warmly on cold days. Wear light-colored, cool clothes on hot days.

Skiing and Snowboarding Safety

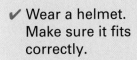

✔ Learn how to use skis and a snowboard.

✔ Ski and snowboard on slopes within your skill level.

✔ Ski and snowboard in designated areas.

✔ Control your speed.

✔ Pay attention to fellow skiers and snowboarders.

✔ When you stop on the trail, move to the side. Avoid blocking the trail.

✔ Use safety equipment such as wrist guards and goggles.

✔ Make sure equipment is in good shape and fits correctly.

✔ Wear warm clothes. Dress in layers, and wear a hat and gloves.

Mountain Biking Safety

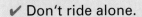

✔ Wear a helmet. Make sure it fits correctly.

✔ Don't ride alone.

✔ Don't ride trails that are too difficult for you.

✔ Develop your bike-handling skills.

✔ Watch where you're going.

✔ Learn safe riding practices. Watch out for other cyclists and hikers on the trail.

✔ Carry plenty of water.

✔ Make sure your bike is the right size for you.

✔ Tune up your bike regularly. Make sure brakes work correctly and tires are inflated.

Lesson Review

Using Vocabulary

1. What are hypothermia and frostbite?

2. Compare heat exhaustion and heatstroke.

Understanding Concepts

3. What are three ways to stay safe whenever you're outside?

Critical Thinking

4. Making Inferences According to the weather report, the temperature outside is 60°F right now. Later, the temperature will be close to 90°F. If you and your friends want to play soccer in the park, what should you wear? What should you bring?

Natural Disasters

What You'll Do

- **Describe** four types of natural disasters.

- **Describe** how you can prepare for natural disasters.

Terms to Learn

- earthquake
- tornado
- hurricane
- flood

Start Off
Write

What can you and your family do to prepare for a natural disaster?

Ryo goes to school in southern California. His school sometimes has earthquake drills. Students get under their desks during the drills.

Have you ever been in an earthquake? An **earthquake** is a shaking of the Earth's surface caused by movement along a break in the Earth's crust. One way to stay safe during an earthquake is to hide under a table or a desk. Because earthquakes are common in southern California, many schools there have earthquake drills.

Earthquakes

Sometimes, earthquakes cause a lot of damage. In fact, some earthquakes are called natural disasters. *Natural disasters* are natural events that cause widespread injury, death, and property damage. Severe earthquakes damage buildings and roads. Earthquakes can cause landslides. Earthquakes may start fires by breaking gas lines.

During an earthquake, stay away from windows and glass. If you are outside, move away from any tall structures. Avoid power lines and trees. If you are in a car, ask the driver to pull over in an open area. Stay in the car until the earthquake is over.

After an earthquake is over, you may not have electricity or water. Watch out for broken glass and debris. Avoid downed power lines. If you think your building has been damaged, go outside until you're sure it is safe.

Figure 14 This earthquake in San Francisco destroyed homes, businesses, and other structures.

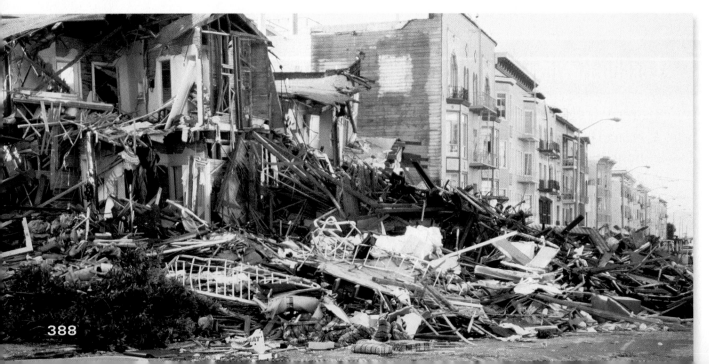

Figure 15 The Anatomy of a Hurricane

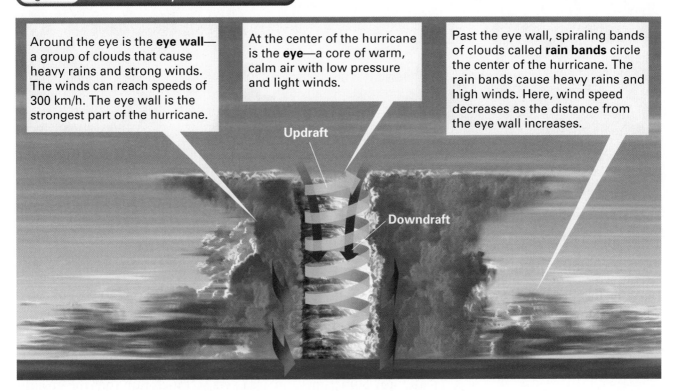

Around the eye is the **eye wall**—a group of clouds that cause heavy rains and strong winds. The winds can reach speeds of 300 km/h. The eye wall is the strongest part of the hurricane.

At the center of the hurricane is the **eye**—a core of warm, calm air with low pressure and light winds.

Past the eye wall, spiraling bands of clouds called **rain bands** circle the center of the hurricane. The rain bands cause heavy rains and high winds. Here, wind speed decreases as the distance from the eye wall increases.

Updraft

Downdraft

Tornadoes and Hurricanes

A **tornado** is a spinning column of air that has a high wind speed and touches the ground. Tornadoes can pick up objects, such as trees, cars, and houses. Most tornadoes are short lived and travel only a few miles. If there is a tornado in your area, go to the basement or the cellar. If you don't have a basement or cellar, go to the bathroom or a closet in the center of your house. If you are outside when a tornado approaches, go indoors. If you can't go indoors, lie down in a large open field or deep ditch.

A **hurricane** is a large, spinning tropical weather system with wind speeds of at least 74 miles per hour. The figure above shows the structure of a hurricane. These storms usually form over warm tropical waters in the Gulf of Mexico or Caribbean Sea. Hurricanes can last for a few days. They often produce high winds, heavy rains, and high surf. Areas near the coast are often evacuated during a hurricane.

New technology has made storm prediction more accurate. There are two kinds of weather alerts. A *watch* is a forecast that alerts people that severe weather may happen. A *warning* is a forecast that tells people that severe weather has developed. Watches and warnings alert people about tornadoes, hurricanes, thunderstorms, floods, and winter storms.

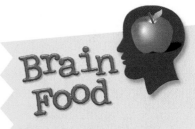

Brain Food

Hurricanes that occur in the northwestern part of the Pacific Ocean near the South China Sea are called *typhoons* (tie FOONZ). Hurricanes that occur in the Indian Ocean are called *cyclones* (SIE KLOHNZ).

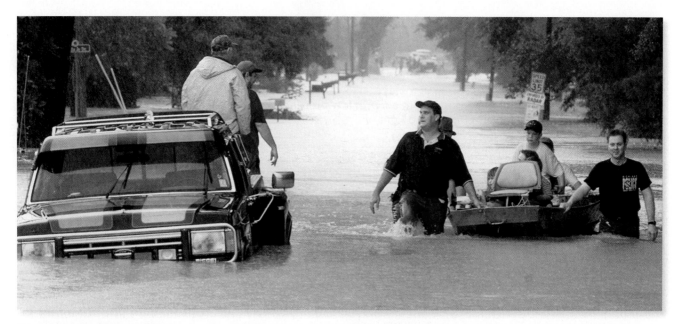

Figure 16 This flood caused a lot of damage around the Mississippi River. Many homes, businesses, and vehicles were caught in its path.

Floods

Storms often produce a lot of rain, hail, or snow. Storms can also cause large waves along the coast. Where does all of this water go? Sometimes, an area gets so much rain that the ground can't absorb any more moisture. So, the area begins to flood. A **flood** is an overflowing of water into areas that are normally dry. Floods tend to occur near rivers or creeks. Some flooding also occurs around lakes and oceans.

Usually, floods can be predicted. But sometimes a flash flood occurs. A *flash flood* is a flood that rises and falls with little or no warning. Flash floods usually happen because of a sudden, intense rainfall, a failed dam, or melting ice.

Floodwater can move very quickly. The water doesn't have to be very deep to pick up a vehicle. People should not drive through floodwater. Many people die each year because they try to drive through a flooded section of road. The best thing to do during a flood is to find high ground and wait until the water goes down.

LIFE SKILLS ACTIVITY

COMMUNICATING EFFECTIVELY

Design an emergency warning system. You can use radio, TV, or emergency sirens. Describe a way you can warn people about different kinds of weather emergencies. Include watches and warnings in your emergency warning system. Share your ideas with the class.

Be Prepared

The best way to stay safe during a storm or natural disaster is to be prepared. Your family should have an emergency kit. Include the following in your kit:

- a battery-operated radio, a flashlight, and batteries
- a first-aid kit and medicine
- canned or freeze-dried food and bottled water
- clothes, shoes, and bedding for everyone

Store your kit in the place where you will seek shelter during an emergency. And remember to stay calm during an emergency.

Myth & Fact

Myth: You don't have to replace anything in your emergency kit except when you use it.

Fact: Food, batteries, medicine, and water can go bad after a long period of time. You should replace most of these items after their expiration dates. Water should be replaced every 6 months.

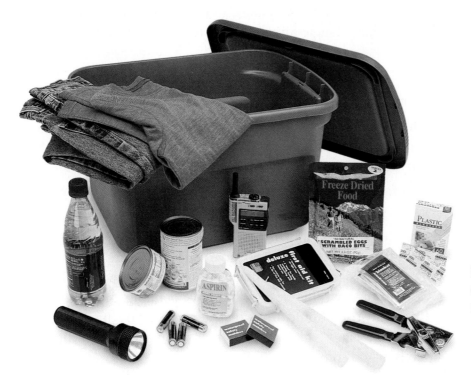

Figure 17 An emergency kit can keep you safe during a natural disaster.

Lesson Review

Using Vocabulary

1. Describe four kinds of natural disasters.

Understanding Concepts

2. What is a natural disaster?

3. Compare a watch and a warning.

4. What should you include in your emergency kit?

Critical Thinking

5. **Applying Concepts** Are all earthquakes, tornadoes, hurricanes, and floods considered natural disasters? Explain your answer.

6. **Making Inferences** Why should emergency kits include a battery-operated radio and a flashlight?

Deciding to Give First Aid

What You'll Do

- **Describe** the three steps of handling an emergency.
- **List** four things you need to say during an emergency phone call.

Terms to Learn

- emergency
- first aid

Start Off Write

What information do you need to provide when you make an emergency phone call?

Maggie's parents posted an emergency phone-number list next to the phone. Maggie's parents included 911, local emergency numbers, and their work numbers on the emergency phone-number list.

An **emergency** is a sudden event that demands immediate action. Maggie's parents keep an emergency phone-number list near the phone so that Maggie knows whom to call during an emergency.

Handling an Emergency

Do you know what to do in an emergency? Follow these steps:

1. **Check out the situation.** Make sure you're safe. If you're not sure you're safe, leave the area. If someone is hurt, try to find out what's wrong. Stay calm, and don't panic.

2. **Call for help.** Yell for help, or use the phone to call for emergency services.

3. **Care for the victim.** During some emergencies, someone may be hurt. You may need to give first aid until help arrives. **First aid** is emergency medical care for someone who has been hurt or who is sick. If you have training, give the victim first aid. You should not give first aid if you haven't taken a first-aid class. Taking a class helps you act quickly and correctly when someone is hurt.

Figure 18 Taking a first-aid class can help you take care of people when they are hurt.

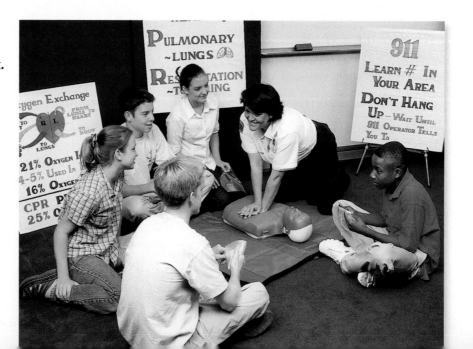

Making an Emergency Phone Call

In most areas of the United States, dialing 911 will get you help during an emergency. If your area doesn't have 911, be sure to know your local emergency number. The operator will need the following information when you call:

- your name and location
- the type of emergency
- the condition of anyone who is hurt
- what you've done to help the victim

Stay as calm as possible. Don't hang up until the operator does. He or she may have special instructions for you.

Your family should keep an emergency phone-number list next to every phone in the house. That way, everyone knows whom to call during an emergency. The table below lists some of the numbers that should be on an emergency phone-number list.

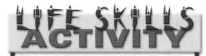

PRACTICING WELLNESS

In pairs, practice making an emergency phone call. One person should act as the operator. The other should give information.

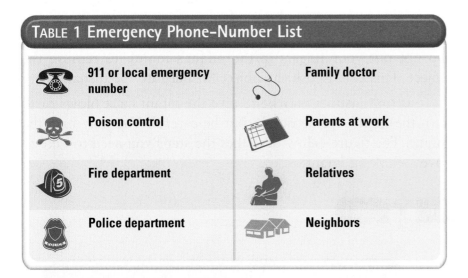

TABLE 1 Emergency Phone–Number List

	911 or local emergency number		Family doctor
	Poison control		Parents at work
	Fire department		Relatives
	Police department		Neighbors

Lesson Review

Using Vocabulary

1. What is first aid?

Understanding Concepts

2. What are the three steps of handling emergencies?

3. What four things should you tell an operator during an emergency phone call?

Critical Thinking

4. Making Inferences Why is it a good idea to include your neighbors' phone numbers and your relatives' phone numbers on your emergency phone-number list?

Lesson 7

Abdominal Thrusts and Rescue Breathing

What You'll Do

- **Describe** how to give abdominal thrusts to adults and to infants.

- **Explain** how to give rescue breathing to adults and to small children.

Terms to Learn

- abdominal thrusts
- rescue breathing
- cardiopulmonary resuscitation (CPR)

Start Off Write

How do you save someone who is choking?

Rashid went out to dinner with his parents. While they were eating, Rashid saw a waiter save a choking man's life. The waiter gave the choking man abdominal thrusts (ab DAHM uh nuhl THRUHSTS).

Abdominal thrusts are actions that apply pressure to a choking person's stomach to force an object out of his or her throat.

First Aid for Choking Infants

You can easily tell when an adult is choking. Adults usually grab their throats. But you may have a hard time telling when an infant is choking. A choking infant won't make any noise and may turn blue. Call for help if an infant appears to be choking. Do not put your fingers in the infant's mouth to remove the object. This could push the object farther into the throat.

Your first instinct may be to give the infant back blows or to turn the infant upside down. But be careful. You may hurt the infant. The figure below describes the steps you need to take to save a choking infant.

Figure 19 Saving a Choking Infant FIRST AID Certification required

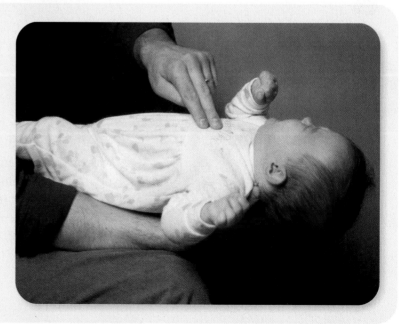

1. Put the infant face up on your forearm. Place your other arm over the infant, and hold his or her jaw. Turn the infant over.

2. Support your arm on your thigh or knee so the infant's head is lower than his or her chest. Give the infant five firm back blows with the heel of your hand.

3. If the object doesn't come loose, turn the infant over. Place two fingers on the infant's breastbone, between and just below the infant's nipples. Push the breastbone in five times.

4. Repeat back blows and chest thrusts until the object comes loose.

First Aid for Choking Adults

Sometimes, someone who seems to be choking may not be in danger. If the victim can speak, breathe, or cough, do not give abdominal thrusts. Let the victim cough until the object comes out.

If the choking person cannot speak or breathe, call for help. Begin abdominal thrusts. Abdominal thrusts compress the victim's abdomen. This increases the pressure in the victim's lungs. This pressure forces the object out of the victim's airway. You can even do abdominal thrusts on yourself. Take a look at the figure below to learn how to give abdominal thrusts to adults and to yourself.

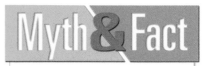

Myth: You should slap a choking person on the back.

Fact: Slapping a person on the back can lodge an object deeper in the throat, making the object more difficult to remove.

Figure 20 Saving an Adult Choking Victim 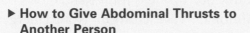 FIRST AID Certification required

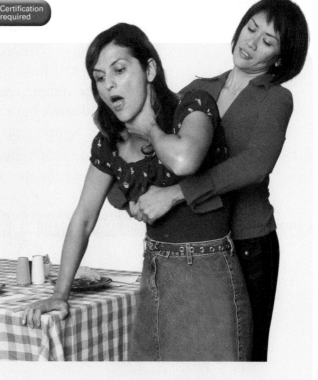

▶ **How to Give Abdominal Thrusts to Another Person**

1. The victim may be standing or sitting. Stand or kneel behind the victim. Wrap your arms around the victim.

2. Make one hand into a fist. Place the thumb side of your fist against the victim's stomach, between the belly button and the end of the breastbone.

3. Cover your fist with your other hand. Give five quick upward thrusts into the victim's stomach.

4. Repeat thrusts until the object comes loose.

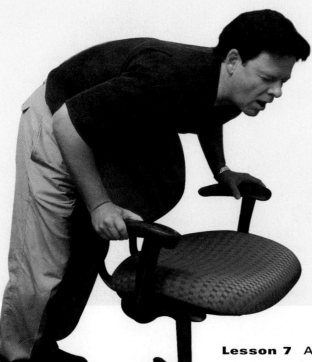

◀ **How to Give Abdominal Thrusts to Yourself**

1. If other people are around, let them know that you need help.

2. Use a chair back, counter, or any other high, solid object. Lean forward and press your stomach against the object.

3. You can also make your hand into a fist. Place it against your stomach, between your belly button and your breastbone. Cover your fist with your other hand. Quickly pull in and upward.

Rescue Breathing for Adults

Sometimes, a person stops breathing. You should act quickly when you find someone who isn't breathing. When someone doesn't breathe for several minutes, permanent injuries or even death can happen. A person who isn't breathing needs rescue breathing. **Rescue breathing** is an emergency technique in which a rescuer gives air to someone who is not breathing.

Don't move the victim unless you're sure doing so is safe. Lay the victim on his or her back. See if the victim is breathing. Tilt the victim's head back. Clear any objects out of the victim's mouth. Look, listen, and feel for breathing. Never give rescue breathing to someone who can still breathe. Before you give rescue breathing, call for help. The figure below shows you how to give rescue breathing.

Sometimes, a victim needs CPR. CPR stands for cardiopulmonary resuscitation (KAHR dee oh PUL muh NER ee ri SUHS uh TAY shuhn). **Cardiopulmonary resuscitation** is an emergency technique used to save a victim who isn't breathing and who doesn't have a heart beat.

CPR and rescue breathing require special training. You shouldn't give either unless you have been trained. The YMCA and the Red Cross offer first-aid and CPR training.

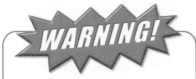

Breathing Mask

If you have a breathing mask, you should use it while giving rescue breathing. A breathing mask can protect you and the victim from disease.

Figure 21 Rescue Breathing for Adults FIRST AID Certification required

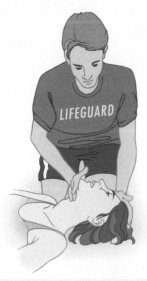

1 Open the victim's airway. Tilt the victim's head back gently. Use your finger to clear any objects out of the victim's mouth. Look at the victim's chest for movement. Also, listen for the sounds of breathing, and feel for breath on your cheek.

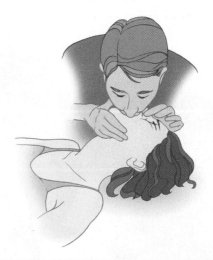

2 If the victim is not breathing, put your mouth around the victim's mouth, and pinch the victim's nose shut. Breathe out, into the victim's mouth. Give two slow rescue breaths. Look to see if the victim's chest is moving up and down in response to your breathing.

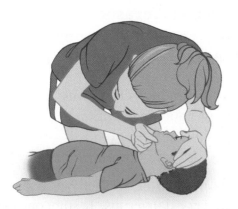

1 Position the victim on his or her back, and tilt the victim's head back. Clear any objects out of the victim's mouth, and check for signs of breathing. Look at the victim's chest for movement, listen for sounds of breathing, and feel for breath on your cheek.

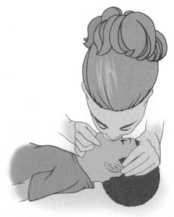

2 If the victim is not breathing, give two slow rescue breaths. Place your mouth over the victim's nose and mouth. Form a tight seal, and breathe out, into the victim's mouth and nose. Look at the victim's chest for movement to see if your breaths are going into the victim's lungs.

Rescue Breathing for Small Children

Rescue breathing is different for adults and small children. First, you don't breathe only into a small child's mouth. You need to breathe into both the child's nose and the child's mouth. Second, you need to remember that small children have smaller lungs than an adult. When giving a small child air, you should give him or her less air than you would give an adult. The figure above shows rescue breathing for small children. The same techniques can be used for an infant. You should get special training before giving rescue breathing to a small child or infant.

Lesson Review

Using Vocabulary

1. What are abdominal thrusts?

2. What does CPR stand for?

Understanding Concepts

3. Describe how to give abdominal thrusts to infants and to adults.

4. Describe how to give rescue breathing to small children and to adults.

Critical Thinking

5. Applying Concepts Explain why you need to breathe into an infant's nose as well as into his or her mouth when you perform rescue breathing.

6. Making Inferences Why is it so important to take a class before giving abdominal thrusts or rescue breathing?

First Aid for Injuries

Paz cut her arm when she crashed her bike. Her mother took her to the emergency room. She had to get 10 stitches to close the cut!

Most cuts and scrapes aren't as serious as Paz's was. But you still need to clean and take care of your small cuts.

Bleeding

Most cuts and scrapes only need to be washed with soap and water. But deep cuts can be very dangerous. If someone gets a cut, stop the bleeding right away. Put a piece of sterile gauze over the cut. Use your hand to put pressure on the cut. If the cut is on an arm or a leg, elevate the limb above the heart. But don't elevate the limb if doing so may cause more injury. Don't remove the gauze if it is soaked. Just add more gauze and apply more pressure. If the bleeding doesn't stop within a few minutes, or if the wound is very large, call for help. You should visit the emergency room for a deep cut, even if the bleeding has stopped. The cut may need stitches.

If you need to help someone who has a cut, use sterile gloves. The gloves will protect you from diseases carried in the blood. They will also protect the victim from any diseases you have. If you don't have gloves, be sure to wash exposed areas with soap and water as soon as you can.

What You'll Do

- **Describe** the treatment for bleeding.
- **Explain** how to care for burns.
- **Describe** how to care for a poisoning victim.
- **Describe** how to care for broken bones and dislocations.
- **Explain** how to care for someone who has a head, neck, or back injury.

Terms to Learn

- fracture
- dislocation

Start Off
Write

What is the proper first aid for a third-degree burn?

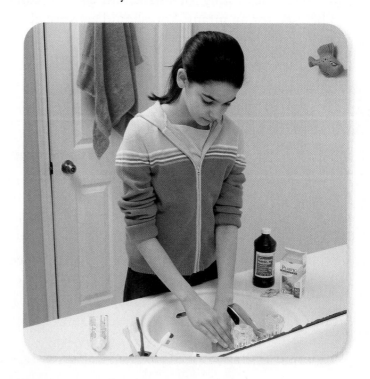

Figure 23 If you cut your hand, wash it with soap and water. Put pressure on the cut until it stops bleeding. Tell your parents about your injury.

TABLE 2 Treating Burns

Type of burn	Description	Treatment
First-degree burns	The burned area is red. Only the top layer of skin is affected.	Run cool water over the burn. Use antibiotic cream on the burn until it heals. If the burn covers most of the body, call a doctor.
Second-degree burns	The top two layers of skin are affected. The skin blisters. The burns are very painful.	Run cool water over the skin or use a wet cold compress. Cover the burn with a sterile bandage. If the burn is larger than 2 inches, go to the emergency room.
Third-degree burns	All three layers of skin are affected. Some muscle and bone may also be burned. Skin will look dark, dry, and leathery. There may be little pain because nerve endings have been damaged.	Call for help immediately. Cover the burn with a clean, wet cloth. Do not remove any clothing stuck to the burn.

Burns

Have you ever burned your hand on the stove? Most burns are caused by heat. Open flames, hot objects, or boiling liquids can cause burns. Some chemicals also cause burns. There are three types of burns. The table above describes each type of burn.

The severity and location of a burn determine whether you should go to the hospital. You should see a doctor if you have a large burn. Also, if you have a burn on your face, hands, feet, or groin, you should see a doctor, even if the burn is small. If a burn isn't cared for properly, it could become infected or leave a scar. Some burns will leave scars anyway. But getting proper care may ensure that scars are smaller and less severe.

Poisoning

Poisons can be eaten, drunk, inhaled, or absorbed through the skin. Many poisonings are accidental. Some poisons are obvious. Pesticides, cleaning products, and automobile fluids all have warning labels. Some substances don't seem so harmful. But some medicines, such as aspirin, can cause poisoning if you take too much of them.

If you find someone who has been poisoned, try to find out what the poison is. Ask the victim or look for bottles and packages in the area. How a victim is cared for depends on the poison. Call 911. Then, call your local poison control center. The operator at the poison control center can tell you what to do for the victim until help arrives.

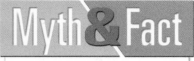

Myth: You can use butter to treat a burn.

Fact: Butter and other oil-based products can retain heat and cause an infection. You should use water and a sterile bandage to treat a burn.

Fractures

Your bones are very strong. But they can be broken in an accident. A **fracture** is a broken or cracked bone. Falls, rough sports, and car accidents all cause fractures. The area around a fractured bone swells and is painful. An injured limb may also look odd or be hard to move.

If you find someone who has a fracture, call for help. In the meantime, avoid moving the injured bone. Moving a broken bone can make the injury worse. Don't try to straighten the fracture. You can use ice to reduce swelling, but be careful. For some fractures, you can use a splint. A splint is a stiff object, such as a stick or a board, that you can use to keep the injured area from moving.

Dislocations

Elbows, fingers, and shoulders are common areas for dislocations. A **dislocation** is an injury in which a bone has been forced out of its normal position in a joint. Dislocations happen when a person falls or runs into something. Dislocations are painful. A dislocated joint may swell and bruise. The injured joint may look unusual.

Victims who have dislocations should go to the emergency room. Call for help, or ask an adult to take the victim to the hospital. Don't move the dislocated limb. Make sure the victim is as comfortable as possible. Stay calm, and wait for help to arrive.

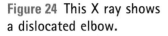
Figure 24 This X ray shows a dislocated elbow.

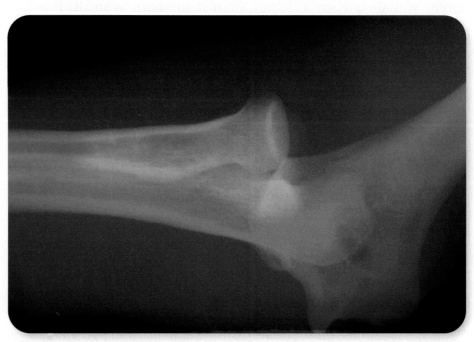

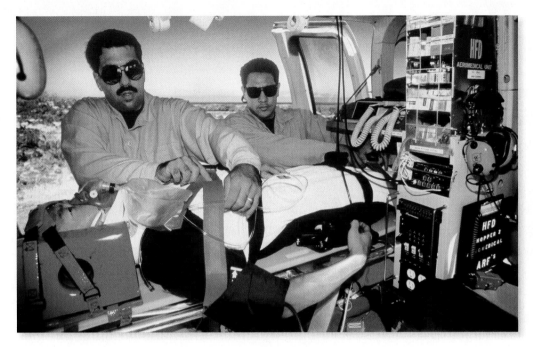

Figure 25 Special equipment keeps a victim's head and neck still after an accident.

Head, Neck, and Back Injuries

Maybe you've bumped your head. You probably had a lump that went away pretty quickly. But some head, neck, and back injuries are very serious. Your brain and nerves in your neck and back control how you move and breathe. If these areas are injured, the damage may not be reversible. Some people who hurt their heads, necks, or backs never recover.

So what do you do for someone who has hurt his or her head, neck, or back? First, don't move the victim. Moving a victim can make the injury worse. The victim may be unconscious. Check to make sure the victim is breathing. Call for help. Keep the victim warm. If the victim is conscious, do your best to keep him or her awake until help arrives. Tell the victim not to move.

Lesson Review

Using Vocabulary

1. Compare fractures and dislocations.

Understanding Concepts

2. What should you do for someone who has a cut?

3. Describe how to take care of burns.

4. What should you do for a poisoning victim?

Critical Thinking

5. **Making Good Decisions** Imagine you found someone unconscious on the floor. There is a bruise on the victim's forehead. What should you do?

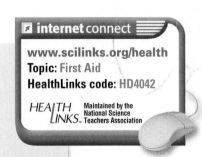

internet connect

www.scilinks.org/health
Topic: First Aid
HealthLinks code: HD4042

HEALTH LINKS™ Maintained by the National Science Teachers Association

Chapter Summary

■ An accident is an unexpected event that may lead to injury. ■ Violence is using physical force to hurt someone or cause damage. ■ A smoke detector is an alarm that detects smoke from a fire. ■ A fire extinguisher is a device that releases chemicals to put out a fire. ■ Helmets protect cyclists and skaters from head injuries. ■ Seat belts and air bags protect people travelling in a car. ■ Hypothermia and frostbite are injuries caused by cold weather. ■ Heat exhaustion and heatstroke are injuries caused by hot weather. ■ One way to be prepared for a natural disaster is to have an emergency kit. ■ The first thing to do during an emergency is to make sure you're safe. ■ You should not give first aid unless you have had special training.

Using Vocabulary

For each pair of terms, describe how the meanings of the terms differ.

1 smoke detector/fire extinguisher

2 hypothermia/frostbite

3 heat exhaustion/heatstroke

4 tornado/hurricane

5 rescue breathing/CPR

For each sentence, fill in the blank with the proper word from the word bank provided below.

fracture	emergency
first aid	dislocation
violence	abdominal thrust

6 An injury in which a bone has been forced out of joint is called a(n) ___.

7 ___ is emergency medical care for someone who is hurt or sick.

8 ___ is using physical force to hurt someone.

9 Actions that apply pressure to a person's stomach to force an object out of the throat are called ___.

Understanding Concepts

10 List four common accidents and ways to avoid them.

11 What are five ways to avoid violence?

12 What should you do if you find a gun?

13 How should you put out a grease fire?

14 If you are walking, riding your bike, or skating after dark, what should you do to stay safe?

15 How does drinking plenty of water keep you safe when you're outside?

16 List four types of natural disasters. How can you prepare for a natural disaster?

17 Arrange the following steps of handling an emergency in the correct order.

   a. Care for the victim.

   b. Check out the situation.

   c. Call for help.

18 What should you do for someone who has a head, neck, or back injury?

19 How can you stay safe in a car? on the bus?

20 What is the first aid for the three types of burns?

Critical Thinking

Applying Concepts

21 Your friend just bought in-line skates and wants to know what kind of safety equipment to get. What would you recommend?

22 Imagine that you are listening to the radio when you hear that a tornado warning has been issued for your area. What should you do?

23 You should see a doctor if you have a burn on your hands, feet, or face. Why is it important to see a doctor for these burns?

24 Sam walks to school in the morning. His first class is wood shop. Then he has a lab class. After school, he goes skateboarding with his friends. They like to try some pretty hard tricks. How can Sam use some of the seven ways to stay safe to make sure that he doesn't have an accident?

Making Good Decisions

25 Imagine that you are at a friend's house. You go into the kitchen and find your friend's younger brother unconscious on the floor. You notice that there is an empty bottle of antifreeze on the floor. What should you do?

26 It is a cold winter day. Maria and Sarah are hiking when Maria notices that Sarah is shivering. Maria asks Sarah if she is OK. Sarah seems confused and her speech is slurred. What should Maria do?

27 George and several friends are at his friend Ben's house. Ben wants to show everyone his parents' gun. George's friends want to see it. What should George do?

28 Imagine that you and a friend are out riding bikes. You're both wearing your helmets. Your friend has an accident. Your friend has several cuts that are bleeding, and his arm is twisted at an odd angle. How should you help your friend?

Interpreting Graphics

Trampoline Injuries Each Year

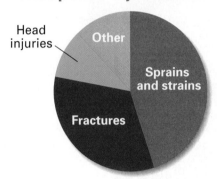

Use figure above to answer questions 29–32.

29 What is the most common type of trampoline-related injury each year?

30 Which injury is the least common type of trampoline-related injury each year?

31 About what percentage of the injuries are strains and sprains?

32 What two types of injuries make up more than 75 percent of all trampoline-related injuries each year?

Reading Checkup

Take a minute to review your answers to the Health IQ questions at the beginning of this chapter. How has reading this chapter improved your Health IQ?

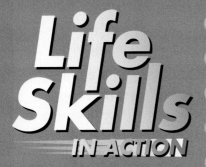

Life Skills IN ACTION

The **5** Steps of Being a Wise Consumer

1. List what you need and want from a product or a service.

2. Find several products or services that may fit your needs.

3. Research and compare information about the products or services.

4. Use the product or the service of your choice.

5. Evaluate your choice.

Being a Wise Consumer

Going shopping for products and services can be fun, but it can be confusing, too. Sometimes, there are so many options to choose from that finding the right one for you can be difficult. Being a wise consumer means evaluating different products and services for value and quality. Complete the following activity to learn how to be a wise consumer.

The Best Baby Seat

ACT 1

Setting the Scene

Beth's mother is having a baby. Beth is very excited and wants to help her mother get ready for the baby. Her mother asked Beth to help her research a baby seat to use in the car. Beth wants to find the best baby seat possible because she knows that the baby's safety is very important. She decides to start researching baby seats on the Internet.

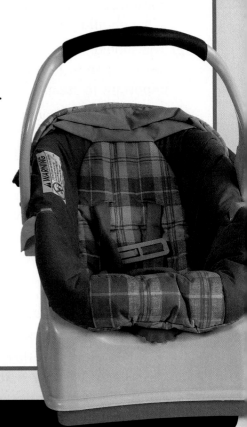

Guided Practice

Practice with a Friend

Form a group of two. Have one person play the role of Beth, and have the second person be an observer. Walking through each of the five steps of being a wise consumer, role-play Beth selecting and evaluating a baby seat for her mother's baby. The observer will take notes, which will include observations about what the person playing Beth did well and suggestions of ways to improve. Stop after each step to evaluate the process.

Independent Practice

Check Yourself

After you have completed the guided practice, go through Act 1 again without stopping at each step. Answer the questions below to review what you did.

1. What are some things that Beth may look for in a baby seat?

2. Other than the Internet, where can Beth find information about baby seats?

3. What are some ways Beth can evaluate the baby seat she selects?

4. When you are looking for safety equipment, why is it important to research several products before buying one?

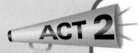

On Your Own

Beth's mother loves the baby seat Beth selected and is impressed that Beth put a lot of effort in picking a good one. She takes Beth out to buy her a present as a thank you for finding the baby seat. Beth decides that she wants a camera so that she can take pictures of the baby when it arrives. Draw a comic strip that shows how Beth can use the five steps of being a wise consumer to find a good camera.

Appendix

The Food Guide Pyramid

Do you know which foods you need to eat to stay healthy? How much of each food do you need to eat? The Food Guide Pyramid is a tool you can use to make sure you're eating healthfully. Each of the major food groups has its own block on the pyramid. The larger the block, the more you need to eat from that food group. The smaller the block, the less you need to eat from that food group. Use the Food Guide Pyramid as a guide for choosing a healthy diet!

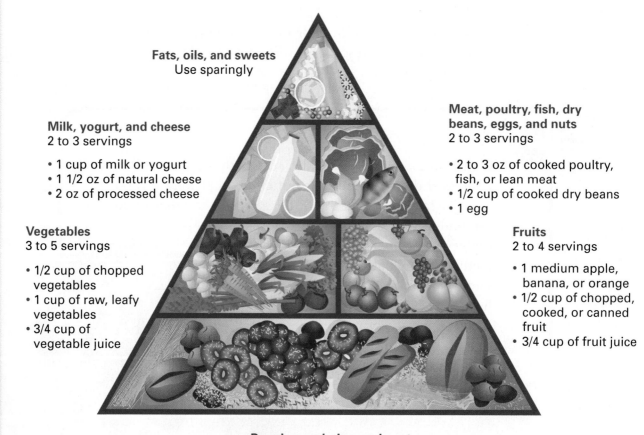

Fats, oils, and sweets
Use sparingly

Milk, yogurt, and cheese
2 to 3 servings

• 1 cup of milk or yogurt
• 1 1/2 oz of natural cheese
• 2 oz of processed cheese

Meat, poultry, fish, dry beans, eggs, and nuts
2 to 3 servings

• 2 to 3 oz of cooked poultry, fish, or lean meat
• 1/2 cup of cooked dry beans
• 1 egg

Vegetables
3 to 5 servings

• 1/2 cup of chopped vegetables
• 1 cup of raw, leafy vegetables
• 3/4 cup of vegetable juice

Fruits
2 to 4 servings

• 1 medium apple, banana, or orange
• 1/2 cup of chopped, cooked, or canned fruit
• 3/4 cup of fruit juice

Bread, cereal, rice, and pasta
6 to 11 servings

• 1 slice of bread
• 1 oz of ready-to-eat cereal
• 1/2 cup of rice or pasta
• 1/2 cup of cooked cereal

Alternative Food Guide Pyramids

The Vegetarian Food Guide Pyramid

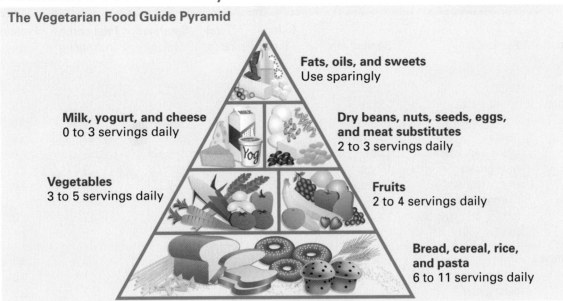

Fats, oils, and sweets
Use sparingly

Milk, yogurt, and cheese
0 to 3 servings daily

Dry beans, nuts, seeds, eggs, and meat substitutes
2 to 3 servings daily

Vegetables
3 to 5 servings daily

Fruits
2 to 4 servings daily

Bread, cereal, rice, and pasta
6 to 11 servings daily

The Mediterranean Food Guide Pyramid

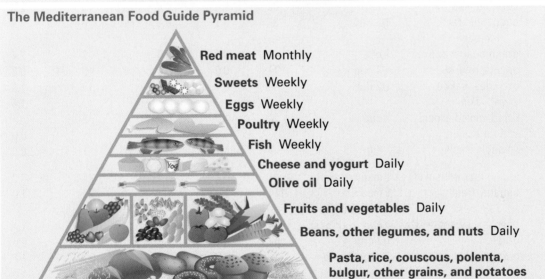

Red meat Monthly

Sweets Weekly

Eggs Weekly

Poultry Weekly

Fish Weekly

Cheese and yogurt Daily

Olive oil Daily

Fruits and vegetables Daily

Beans, other legumes, and nuts Daily

Pasta, rice, couscous, polenta, bulgur, other grains, and potatoes Daily

The Asian Food Guide Pyramid

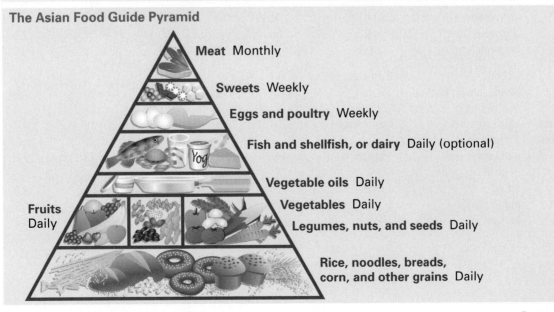

Meat Monthly

Sweets Weekly

Eggs and poultry Weekly

Fish and shellfish, or dairy Daily (optional)

Vegetable oils Daily

Vegetables Daily

Fruits Daily

Legumes, nuts, and seeds Daily

Rice, noodles, breads, corn, and other grains Daily

TABLE 1 Calorie and Nutrient Content of Common Foods

Food group	Food	Serving size	Calories (kcal)	Total fat (g)	Saturated fat (g)	Total carbo-hydrate (g)	Protein (g)
Bread, cereal, rice and pasta	bagel, plain	1 bagel	314	1.8	0.3	51	10.0
	biscuit	1 biscuit	101	5.0	1.2	13	2.0
	bread, white	1 slice	76	1.0	0.4	14	2.0
	bread, whole wheat	1 slice	86	1.0	0.3	16	3.0
	matzo	1 matzo	111	0.2	0.0	22	3.5
	pita bread, wheat	1 pita	165	1.0	0.1	33	5.0
	rice, brown	1/2 cup	110	1.0	0.2	23	2.0
	rice, white and enriched	1/2 cup	133	0.0	0.1	29	2.0
	tortilla, corn and plain	1 tortilla, 6 in.	58	0.7	0.1	12	2.0
	tortilla, flour	1 tortilla, 8 in.	104	2.3	0.6	18	3.0
Vegetables	broccoli, cooked	1 cup	27	0.0	0.0	5	3.0
	carrots, raw	1 baby carrot	4	0.0	0.0	1	0.0
	celery, raw	4 small stalks	10	0.1	0.0	2	0.5
	corn, cooked	1 ear	83	1.0	0.0	19	2.6
	cucumber, raw with peel	1/8 cup	25	0.1	0.0	6	0.6
	green beans, cooked	1 cup	44	0.4	0.0	10	2.4
	onions, raw, sliced	1/4 cup	11	0.0	0.0	3	0.3
	potatoes, baked with skin	1/2 cup	66	0.1	0.0	15	1.0
							1.4
	salad, mixed green, no dressing	1 cup	10	1.0	0.0	2	0.0
	spinach, fresh	1 cup	7	0.1	0.0	1	0.9
Fruits	apple, raw, with skin	1 medium apple	81	0.1	0.1	21	0.2
	banana, fresh	1 medium banana	114	1.0	0.2	27	1.0
	cherries, sweet, fresh	1 cup, with pits	84	0.3	0.0	19	1.4
	grapes	1/2 cup	62	0.1	0.0	16	0.6
	orange, fresh	1 large orange	85	0.0	0.0	21	1.7
	peach, fresh	1 medium peach	37	0.0	0.0	9	1.0
	pear, fresh	1 medium pear	123	1.0	0.0	32	0.8
	raisins, seedless, dry	1 cup	495	0.2	0.0	131	5.3
	strawberries, fresh	1 cup	46	0.0	0.0	11	0.9
	tomatoes, raw	1 cup	31	0.5	0.0	7	1.3
	watermelon	1/2 cup	26	0.0	0.0	6	0.0
Meat, poultry, fish, dry beans, eggs, and nuts	bacon	3 pieces	109	9.0	3.3	0	6.0
	beans, black, cooked	1/2 cup	114	0.0	0.1	20	7.6
	beans, refried, canned	1/2 cup	127	1.0	0.1	23	8.0
	chicken breast, fried meat and skin	1 split breast	364	18.5	4.9	13	34.8
	chicken breast, skinless, grilled	1 split breast	142	3.0	0.9	73	27.0
	chorizo	1 link	273	23.0	8.6	1	14.5
	egg, boiled	1 large egg	78	5.3	1.0	0	6.0
	humus	1/4 cup	106	5.2	0.0	13	3.0

TABLE 1 Calorie and Nutrient Content of Common Foods *(continued)*

Food group	Food	Serving size	Calories (kcal)	Total fat (g)	Saturated fat (g)	Total carbohydrate (g)	Protein (g)
Meat, poultry, fish, dry beans, eggs, and nuts *(continued)*	peanut butter	2 Tbsp	190	16.0	3.0	7	8.0
	pork chop	3 oz	300	24.0	9.7	0	19.7
	roast beef	3 oz	179	6.5	2.3	0	28.1
	shrimp, breaded and fried	4 large shrimp	73	3.5	0.6	3	6.4
	steak, beef, broiled	6 oz	344	14.0	5.2	0	52.0
	sunflower seeds	1/4 cup	208	19.0	2.0	5	7.0
	tofu	1/2 cup	97	5.6	0.8	4	10.1
	tuna, canned in water	3 oz	109	2.5	0.7	0	20.1
	turkey, roasted	3 oz	145	4.2	1.4	0	24.9
Milk, yogurt, and cheese	cheese, American, prepackaged	1 slice	70	5.0	2.0	2	4.0
	cheese, cheddar	1 oz	114	9.0	6.0	0	7.1
	cheese, cottage, lowfat	1/2 cup	102	1.4	0.9	4	7.0
	cheese, cream	1 Tbsp	51	5.0	3.2	0	1.1
	milk, chocolate, reduced fat (2%)	1 cup	179	5.0	3.1	26	8.0
	milk, lowfat (1%)	1 cup	102	3.0	1.6	12	8.0
	milk, reduced fat (2%)	1 cup	122	5.0	2.9	12	8.1
	milk, skim, fat free	1 cup	91	0.0	0.0	12	8.0
	milk, whole	1 cup	149	8.0	5.1	11	8.0
	yogurt, lowfat, fruit flavored	1 cup	231	3.0	2.0	47	12.0
Fats, oils, and sweets	brownie	1 square	227	10.0	2.0	30	1.5
	butter	1 tsp	36	3.7	2.4	0	0.0
	candy, chocolate bar	1.3 oz	226	14.0	8.1	26	3.0
	soda, no ice	12 oz	184	0.0	0.0	38	0.0
	cheesecake	1 piece	660	46.0	28.0	52	11.0
	cookies, chocolate chip	1 cookie	59	2.5	0.8	8	0.6
	cookies, oatmeal	1 cookie	113	3.0	0.8	20	1.0
	gelatin dessert, flavored	1/2 cup	80	0.0	0.0	19	2.0
	ice-cream cone, one scoop regular ice cream	1 cone	178	8.0	4.9	22	3.0
	margarine, stick	1 tsp	34	3.8	0.7	0	0.0
	mayonnaise, regular	1 Tbsp	57	4.9	0.7	4	0.1
	pie, apple, double crust	1 piece	411	18.0	4.0	58	3.7
	popcorn, microwave, with butter	1/3 bag	170	12.0	2.5	26	2.0
	potato chips	1 oz	150	10.0	3.0	10	1.0
	pretzels	10 twists	229	2.1	0.5	48	5.5
	tortilla chips, plain	1 oz	140	7.3	1.4	18	2.0

APPENDIX

Food Safety Tips

Few things taste better than a hot, home-cooked meal. It looks good and it smells good, but how do you know if it is safe to eat? Food doesn't have to look or smell bad to make you ill. To protect yourself from food-related illnesses, follow the food safety tips listed below.

Tips for Preparing Food

- Wash your hands with hot, soapy water before, during, and after you prepare food.

- Do not defrost food at room temperature. Always defrost food in the refrigerator or in the microwave.

- Always use a clean cutting board. If possible, use two cutting boards when preparing food. Use one cutting board for fruits and vegetables and the other cutting board for raw meat, poultry, and seafood.

- Wash cutting boards and other utensils with soap and hot water, especially those that come in contact with raw meat, poultry, and seafood.

- Keep raw meat, poultry, seafood, and their juices away from other foods.

- Marinate food in the refrigerator. Do not use leftover marinade sauce on cooked foods unless it has been boiled.

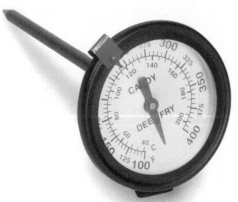

Tips for Cooking Food

- Use a food thermometer when cooking to ensure that food is cooked to a proper temperature.

- Red meats should be cooked to a temperature of 160°F.

- Poultry should be cooked to a temperature of 180°F.

- When cooked completely, fish flakes easily with a fork.

- Eggs should be cooked until the yolk and the white are firm.

Tips for Cleaning the Kitchen

- Wash all dishes, utensils, cutting boards, and pots and pans with hot, soapy water.

- Clean countertops with a disinfectant, such as a household cleaner that contains bleach. Wipe the countertop with paper towels, which can be thrown away. If you use a cloth towel, put it in the wash after using it.

- Refrigerate or freeze leftovers within 2 hours of cooking. Leftovers should be stored in small, shallow containers.

BMI

What Is BMI?

The body mass index (BMI) is a calculation that you can use to determine your healthy weight range. It is a mathematical formula that uses height and weight to evaluate body composition. A high BMI indicates that the person being evaluated may be overweight or obese.

How Do You Calculate BMI?

BMI can be calculated by using the following formula:

$$\text{BMI} = \text{weight in pounds} \times 704.3 \div \text{height in inches}^2$$

For example, a 14-year-old girl who is 4 feet 8 inches tall and weighs 98 pounds would calculate her BMI as follows:

$$\text{BMI} = 98 \times 704.3 \div 56^2 = 22.0$$

Is BMI Accurate?

While BMI works well for many people, it is not perfect. The following are some of the limitations of BMI:

- BMI does not account for frame size. So, someone who is stocky may be considered overweight based on BMI even when that person has a healthy amount of body fat.

- Despite being very fit, athletic people who have low body fat and a lot of muscle may be considered overweight by the BMI. Muscle weighs more than fat which results in a higher BMI measurement.

- Most BMI tables are inaccurate for children and teens because they are based on adult heights. However, some tables have been adjusted to be more accurate for children and teens.

TABLE 2 Healthy BMI Ranges for Ages 10 to 17		
Age	Boys	Girls
10	15.3–21.0	16.2–23.0
11	15.8–21.0	16.9–24.0
12	16.0–22.0	16.9–24.5
13	16.6–23.0	17.5–24.5
14	17.5–24.5	17.5–25.0
15	18.1–25.0	17.5–25.0
16	18.5–26.5	17.5–25.0
17	18.8–27.0	17.5–26.0

Source: *FITNESSGRAM.*

The Physical Activity Pyramid

How often do you exercise during the week? Do you think you get enough exercise to stay fit? Take a look at the Physical Activity Pyramid to find out if you're exercising enough to stay fit!

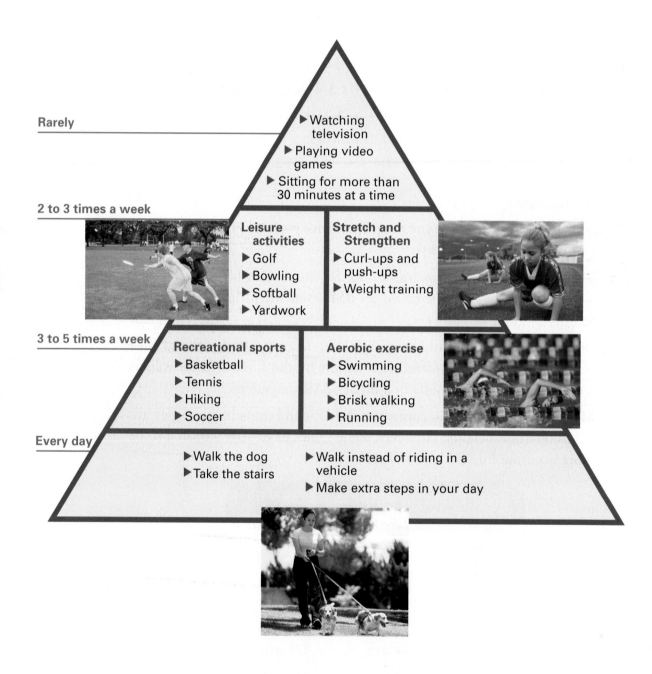

Rarely

- ▶ Watching television
- ▶ Playing video games
- ▶ Sitting for more than 30 minutes at a time

2 to 3 times a week

Leisure activities
- ▶ Golf
- ▶ Bowling
- ▶ Softball
- ▶ Yardwork

Stretch and Strengthen
- ▶ Curl-ups and push-ups
- ▶ Weight training

3 to 5 times a week

Recreational sports
- ▶ Basketball
- ▶ Tennis
- ▶ Hiking
- ▶ Soccer

Aerobic exercise
- ▶ Swimming
- ▶ Bicycling
- ▶ Brisk walking
- ▶ Running

Every day

- ▶ Walk the dog
- ▶ Take the stairs
- ▶ Walk instead of riding in a vehicle
- ▶ Make extra steps in your day

Water Safety

Water activities can be refreshing, fun, and exciting. But water can also be dangerous. Thousands of people drown each year. In fact, drowning is the second-leading cause of accidental death for people under the age of 15. But you can make sure you're safe around water. Keep the following tips in mind.

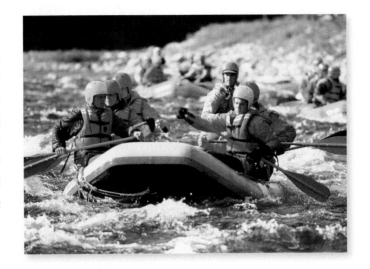

Swimming

- One of the best ways to stay safe in the water is to learn how to swim.
- Always swim with other people.
- Obey posted safety warnings. Signs around swimming areas let you know about safety risks.
- Swim in designated areas.
- Avoid areas that don't have a lifeguard on duty.
- Watch out for boats. Boaters often can't see swimmers.
- Don't swim away from shore. Swim parallel to shore. That way you can get back to shore more easily if you get tired.
- Avoid swimming in rough water and bad weather.

Diving

- Don't dive into unfamiliar bodies of water. If the water is shallow, you could injure your head, neck, or back.
- Get into water feet first until you know the water is deep enough to dive safely.
- Lower yourself into the water. Jumping feet first into shallow water could lead to foot, leg, and spine injuries.

Boating

- Always wear a life jacket. A life jacket can keep your head above water if you have an accident while boating.
- Always go boating with an experienced person.
- Don't stand in the boat. The boat may tip over, or you may fall out.
- Avoid boating in bad weather.
- Avoid rough water unless you know how to handle it. If you are white-water rafting, wear your life jacket and wear a helmet to protect your head.

Staying Home Alone

It is not unusual for teens to spend time home alone after school. Their parents may still be at work. Or they may be running errands. If you spend time at home alone, remember the following safety tips:

- Lock the doors and make sure your windows are locked.

- Never let anyone who calls or comes to your door know that you are home alone.

- Don't open the door for anyone you don't know or for anyone that isn't supposed to be at your home. If the visitor is delivering a package, ask him or her to leave it at the door. If the visitor wants to use the phone, send him or her to a phone booth. If the visitor is selling something, you can tell him or her through the door, "We're not interested."

- If a visitor doesn't leave or you see someone hanging around your home, call a trusted neighbor or the police for help.

- If you answer the phone, don't tell the caller anything personal. Offer to take a message without revealing you're alone. If the call becomes uncomfortable or mean, hang up the phone and tell your parents about it when they get home. You can also avoid answering the phone altogether when you're alone. Then, the caller can leave a message on the answering machine.

- Keep an emergency phone number list next to every phone in your home. If there is an emergency, call 911. Don't panic. Follow the operator's instructions. If the emergency is a fire, immediately leave the building and go to a trusted neighbor's home to call for help.

- Find an interesting way to spend your time. Time passes more quickly when you're not bored. Get a head start on your homework, read a book or magazine, clean your room, or work on a hobby. Avoid watching television unless your parents have given you permission to watch a specific program.

- Consider having a friend stay with you. But do so only if your parents have given you permission to have your friend over. That way, you won't be alone and you will have someone to pass the time with you.

- Remember your safety behaviors. By practicing them, you can make sure you stay safe.

☑ Think before you act. ☑ Use safety equipment.

☑ Pay attention. ☑ Change risky behavior.

☑ Know your limits. ☑ Change risky situations.

☑ Practice refusal skills.

Emergency Kit

A disaster can happen anytime and anywhere. During a disaster, people lose power, gas, and water. Sometimes, people are not able to get help for a few days. You can prepare for disasters by making an emergency kit. There are six basic things you should keep stocked in your emergency kit.

1. **Water** Store water in plastic containers. You'll need water for drinking, food preparation, and cleaning. Store a gallon of water per person per day. Have at least three days' worth of water in your kit.

2. **Food** Store at least three days' worth of nonperishable food. These foods include canned foods, freeze-dried foods, canned juices, and high-energy foods, such as nutrition bars. You should also keep vitamins in your emergency kit.

3. **First-Aid Kit** Someone may get hurt, so you'll want to have plenty of first-aid supplies. Include the following supplies in your first-aid kit:

   - self-adhesive bandages
   - gauze pads
   - rolled gauze
   - adhesive tape
   - antibacterial ointment and cleansers
   - thermometer
   - scissors, tweezers, and razor blades
   - sterile gloves and breathing mask
   - over-the-counter medicines

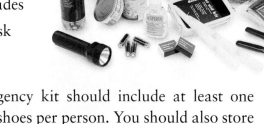

4. **Clothing and Bedding** An emergency kit should include at least one complete change of clothing and shoes per person. You should also store blankets or sleeping bags, rain gear, and thermal underwear.

5. **Tools and Supplies** Always keep your emergency kit stocked with a flashlight, battery-operated radio, and extra batteries. Also, include a can opener, cooking supplies, candles, waterproof matches, fire extinguisher, tape, and hardware tools. You should also store emergency signal supplies, such as signal flares, whistles, and signal mirrors.

6. **Special Items** Be sure to remember family members who have special needs. For example, store formula, baby food, and diapers for infants. For adults, you might keep contact lens supplies, special medications, and extra eyeglasses in your emergency kit.

Internet Safety

The Internet is a wonderful tool. It allows you to communicate with people, access information, and educate yourself. You can also use it to have fun. But when using any tool, there are certain precautions or safety measures you must take. Using the Internet is no different. Listed below are some rules to follow to make sure you stay safe when you are using the Internet.

Rules for Internet Safety

- Set up rules with your parents or another trusted adult about what time of day you can use the Internet, how long you can use the Internet, and what sites you can visit on the Internet. Follow the rules that have been set.

- Do not give out personal information, such as your address, telephone number, or the name and location of your school.

- If you find any information that makes you uncomfortable, tell a parent or another trusted adult immediately.

- Do not respond to any messages that make you uncomfortable. If you receive such a message, tell your parents or another trusted adult immediately.

- Never agree to meet with anyone before talking to your parents or another trusted adult. If your parents give you permission to meet someone, make sure you do so in a public place. Have an adult come with you.

- Do not send a picture of yourself or any other information without first checking with your parents or a trusted adult.

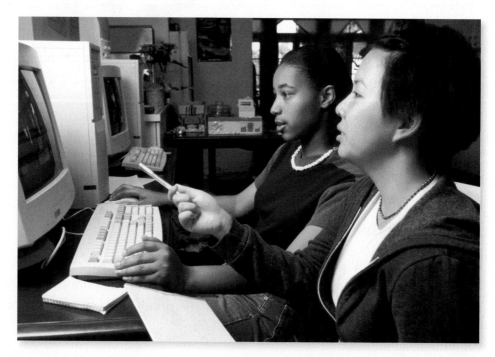

Baby Sitter Safety

Baby-sitting is an important job. You're responsible for taking care of another person's children. You have to make decisions not only for yourself but also for other people. So, you have to make good decisions. Keep the following tips in mind when you baby-sit.

Before you Baby-Sit

- Take a baby-sitting course or first-aid class.
- Find out what time you should arrive and arrange for your transportation to and from the home.
- Ask the parents how long they plan to be away.
- Find out how many children you will be caring for and what your responsibilities are.
- Settle on how much the parents will pay you for your work.
- Consider visiting the family while the parents are home so you can get to know the children a few days before you baby-sit.

When You Arrive

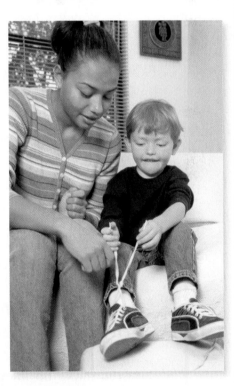

- Arrive early so the parents can give you information about caring for the children. Ask the parents about the children's eating habits, TV habits, and bedtime routine.
- Find out where the parents are going. Write down the address and phone number for where they will be and put it next to the phone. Find out when they plan to return. If the parents have a cellular phone, be sure to get that number, too.
- Know where the emergency numbers are posted. Also, make sure you have the address for the home so that you can give it to an operator in the event of an emergency.
- If you are watching toddlers or infants, find out where their formula and diaper supplies are stored.
- Learn where the family keeps their first-aid supplies. If the children need any medicine while you care for them, make sure you know how to give it to them. Remember that you shouldn't give children medicine unless you have the parents' permission to do so.
- Ask if the children have any special needs. For example, some children are diabetic or asthmatic. Make sure you know what to do if they have any trouble.

While You Are Baby-Sitting

- Never leave a child alone, even for a short time.

- Don't leave an infant alone on a changing table, sofa, or bed.

- Check on the children often, even when they're sleeping.

- Don't leave children alone in the bathtub or near a pool.

- Keep breakable and dangerous objects out of the reach of children.

- Keep the doors locked. Unless the parents have given you permission, do not open the door for anyone.

- If the phone rings, take a message. Do not let the caller know that you are the baby sitter and that the parents are not home.

- If the child gets hurt or sick, call the parents. Don't try to take care of it yourself. In case of a serious emergency, call 911. Then, call the parents.

FUN THINGS YOU CAN DO WHILE YOU BABY-SIT

Baby-sitting is a huge responsibility. But it is also very rewarding. Children love it when you pay attention to them and when you play with them. Don't be afraid to get down on the floor with them. They like you to play at their level. Consider doing the following fun activities, but remember to always get the parents' permission, first!

- Take children outside or to a local park to play.

- Read stories to each other. Let the children pick their favorite story.

- Go to story time at the local library.

- Draw pictures, or color in coloring books. Take this a step further by pretending there is an art gallery in the house. Hang up the pictures, and pretend to be visiting the gallery.

- Pretend you are at a restaurant during mealtimes. Have the children make up menus and pretend to be waiters.

- Plan a scavenger hunt.

- Bring some simple craft items for the children, and let them get creative.

- Play board games or card games.

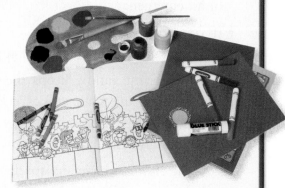

The Body Systems

The Nervous System

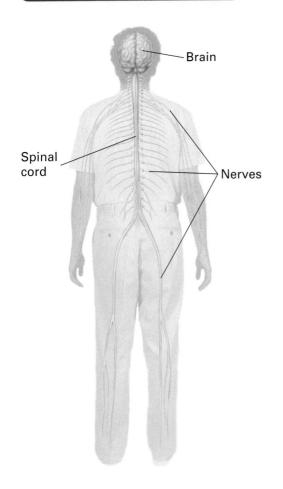

Brain

Spinal cord

Nerves

The Endocrine System

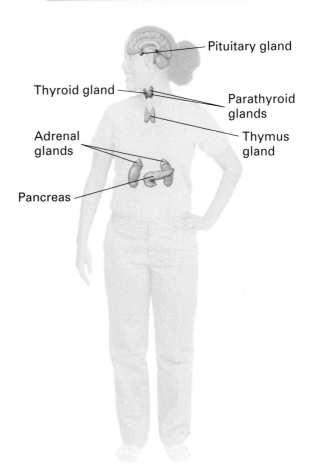

Pituitary gland

Thyroid gland

Parathyroid glands

Adrenal glands

Thymus gland

Pancreas

The Nervous System

The nervous system controls all of your body's functions. The nervous system is composed of the brain, the spinal cord, nerves, and sensory organs, such as your eyes, ears, and taste buds. The nervous system controls voluntary activities, such as walking, and involuntary activities, such as the beating of your heart. The nervous system also allows you to hear, see, smell, taste, and detect pain and pressure.

The Endocrine System

The endocrine system helps the nervous system control your body's functions. The endocrine system also helps regulate growth. The endocrine system is a network of tissues and organs that make and release hormones. Hormones are chemicals that cause changes in the body. Some hormones control how your body grows. Other hormones control how your body responds to stress.

The Skeletal System

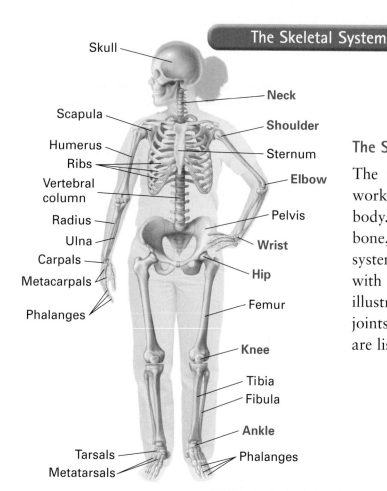

Skull
Neck
Scapula
Shoulder
Humerus
Sternum
Ribs
Elbow
Vertebral column
Radius
Pelvis
Ulna
Wrist
Carpals
Hip
Metacarpals
Phalanges
Femur
Knee
Tibia
Fibula
Ankle
Tarsals
Phalanges
Metatarsals

The Skeletal System

The skeletal system provides a framework that supports and protects your body. The skeletal system is made up of bone, cartilage, and joints. The skeletal system also stores minerals and works with muscles to help you move. The illustration at left lists the bones and joints of your skeletal system. The joints are listed in blue.

The Muscular System

The Muscular System

The muscular system works with the skeletal system to allow you to move. The muscular system is made up of muscles, or tissue composed of cells that contract and expand to cause movement. There are three types of muscle in the body. Smooth muscle is found in the digestive tract, blood vessels, and reproductive organs. Cardiac muscle is found in the heart. Skeletal muscle attaches to bones. The illustration at right shows the skeletal muscles of the muscular system.

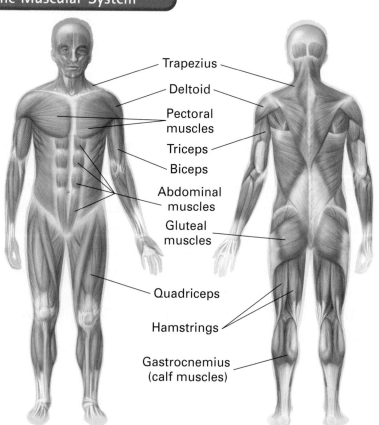

Trapezius
Deltoid
Pectoral muscles
Triceps
Biceps
Abdominal muscles
Gluteal muscles
Quadriceps
Hamstrings
Gastrocnemius (calf muscles)

The Digestive System

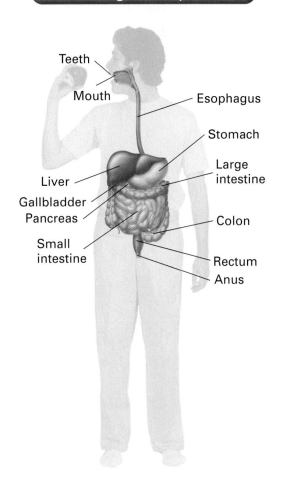

Teeth

Mouth

Esophagus

Stomach

Liver

Large intestine

Gallbladder

Pancreas

Colon

Small intestine

Rectum

Anus

The Urinary System

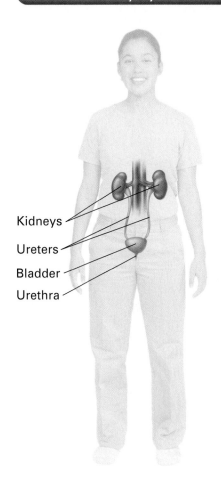

Kidneys

Ureters

Bladder

Urethra

The Digestive System

The digestive system breaks down food into simpler substances, transfers nutrients to the blood, and removes solid waste from your body. The digestive system is composed of organs, such as the stomach and intestines, and glands, such as the liver and gallbladder, that work together to digest food.

The Urinary System

The urinary system filters liquid waste products from the blood and eliminates them from your body. Waste products are filtered from the blood by the kidneys. The waste products are moved from the kidneys to the bladder. Wastes are then eliminated from the body through urination.

The Circulatory System

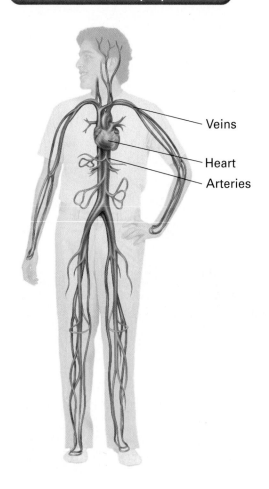

Veins

Heart

Arteries

The Respiratory System

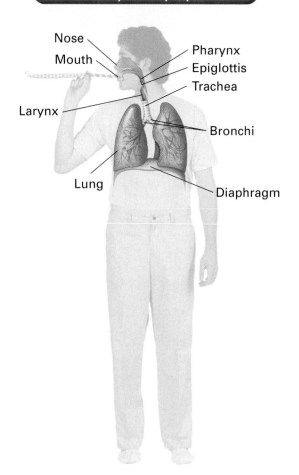

Nose

Mouth

Pharynx

Epiglottis

Trachea

Larynx

Bronchi

Lung

Diaphragm

The Circulatory System

The circulatory system is responsible for transporting and distributing gases, nutrients, and hormones throughout your body. The circulatory system also collects and transports waste products for elimination from your body and protects your body from disease. The circulatory system is made up of your heart, blood vessels, and blood.

The Respiratory System

The respiratory system transfers oxygen from the air into your body and removes carbon dioxide from your body. The gases move into and out of the body through the action of breathing. Air enters the body through the mouth and nose. The air moves through the throat and into the lungs. In the lungs, oxygen and carbon dioxide are exchanged between the blood and the lungs.

Glossary

abdominal thrusts (ab DAHM uh nuhl THRUHSTS) the act of applying pressure to a choking person's stomach to force an object out of the throat (394)

abstinence the refusal to take part in an activity that puts your health or the health of others at risk; in particular the refusal to engage in sexual activity (314)

abuse the harmful or offensive treatment of one person by another person (182)

accident an unexpected event that may lead to injury or death (374)

active listening the act of hearing and showing that you understand what a person is communicating (138)

active rest a way to recover from exercise by reducing the amount of activity you do (86)

acute injury (uh KYOOT IN juh ree) an injury that happens suddenly (82)

additives the chemicals that help tobacco stay moist, burn longer, and taste better (220)

adolescence the stage of development during which humans grow from childhood to adulthood (364)

adulthood the period of life that follows adolescence and that ends at death (365)

aerobic exercise (er OH bik EK suhr SIEZ) exercise that lasts a long time and uses oxygen to get energy (72)

aggression any action or behavior that is hostile or threatening to another person (210)

AIDS acquired immune deficiency syndrome (uh KWIERD im MYOON dee FISH uhn see SIN DROHM), an illness that is caused by HIV infection and that makes an infected person more likely to get unusual forms of cancer and infection because HIV attacks the body's immune system (312)

alcohol abuse the failure to drink in moderation or at appropriate times (251)

alcoholism a disease caused by addiction to alcohol; a physical and psychological dependence on alcohol (258)

Alzheimer's disease (AHLTS HIE muhrz di ZEEZ) a brain disease that affects thinking, memory, and behavior; people who have Alzheimer's may lose their ability to speak and to control their bodies (330)

anaerobic exercise (an er OH bik EK suhr SIEZ) exercise that does not use oxygen to get energy and that lasts a very short time (72)

anorexia nervosa (AN uh REKS ee uh nuhr VOH suh) an eating disorder that involves self-starvation, an unhealthy body image, and extreme weight loss (122)

antibiotic a drug that kills bacteria or slows the growth of bacteria (309)

asthma a respiratory disorder that causes the small bronchioles in the lung to narrow; asthma causes shortness of breath, wheezing, coughing, or breathing with a whistling sound (329)

attitude the way in which you act, think, or feel that causes you to make particular choices (10)

B

bacteria (bak TIR ee uh) extremely small, single-celled organisms that do not have a nucleus; single-celled microorganisms that are found everywhere (306)

behavior the way that a person chooses to respond or act (179)

binge drinking for men, drinking five or more drinks in one sitting; for women, drinking four or more drinks in one sitting (253)

binge eating disorder an eating disorder in which a person has difficulty controlling how much food he or she eats (123)

blood alcohol concentration (BAC) the percentage of alcohol in a person's blood (249)

body image the way that you see yourself and imagine your body (116)

body language a way of communicating by using facial expressions, hand gestures, and posture (138, 178, 203)

body system a group of organs that work together to complete a specific task in the body (322)

brainstorming the act of thinking of all of the ways to carry out a decision (25)

bulimia nervosa (boo LEE mee uh nuhr VOH suh) an eating disorder in which a person eats a large amount of food and then tries to remove the food from his or her body (122)

bullying scaring or controlling another person by using threats or physical force (200)

C

carbohydrate (KAHR boh HIE drayt) a chemical composed of one or more simple sugars; includes sugars, starches, and fiber (99)

carcinogen any chemical or agent that causes cancer (226)

cardiopulmonary resuscitation (CPR) (KAHR dee oh PUL muh NER ee ri SUHS uh TAY shuhn) a life-saving technique that combines rescue breathing and chest compressions (396)

cardiovascular disease a disorder of the circulatory system (225)

cataract a clouding of the natural lens of the eye (341)

celiac disease (SEE lee AK di ZEEZ) a disease of the digestive system that makes the body allergic to the protein gluten (335)

central nervous system (CNS) the brain and spinal cord (330)

chronic injury an injury that develops over a long period of time (83)

collaboration a solution to a conflict in which both parties get what they want without having to give up anything important (205)

communication the ability to exchange information and the ability to express one's thoughts and feelings clearly (40)

community a group of people who have a common background or location or who share similar interests, beliefs, or goals (184)

competition a contest between two or more individuals or teams (74)

compromise a solution to a conflict in which both sides give up things to come to an agreement (205)

conflict any situation in which ideas or interests go against one another (198)

congenital disorder any disease, abnormality, or disorder that is present at birth but that is not inherited (325)

consequence a result of one's actions and decisions (23)

coping dealing with problems and troubles in an effective way (39)

creative expression the use of an art to express emotion (139)

deafness the partial or total loss of the ability to hear (341)

defense mechanism an automatic, short-term behavior to cope with distress (141, 164)

depressant (dee PREHS uhnt) any drug that decreases activity in the body (248, 285)

depression a mood disorder in which a person is extremely sad and hopeless for a long period of time (145)

diet a pattern of eating that includes what a person eats, how much a person eats, and how often a person eats (96)

Dietary Guidelines for Americans a set of suggestions designed to help people develop healthy eating habits and increase physical activity levels (102)

digestion the process of breaking down food into a form that the body can use (95)

dislocation an injury in which a bone has been forced out of its normal position in a joint (400)

distress any stress response that keeps you from reaching your goals or that makes you sick; the negative physical, mental, or emotional strain in response to a stressor (159)

driving under the influence (DUI) the driving of a motor vehicle by a person who is legally intoxicated or who is using illegal drugs (256)

drug any chemical substance that causes a change in a person's physical or psychological state (248, 270)

drug abuse the purposeful misuse of a legal drug or the use of an illegal drug (277)

drug addiction the condition in which a person can no longer control his or her need or desire for a drug (230, 278)

drug misuse use of a drug that differs from the intended use (276)

earthquake a shaking of the Earth's surface that is caused by movement along a break in the Earth's crust (388)

eating disorder a disease in which a person has an unhealthy concern for his or her body weight and shape (121)

egg the sex cell made by females (354)

embryo a developing human, from fertilization until the end of the eighth week of pregnancy (360)

emergency a sudden event that demands immediate action (392)

emotion a feeling that is produced in response to a life event (134)

emotional health the way that a person experiences and deals with feelings (135)

emphysema a respiratory disease in which oxygen and carbon dioxide have difficulty moving through the alveoli because the alveoli are thin and stretched out or have been destroyed (329)

endocrine gland a group of cells or an organ that produces hormones (332)

endocrine system (EN doh krin SIS tuhm) a network of tissues and organs that release chemicals that control certain body functions (358)

endurance (en DOOR uhns) the ability to do activities for more than a few minutes (66)

environment all of the living and nonliving things around you (9, 349)

environmental tobacco smoke (ETS) the mixture of exhaled smoke and smoke from the ends of burning cigarettes (223)

exercise any physical activity that maintains or improves your physical fitness (68)

fad diet a diet that promises quick weight loss with little effort (120)

fatigue physical or mental exhaustion; a feeling of extreme tiredness (162)

fats an energy-storage nutrient that helps the body store some vitamins (99)

fetal alcohol syndrome (FAS) a group of birth defects that affect an unborn baby that has been exposed to alcohol (255)

fetus the developing human in a woman's uterus, from the start of the ninth week of pregnancy until birth (360)

fire extinguisher a device that releases chemicals to put out a fire (379)

first aid emergency medical care for someone who has been hurt or who is sick (392)

flexibility (FLEKS uh BIL uh tee) the ability to bend and twist joints easily (67)

flood an overflowing of water into areas that are normally dry (390)

Food Guide Pyramid a tool for choosing what kinds of foods to eat and how much of each food to eat every day (103)

fracture a crack or break in a bone (400)

friendship a relationship between people who enjoy being together, who care about each other and who often have similar interests (186)

frostbite damage to skin and other tissues caused by extreme cold (384)

genes (JEENZ) a set of instructions found in every cell of a person's body that describe how that person's body will look, grow, and function (348)

gland a tissue or group of tissues that makes and releases chemicals such as hormones (332, 358)

glaucoma a disease that causes pressure in the fluid inside the eye; the high pressure damages the optic nerve and causes a permanent loss of vision (341)

goal something that someone works toward and hopes to achieve (32)

good decision a decision in which a person carefully considers the outcome of each choice (22)

grief a feeling of deep sadness about a loss (367)

hallucinogen (huh LOO si nuh juhn) any drug that causes the user to see or hear things that are not real (288)

health a condition of physical, emotional, mental, and social well-being (4)

healthy weight range an estimate of how much one should weigh depending on one's height and body frame (124)

heart attack a condition in which the heart does not receive enough blood and the heart tissue is damaged or killed, which causes the heart not to pump well (325)

heat exhaustion (HEET eg ZAWS chuhn) a condition caused by losing too much water through sweating on a hot day (385)

heatstroke a failure of the body's heat-regulation systems (385)

heredity (huh RED i tee) the passing down of traits from parents to their biological child (8, 348)

HIV human immunodeficiency virus (HYOO muhn IM myoo NOH dee FISH uhn see VIE ruhs), a virus that attacks the human immune system and that causes AIDS (312)

hobby something that you like to do or to study in your spare time (262)

hormone a chemical made in one part of the body that is released into the blood, that is carried through the bloodstream, and that causes a change in another part of the body; controls growth and development and many other body functions (134, 332, 358)

hurricane a large, spinning tropical weather system that has wind speeds of at least 74 miles per hour (389)

hypertension (HIE puhr TEN shuhn) a condition in which the pressure inside the large arteries is too high; also called *high blood pressure* (326)

hypothermia (HIE poh THUHR mee uh) a below-normal body temperature (384)

I

infectious disease (in FEK shuhs dih ZEEZ) any disease that is caused by an agent or pathogen that invades the body (304)

inhalant (in HAY luhnt) any drug that is inhaled and that is absorbed into the bloodstream through the lungs (289)

interest something that one enjoys and wants to know more about (33)

intoxication (in TAHKS i KAY SHUHN) the physical and mental changes produced by drinking alcohol (250)

K

kidneys organs that filter blood and remove liquid wastes and extra water from the blood (336)

L

leukemia (loo KEE mee uh) cancer of the tissues of the body that make white blood cells (327)

life skills tools that help you deal with situations that can affect your health (12)

lifestyle a set of behaviors by which you live your life (10)

M

marijuana (mar uh WAH nuh) the dried flowers and leaves of the *Cannabis* plant (286)

mediation a process in which a third party, called a *mediator,* becomes involved in a conflict, listens to both sides of the conflict, and then offers solutions to the conflict (207)

medicine a drug that is used to cure, prevent, or treat pain, disease, or illness (274)

menstruation (MEN STRAY shuhn) the monthly breakdown and shedding of the lining of the uterus during which blood and tissue leave the woman's body through the vagina (355)

mental health the way that people think about and respond to events in their lives (134)

mental illness a disorder that affects a person's thoughts, emotions, and behaviors (144)

mineral (MIN uhr uhlz) an element that is essential for good health (100)

muscular dystrophy a group of hereditary muscle diseases that cause muscles to become weak and disabled gradually (339)

N

negative thinking focusing on the bad parts of a situation (140)

neglect the failure of a parent or other responsible adult to provide for basic needs, such as food, clothing, or love (182)

negotiation discussion of a conflict to reach an agreement (204)

nicotine a highly addictive drug that is found in all tobacco products (221)

nicotine replacement therapy (NRT) a form of medicine that contains safe amounts of nicotine (235)

noninfectious disease a disease that is not caused by a pathogen (322)

nurturing (NUR chuhr ing) providing the care and other basic things that people need in order to grow (181)

nutrient a substance in food that the body needs in order to work properly (95)

Nutrition Facts label a label that is found on the outside packages of food and that states the number of servings in the container, the number of Calories in each serving, and the amount of nutrients in each serving (104)

O

option a choice that you can make (25)

organ two or more tissues that work together to perform a special function (322)

osteoporosis a bone disease that causes loss of bone density (339)

over-the-counter (OTC) medicine any medicine that can be bought without a prescription (275)

overtraining a condition caused by too much exercise (81)

ovulation (AHV yoo LAY shuhn) the process in which the ovaries release a mature ovum every month (355)

P

peer pressure a feeling that you should do something because your friends want you to (29, 232, 246)

peripheral nervous system (PNS) the nerves that connect the brain and spinal cord to all other parts of the body (330)

persistence the commitment to keep working toward a goal even when things make a person want to quit (37)

phobia (FOH bee uh) a strong, abnormal fear of something (147)

physical dependence a state in which the body chemically needs a drug in order to function normally (279)

physical fitness the ability to perform daily physical activities without becoming short of breath, sore, or overly tired (66)

positive self-talk thinking about the good parts of a bad situation (140)

positive stress stress response that makes a person feel good; the stress response that happens when a person wins, succeeds, and achieves (169)

pregnancy the time when a woman carries a developing fetus in her uterus (360)

prescription medicine (pree SKRIP shuhn MED i suhn) a medicine that can be bought only with a written order from a doctor (274)

preventive healthcare taking steps to prevent illness and accidents before they happen (11)

protein (PROH TEEN) a nutrient that supplies the body with energy for building and repairing tissues and cells (99)

psychiatrist (sie KIE uh trist) a medical doctor who specializes in how illnesses of the brain and body are related to emotions and behavior (150)

psychological dependence (SIE kuh LAHJ it kuhl dee PEN duhns) the state of emotionally or mentally needing a drug in order to function (279)

puberty the period of time during adolescence when the reproductive system becomes mature (364)

R

reaction time the amount of time that passes from the instant when the brain detects an external stimulus until the moment a person responds (250)

recovery the process of learning to live without alcohol (259)

redirection taking energy from your stress response and directing it into an activity that is not stressful (167)

reframing looking at a situation from another point of view and changing one's emotional response to the situation (167)

refusal skill a strategy to avoid doing something that you don't want to do (42)

relationship an emotional or social connection between two or more people (176)

relaxation the state of doing something to take one's mind off a problem and to focus on something else that is not stressful (167)

rescue breathing an emergency technique in which a rescuer gives air to someone who is not breathing (396)

resting heart rate (RHR) the number of times that the heart beats per minute while the body is at rest (71)

S

self-concept a measure of how you see and imagine yourself as a person (54)

self-esteem a measure of how much you value, respect, and feel confident about yourself (32, 50)

sex cell a parent cell that joins with another sex cell to create a new cell that contains all of the information needed to develop into a new human being (348)

sexual abstinence (SEK shoo uhl AB stuh nuhns) the refusal to take part in sexual activity (190)

sexually transmitted disease (STD) any of a number of infections that are spread from one person to another by sexual contact (314)

smoke detector a small, battery-operated alarm that detects smoke from a fire (378)

social strain the awkwardness of a situation or the tension among family members and friends because of the use of tobacco (229)

sperm the sex cell made by males (350)

sportsmanship the ability to treat all players, officials, and fans fairly during competition (74)

stimulant (STIM yoo luhnt) any drug that increases the body's activity (284)

strength the amount of force that muscles can apply when they are used (66)

stress the combination of a new or possibly threatening situation and the body's natural response to the situation (158)

stress management the ability to handle stress in healthy ways (167)

stress response a set of physical changes that prepare your body to act in response to a stressor; the body's response to a stressor (162)

stressor anything that triggers a stress response (158)

success the achievement of one's goals (36)

suicide the act of killing oneself (145)

targeted marketing advertising aimed at a particular group of people (233)

testes (TES TEEZ) the male reproductive organs that make sperm and the hormone testosterone (350)

THC tetrahydrocannabinol, the active substance in marijuana (286)

therapist a professional who is trained to treat emotional problems by talking about them (150)

tobacco a plant whose leaves can be dried and mixed with chemicals to make products such as cigarettes, smokeless tobacco, and cigars (231)

tolerance (TAHL uhr uhns) the ability to overlook differences and to accept people for who they are (184); a condition in which a person needs more of a drug to feel the original effects of the drug (231)

tornado a spinning column of air that has high wind speed and that touches the ground (389)

trigger a person, situation, or event that influences emotions (142)

type 1 diabetes a disease of the endocrine system in which the body makes little or no insulin (333)

type 2 diabetes a disease of the endocrine system in which the body makes insulin but cannot use insulin properly (333)

vaccine a substance that is used to make a person immune to a certain disease (311)

values beliefs that one considers to be of great importance (25)

verbal communication the act of expressing and understanding thoughts and emotions by talking (138)

violence physical force that is used to harm people or damage property (208, 375)

virus a tiny, disease-causing particle that consists of genetic material and a protein coat and that invades a healthy cell and instructs that cell to make more viruses (310)

vitamin (VIET uh minz) an organic compound that controls many body functions and that is needed in small amounts to maintain health and allow growth (100)

weight training the use of weight to make muscles stronger or bigger (76)

wellness a state of good health that is achieved by balancing physical, emotional, mental, and social health (7)

withdrawal uncomfortable physical and psychological symptoms produced when a person who is physically dependent on drugs stops using drugs (231, 278)

Spanish Glossary

abdominal thrusts/empujes abdominal acción de aplicar presión al estómago de una persona atragantada para lograr que un objeto salga por la garganta (394)

abstinence/abstinencia decisión de no participar en una actividad que ponga en riesgo la salud propia o la de otros; especialmente la decisión de no participar en actividades sexuales (314)

abuse/abuso tratamiento dañino u ofensivo de una persona hacia otra (182)

accident/accidente acontecimiento inesperado que puede provocar lesión o muerte (374)

active listening/escuchar activamente acción de escuchar y demostrar que comprendes lo que una persona intenta comunicar (138)

active rest/descanso activo forma de recuperarse del ejercicio reduciendo la cantidad de actividad que realizas (86)

acute injury/lesión aguda lesión que se produce de manera repentina (82)

additives/aditivos sustancias químicas que permiten que el tabaco se mantenga húmedo, permanezca encendido por más tiempo y tenga un mejor sabor (220)

adolescence/adolescencia etapa del desarrollo en la que los seres humanos pasan de la infancia a la edad adulta (364)

adulthood/edad adulta período de la vida que sigue a la adolescencia y termina con la muerte (365)

aerobic exercise/ejercicio aeróbico ejercicio que se realiza durante un período de tiempo prolongado y utiliza el oxígeno para obtener energía (72)

aggression/agresión toda acción o conducta hostil o amenazante hacia otra persona (210)

AIDS/SIDA síndrome de inmunodeficiencia adquirida, enfermedad producida por la infección del VIH que hace que una persona infectada tenga más posibilidades de contraer formas poco comunes de cáncer e infecciones debido a que el VIH ataca al sistema inmunológico del cuerpo (312)

alcohol abuse/abuso de alcohol la falta de moderación para beber en los momentos apropiados (251)

alcoholism/alcoholismo enfermedad ocasionada por la adicción al alcohol; dependencia física y psicológico al alcohol (258)

Alzheimer's disease/enfermedad de Alzheimer enfermedad del cerebro que afecta el pensamiento, la memoria y la conducta; las personas con la enfermedad de Alzheimer pueden perder la capacidad de hablar y controlar el cuerpo (330)

anaerobic exercise/ejercicio anaeróbico ejercicio que no utiliza el oxígeno para obtener energía y que se realiza durante un período de tiempo corto (72)

anorexia nervosa/anorexia nerviosa trastorno alimenticio en el que la persona deja de comer, tiene una percepción enferma de su cuerpo y sufre una pérdida de peso extrema (122)

antibiotic/antibiótico droga que mata a las bacterias o demora su crecimiento (309)

asthma/asma trastorno respiratorio que hace que los bronquiolos pequeños en los pulmones se estrechen; el asma produce dificultad para respirar, jadeo, tos o un silbido al respirar (329)

attitude/actitud forma particular de actuar, pensar o sentir de una persona (10)

B

bacteria/bacteria organismos unicelulares extremadamente pequeños que no tienen núcleo; microorganismos de una sola célula que se encuentran en todas partes (306)

behavior/conducta la forma en la que una persona decide reaccionar o actuar (179)

binge drinking/beber compulsivamente en el caso de los hombres, beber cinco o más bebidas en una misma ocasión; en el caso de las mujeres, beber cuatro o más bebidas en una misma ocasión (253)

binge eating/disorder trastorno alimenticio compulsivo trastorno alimenticio en el que una persona tiene dificultad para controlar cuánto come (123)

blood alcohol concentration (BAC)/ concentración de alcohol en la sangre (CAS) porcentaje de alcohol en la sangre de una persona (249)

body image/imagen corporal forma en que piensas en ti mismo y en tu cuerpo (116)

body language/lenguaje corporal forma de comunicarse utilizando expresiones de la cara, gestos con la mano y la postura del cuerpo (138, 178, 203)

body system/sistema corporal grupo de órganos que trabajan juntos para cumplir una función específica en el cuerpo (322)

brainstorming/lluvia de ideas acción de pensar en todas las maneras posibles de llevar a cabo una decisión (25)

bulimia nervosa/bulimia nerviosa trastorno alimenticio en el que una persona come una gran cantidad de alimentos y luego intenta eliminar la comida del cuerpo (122)

bullying/gandallismo acción de asustar o manipular a otra persona mediante amenazas o la fuerza física (200)

 C

carbohydrate/carbohidratos sustancia química compuesta por uno o más azúcares simples; incluye azúcares, féculas y fibras (99)

carcinogen/carcinógeno toda sustancia química o agente que causa cáncer (226)

cardiopulmonary resuscitation (CPR)/ resucitación cardiopulmonar (RCP) técnica para salvar la vida que combina la recuperación de la respiración y compresiones en el pecho (396)

cardiovascular disease/enfermedad cardiovascular enfermedades y trastornos originados por el daño progresivo al corazón y los vasos sanguíneos (225)

cataract/catarata opacidad del cristalino natural del ojo (341)

celiac disease/enfermedad celíaca enfermedad del aparato digestivo que hace que el cuerpo se vuelva alérgico a la proteína de gluten (335)

central nervous system (CNS)/sistema nervioso central (SNC) el cerebro y la médula espinal (330)

chronic injury/lesión crónica lesión que se desarrolla durante un largo período de tiempo (83)

collaboration/colaboración solución a un problema en el que ambas partes obtienen lo que desean sin tener que renunciar a nada importante (205)

communication/comunicación capacidad de intercambiar información y de expresar los pensamientos y los sentimientos propios con claridad (40)

community/comunidad grupo de personas que tienen un origen común, residen en la misma zona o comparten intereses, creencias u objetivos similares (184)

competition/competencia enfrentamiento entre dos o más personas o equipos (74)

compromise/convenio solución a un problema en el que ambas partes renuncian a ciertas cosas para lograr un acuerdo (205)

conflict/conflicto toda situación en la que las ideas o los intereses se enfrentan (198)

congenital disorder/trastorno congénito toda enfermedad, anormalidad o trastorno presente al nacer pero no hereditario (325)

consequence/consecuencia resultado de las acciones y las decisiones de una persona (23)

coping/sobrellevar manejar los problemas y los inconvenientes de manera eficaz (39)

creative expression/expresión creativa uso de una actividad artística para expresar emociones (139)

deafness/sordera pérdida total o parcial de la capacidad de oír (341)

defense mechanism/mecanismo de defensa conducta automática que se mantiene durante un período de tiempo corto para sobrellevar dificultades (141, 164)

depressant/depresivo droga que disminuye la velocidad del funcionamiento del cuerpo y el cerebro (248, 285)

depression/depresión tristeza y desesperanza que impiden a una persona realizar las actividades diarias (145)

diet/dieta plan de alimentos que incluye lo que una persona come, cuánto come y cada cuánto come (96)

Dietary Guidelines for Americans/Guía alimenticia para los Estadounidenses conjunto de sugerencias diseñado para ayudar a las personas a crear hábitos alimenticios sanos y aumentar los niveles de actividad física (102)

digestion/digestión proceso de descomponer los alimentos de manera que el cuerpo pueda utilizarlos (95)

dislocation/dislocación lesión en la que un hueso sale de su posición normal en una articulación (400)

distress/alteración toda respuesta nerviosa que hace que una persona no logre alcanzar una meta o se enferme; tensión física, mental o emocional negativa que se manifiesta como respuesta a un factor estresante (159)

driving under the influence (DUI)/conducir bajo efectos (CBE) situación en la que una persona que legalmente está intoxicada o ha consumido drogas ilegales conduce un vehículo motorizado (256)

drug/droga toda sustancia química que provoca un cambio en el estado físico o psicológico de una persona (248, 270)

drug abuse/abuso de drogas uso incorrecto o inseguro de una droga (277)

drug addiction/drogadicción estado en el que una persona ya no puede controlar el consumo de una droga (230, 278)

drug misuse/uso indebido de drogas uso de una droga distinto al uso adecuado (276)

earthquake/terremoto temblor de la superficie de la Tierra producido por un movimiento a lo largo de una ruptura en la corteza terrestre (388)

eating disorder/trastorno alimenticio enfermedad en la que una persona se preocupa de manera negativa por su silueta y su peso corporal (121)

egg/óvulo célula sexual elaborada por las mujeres (354)

embryo/embrión ser humano en desarrollo, desde el momento de la fecundación hasta la octava semana del embarazo (360)

emergency/emergencia hecho repentino que requiere acción inmediata (392)

emotion abuso/emocional uso repetido de acciones y palabras que implican que una persona no tiene valor ni poder (134)

emotional health/intimidad emocional condición de estar emocionalmente relacionado con otra persona (135)

emphysema/enfisema enfermedad respiratoria en la que el oxígeno y el dióxido de carbono no se pueden desplazar fácilmente a través de los alvéolos dado que éstos se afinaron, se distendieron o se han destruido (329)

endocrine gland/glándula endocrina órgano que libera hormonas en el torrente sanguíneo o en el líquido que rodea las células (332)

endocrine system/sistema endocrino red de tejidos y órganos que liberan sustancias químicas que controlan ciertas funciones corporales (358)

endurance/resistencia capacidad de realizar actividades durante más de unos pocos minutos (66)

environment/medio ambiente todos los seres vivos y elementos sin vida que rodean a una persona (9, 349)

environmental tobacco smoke (ETS)/ humo de tabaco ambiental (HTA) mezcla del humo exhalado por los fumadores y el humo de los cigarrillos al consumirse (223)

exercise/ejercicio toda actividad física que mantiene o mejora el estado físico (68)

fad diet/dieta de moda dieta que permite bajar de peso rápidamente con poco esfuerzo (120)

fatigue/fatiga agotamiento físico o mental; sensación de mucho cansancio (162)

fats/grasas nutriente que almacena energía y permite al cuerpo almacenar algunas vitaminas (99)

fetal alcohol syndrome (FAS)/síndrome de alcohol fetal (SAF) grupo de defectos de nacimiento que afectan a un bebé que estuvo expuesto al alcohol durante la gestación (255)

fetus/feto ser humano en desarrollo en el útero de la madre, desde el inicio de la novena semana de embarazo hasta el nacimiento (360)

fire extinguisher/extintor dispositivo que libera sustancias químicas para apagar un incendio (379)

first aid/primeros auxilios atención médica de emergencia para una persona que se lastimó o está enferma (392)

flexibility/flexibilidad capacidad de doblar y girar las articulaciones con facilidad (67)

flood/inundación exceso de agua en zonas normalmente secas (390)

Food Guide Pyramid/Pirámide alimenticia herramienta para escoger qué tipos de alimentos se deben comer y qué cantidad de cada alimento se debe comer cada día (103)

fracture/fractura fisura o rotura de un hueso (400)

friendship/amistad relación entre personas que disfrutan de estar juntas, se cuidan entre sí y suelen tener intereses similares (186)

frostbite/congelación daño a la piel y a otros tejidos provocado por un frío intenso (384)

G

genes/genes conjunto de instrucciones que se encuentran en todas las células del cuerpo de una persona y proporcionan una descripción del cuerpo: qué aspecto tendrá, cómo crecerá y cómo funcionará (348)

gland/glándula tejido o grupo de tejidos que elaboran y liberan sustancias químicas; por ejemplo, las hormonas (332, 358)

glaucoma/glaucoma enfermedad que produce presión en el líquido dentro del ojo; la alta presión daña el nervio óptico y provoca la pérdida permanente de la visión (341)

goal/meta algo por lo que una persona se esfuerza y que espera alcanzar (32)

good decision/buena decisión decisión que toma una persona luego de analizar sus consecuencias detenidamente (22)

grief/duelo sentimiento de profunda tristeza por una pérdida (367)

H

hallucinogen/alucinógeno cualquier droga que hace que el usuario vea o oiga cosas que no son reales (288)

health/salud condición de bienestar físico, emocional, mental y social (4)

healthy weight range/rango de peso saludable cálculo del peso que debería tener una persona según su altura y su estructura corporal (124)

heart attack/ataque al corazón daño y pérdida de la función de una zona del músculo del corazón debido a la falta de suministro de sangre (325)

heat exhaustion/agotamiento por calor condición causada por la pérdida excesiva de agua a través de la transpiración en un día de calor (385)

heatstroke/insolación falla del sistema de regulación de calor del cuerpo (385)

heredity/herencia transmisión de rasgos de padres a hijos (8, 348)

HIV/VIH virus de inmunodeficiencia humana, un virus que ataca al sistema inmunológico del ser humano y causa el SIDA (312)

hobby/prueba de anticuerpo del VIH algo que te gusta hacer o estudiar en el tiempo libre (262)

hormone/hormona sustancia química elaborada en una parte del cuerpo que se libera dentro de la sangre, se transporta a través del torrente sanguíneo y produce un cambio en otra parte del cuerpo; controla el crecimiento y el desarrollo y muchas otras funciones del cuerpo (134, 332, 358)

hurricane/huracán fenómeno del clima tropical que produce una masa grande y giratoria de vientos que se desplazan por lo menos a aproximadamente 74 millas por hora (389)

hypertension/hipertensión condición en la que la presión dentro de las arterias grandes es demasiado alta; también se llama *presión arterial alta* (326)

hypothermia/hipotermia temperatura corporal inferior al valor normal (384)

infectious disease/enfermedad infecciosa toda enfermedad causada por un agente o un patógeno que invade el cuerpo (304)

inhalant/inhalantes drogas que se inhalan en forma de vapor y se absorben en el torrente sanguíneo a través de los pulmones (289)

interest/interés algo que uno disfruta y desea conocer mejor (33)

intoxication/intoxicación cambios físicos y mentales producidos por beber alcohol (250)

kidneys/riñones órganos que filtran la sangre y eliminan los desechos líquidos y la cantidad adicional de agua de la sangre (336)

leukemia/leucemia cáncer de los tejidos del cuerpo que producen glóbulos blancos (327)

life skills/destrezas para la vida herramientas que te ayudan a manejarse en situaciones que pueden afectar tu salud (12)

lifestyle/estilo de vida conjunto de conductas que marcan tu forma de vivir (10)

marijuana/marihuana flores y hojas secas de la planta *Cannabis* (286)

mediation/mediación proceso en el que un tercero, llamado *mediador*, participa en un conflicto, escucha a ambas partes y, luego, ofrece soluciones al conflicto (207)

medicine/medicamento toda droga utilizada para curar, prevenir o tratar enfermedades o molestias (274)

menstruation/menstruación proceso mensual de desprendimiento del recubrimiento interior de la matriz durante el que la sangre y los tejidos salen del cuerpo de la mujer a través de la vagina (355)

mental health/salud mental forma en la que una persona piensa y responde a hechos de su vida (134)

mental illness/enfermedad mental trasforno que afecta los pensamientos, las emociones y la conducta de una persona (144)

mineral/mineral elemento esencial para una buena salud (100)

muscular dystrophy/distrofia muscular grupo de enfermedades musculares hereditarias que hacen que los músculos se debiliten y atrofien poco a poco (339)

negative thinking/pensamiento negativo concentración en los aspectos malos de una situación (140)

neglect/negligencia incumplimiento de un padre u otro adulto responsable en su deber de satisfacer las necesidades básicas, tales como comida, ropa o amor (182)

negotiation/negociación debate sobre un conflicto para llegar a un acuerdo (204)

nicotine/nicotina droga altamente adictiva que se encuentra en todos los productos con tabaco (221)

nicotine replacement therapy (NRT)/ terapia de reemplazo de nicotina (TRN) tratamiento con medicamentos que contienen cantidades seguras de nicotina (235)

noninfectious disease/enfermedad no infecciosa enfermedad que no es causada por un agente patógeno (322)

nurturing/nutrir proporcionar los cuidados y otros elementos básicos que las personas necesitan para crecer (181)

nutrient/nutriente sustancia en los alimentos que el cuerpo necesita para funcionar correctamente (95)

Nutrition Facts label/etiqueta de Valores nutricionales etiqueta que se encuentra en el exterior de los envases de alimentos y en la que se informa el número de porciones que incluye el envase, el número de calorías que contiene cada porción y la cantidad de nutrientes que aporta cada porción (104)

option/opción elección que puedes realizar (25)

organ/órgano dos o más tejidos que trabajan juntos para llevar a cabo una función especial (322)

osteoporosis/osteoporosis enfermedad que produce la pérdida de la densidad de los huesos (339)

over-the-counter (OTC) medicine/ medicamentos de venta sin receta (VSR) todo medicamento que se puede comprar sin receta médica (275)

overtraining/sobreentrenamiento condición causada por el exceso de ejercicio (81)

ovulation/ovulación proceso mensual mediante el cual los ovarios liberan un óvulo maduro (355)

peer pressure/presión de pares sensación de que debes hacer algo que tus amigos quieren que hagas (29, 232, 246)

peripheral nervous system (PNS)/sistema nervioso periférico (SNP) nervios que conectan al cerebro y la médula espinal con todas las demás partes del cuerpo (330)

persistence/persistencia compromiso a seguir trabajando para alcanzar una meta aun cuando las situaciones hacen que se quiera renunciar (37)

phobia/fobia miedo fuerte y anormal a algo (147)

physical dependence/dependencia física condición en la que el cuerpo depende de una droga determinada para funcionar (279)

physical fitness/buen estado físico capacidad de realizar actividades físicas todos los días sin sentir falta de aire, dolor o cansancio extremos (66)

positive self-talk/lenguaje interno positivo pensar sobre los aspectos buenos de una situación mala (140)

positive stress/estrés positivo respuesta de estrés que hace que una persona se sienta bien; respuesta de estrés que se produce cuando una persona experimenta triunfos y logros (169)

pregnancy/embarazo período durante el cual una mujer lleva a un feto en desarrollo dentro de la matriz (360)

prescription medicine/medicamento recetado medicamento que se puede comprar sólo con una orden escrita del médico (274)

preventive healthcare/cuidado preventivo de la salud medidas para prevenir enfermedades y accidentes antes de que ocurran (11)

protein/proteína nutriente que suministra energía al cuerpo para construir y reparar tejidos y células (99)

psychiatrist/psiquiatra médico que se especializa en estudiar cómo se relacionan las enfermedades del cerebro y el cuerpo con las emociones y la conducta (150)

psychological dependence/dependencia psicológica estado de necesidad mental o emocional de una droga para poder funcionar (279)

puberty/pubertad período de tiempo durante la adolescencia en el que se produce la maduración del aparato reproductor (364)

reaction time/tiempo de reacción cantidad de tiempo que transcurre desde el instante en el que el cerebro detecta un estímulo externo hasta el momento de respuesta de la persona (250)

recovery/recuperación proceso de aprender a vivir sin alcohol (259)

redirection/redireccionamiento desviar energía de una respuesta de estrés a una actividad no estresante (167)

reframing/reenfocar analizar una situación desde otro punto de vista y cambiar la respuesta emocional a esa situación (167)

refusal skill/habilidad de negación estrategia para evitar hacer algo que no quieres hacer (42)

relationship/relación conexión emocional o social entre dos o más personas (176)

relaxation/relajación estado de hacer algo para despejar un problema de la mente y concentrarse en otra cosa que no sea estresante (167)

rescue breathing/respiración de rescate técnica de emergencia mediante la cual una persona le proporciona aire a la que no respira (396)

resting heart rate (RHR)/índice de pulsaciones en reposo (IPR) número de veces que el corazón late por minuto mientras el cuerpo está en reposo (71)

self-concept/autoconcepto medición de cómo una persona se ve y se imagina a sí misma como individuo (54)

self-esteem/autoestima medición de cuánto se valora, respeta y cuánta confianza en sí misma tiene una persona (32, 50)

sex cell/célula sexual célula paterna o materna que se une con otra célula sexual para crear una célula nueva que contiene toda la información necesaria para desarrollar un nuevo ser humano (348)

sexual abstinence/abstinencia sexual negación de participar en actividades sexuales (190)

sexually transmitted disease (STD)/ enfermedad de transmisión sexual (ETS) cualquiera de un número de infecciones que se transmiten de una persona a otra a través del contacto sexual (314)

smoke detector/detector de humo
alarma pequeña que funciona con pilas
utilizada para detectar el humo de un
incendio (378)

social strain/tensión social incomodidad
de una situación o la tensión entre
integrantes de una familia y amigos
por el consumo de tabaco (229)

sperm/espermatozoide célula sexual
elaborada por los hombres (350)

sportsmanship/actitud deportiva
capacidad de tratar a todos los
jugadores, funcionarios y espectadores
de manera justa durante una
competencia (74)

stimulant/estimulante toda droga que
aumente la actividad del cuerpo (284)

strength/fuerza cantidad de fuerza empleada
por los músculos al utilizarlos (66)

stress/estrés combinación de una
situación nueva o posiblemente
amenazante y la respuesta natural del
cuerpo a esa situación (158)

stress management/control del estrés
capacidad de manejar el estrés de forma
sana (167)

stress response/respuesta de estrés
conjunto de cambios físicos que preparan
el cuerpo para actuar en respuesta a un
factor estresante; respuesta del cuerpo a
un factor estresante (162)

stressor factor/estresante cualquier factor
que origine una respuesta de estrés (158)

success/éxito logro de las metas
propuestas (36)

suicide/suicidio acción de matarse a uno
mismo (145)

T

**targeted marketing/comercialización
dirigida** publicidad que apunta a un
grupo de personas en particular (233)

testes/testículos órganos reproductores
masculinos que producen
espermatozoides y la hormona
testosterona (350)

THC/THC tetrahidrocanabinol, sustancia
activa en la marihuana (286)

therapist/terapeuta profesional capacitado
en el tratamiento de problemas
emocionales a través de charlas (150)

tobacco/tabaco planta cuyas hojas se
secan y mezclan con sustancias químicas
para hacer productos tales como
cigarrillos, tabaco rapé y puros (231)

tolerance/tolerancia capacidad de aceptar
a las personas por lo que son a pesar
de las diferencias (184); condición en la
que una persona necesita más cantidad
de una droga para sentir sus efectos
originales (231)

tornado/tornado columna giratoria de
aire que tiene vientos de alta velocidad
y cuyo extremo toca el suelo (389)

trigger/disparador persona, situación
o acontecimiento que afecta a las
emociones (142)

type 1 diabetes/diabetes tipo 1 enfermedad
del sistema endocrino en la que el
cuerpo produce poca cantidad o nada
de insulina (333)

type 2 diabetes/diabetes tipo 2 enfermedad
del sistema endocrino en la que el
cuerpo produce insulina pero no puede
utilizarla correctamente (333)

vaccine/vacuna sustancia que generalmente se prepara a partir de patógenos débiles o sin vida o material genético y se introduce en un cuerpo para proporcionar inmunidad (311)

values/valores creencias que uno considera de mucha importancia (25)

verbal communication/comunicación verbal acción de expresarse y comprender los pensamientos y las emociones mediante el habla (138)

violence/violencia fuerza física que se utiliza para dañar a una persona o una propiedad (208, 375)

virus/virus partícula pequeña, capaz de causar enfermedades, formada por material genético y un revestimiento de proteína que invade a una célula sana y le indica que produzca más virus (310)

vitamin/vitamina compuesto orgánico que controla muchas funciones del cuerpo y que es necesario en pequeñas cantidades para mantener la salud y permitir el crecimiento (100)

weight training/entrenamiento con pesas uso de pesas para fortalecer y agrandar los músculos (76)

wellness/bienestar estado de buena salud que se logra mediante el equilibrio de la salud física, emocional, mental y social (7)

withdrawal/supresión síntomas psicológicos y físicos molestos que se producen cuando una persona que tiene dependencia a una droga deja de consumirla (231, 278)

Index

Note: Page numbers followed by *f* refer to figures. Page numbers followed by *t* refer to tables. Boldface page numbers refer to the main discussions.

INDEX

Acknowledgments continued from page iv.

Academic Reviewers
(continued)

Marianne Suarez, Ph.D.
Postdoctoral Psychology Fellow
Center on Child Abuse and Neglect
The University of Oklahoma
  Health Sciences Center
Oklahoma City, Oklahoma

Nathan R. Sullivan, M.S.W.
Associate Professor
College of Social Work
The University of Kentucky
Lexington, Kentucky

Josey Templeton, Ed.D.
Associate Professor
Department of Health, Exercise,
  and Sports Medicine
The Citadel, The Military College
  of South Carolina
Charleston, South Carolina

Martin Van Dyke, Ph.D.
Professor of Chemistry Emeritus
Front Range Community College
Westminster, Colorado

Graham Watts, Ph.D.
*Assistant Professor
  of Health and Safety*
The University of Indiana
Bloomington, Indiana

Teacher Reviewers

Dan Aude
Magnet Programs Coordinator
Montgomery Public Schools
Montgomery, Alabama

Judy Blanchard
District Health Coordinator
Newtown Public Schools
Newtown, Connecticut

David Blinn
Secondary Sciences Teacher
Wrenshall School District
Wrenshall, Minnesota

Johanna Chase, C.H.E.S.
Health Educator
California State University
Dominguez Hills, California

JeNean Erickson
*Sports Coach, Physical Education
  and Health Teacher*
New Prague Middle School
New Prague, Minnesota

Stacy Feinberg, L.M.H.C.
Family Counselor for Autism
Broward County School System
Coral Gables, Florida

Arthur Goldsmith
Secondary Sciences Teacher
Hallendale High School
Hallendale, Florida

Jacqueline Horowitz-Olstfeld
Exceptional Student Educator
Broward County School District
Fort Lauderdale, Florida

Kathy LaRoe
Teacher
St. Paul School District
St. Paul, Nebraska

Regina Logan
*Sports Coach, Physical Education
  and Health Teacher*
Dade County Middle School
Trenton, Georgia

Alyson Mike
*Sports Coach, Science
  and Health Teacher*
East Valley Middle School
East Helena, Montana

Elizabeth Rustad
*Sports Coach, Life Science
  and Health Teacher*
Centennial Middle School
Yuma, Arizona

Rodney Sandefur
Principal
Nucla Middle School
Nucla, Colorado

Helen Schiller
Science and Health Teacher
Northwood Middle School
Taylor, South Carolina

Gayle Seymour
Health Teacher
Newton Middle School
Newtown, Connecticut

Bert Sherwood
Science and Health Specialist
Socorro Independent School
  District
El Paso, Texas

Beth Truax, R.N.
Science Teacher
Lewiston-Porter Central School
Lewiston, New York

Dan Utley
Sports Coach and Health Teacher
Hilton Head School District
Hilton Head Island, South
  Carolina

Jenny Wallace
Science Teacher
Whitehouse Middle School
Whitehouse, Texas

Kim Walls
Alternative Education Teacher
Lockhart Independent School
  District
Lockhart, Texas

Alexis Wright
Principal, Middle School
Rye Country Day School
Rye, New York

Joe Zelmanski
Curriculum Coordinator
Rochester Adams High School
Rochester Hills, Michigan

Teen Advisory Board

Teachers

Melissa Landrum
Physical Education Teacher
Hopewell Middle School
Round Rock, Texas

Stephanie Scott
Physical Education Teacher
Hopewell Middle School
Round Rock, Texas

Krista Robinson
Physical Education Teacher
Hopewell Middle School
Round Rock, Texas

Illustration and Photography Credits

Abbreviations used: (t) top, (c) center, (b) bottom, (l) left, (r) right, (bkgd) background

Illustrations

All work, unless otherwise noted, contributed by Holt, Rinehart & Winston.

Chapter One: Chapter One: L1: Page 7 (tr), Leslie Kell; REV: 17 (tr), Leslie Kell.

Chapter Two: L1: Page 22 (b), Marty Roper/Planet Rep; L2: 24 (b), Rita Lascaro; L3: 30 (t), Laura Bailie; L4: 34 (t), Argosy; REV: 45 (tr), Leslie Kell.

Chapter Three: L1: Page 51 (r), Marty Roper/Planet Rep; 52-53 (t), Rita Lascaro; REV: 61 (tr), Leslie Kell; FEA: 62 Laura Bailie.

Chapter Four: L2: Page 68 (b), Marty Roper/Planet Rep; 70 (tl), Argosy; L6: 81 (t), Argosy; L8: 85 (b), Mark Heine.

Chapter Five: L3: Page 104 (c), Argosy; L4: 108 (tr), Argosy; FEA: 112 Argosy.

Chapter Six: L2: Page 118 (bl), (bc), (br), Rick Herman; L4: 125 (b), Argosy; REV: 129 (tr), Leslie Kell.

Chapter Seven: L1: Page 135 (b), Marty Roper/Planet Rep; L5: 150 (tr), Leslie Kell; FEA: 155 Rita Lascaro.

Chapter Eight: L4: Page 168-169 (t), Argosy; FEA: 173 Argosy.

Chapter Nine: L4: Page 187 (tl), Marty Roper/Planet Rep; FEA: 195 Laura Bailie.

Chapter Ten: L1: Page 200 (t), Marty Roper/Planet Rep; L2: 202 (b), Rita Lascaro; 204 (tr), Marty Roper/Planet Rep; L4: 209 (t), Stephen Durke/Washington Artists.

Chapter Eleven: L1: Page 220 (b), Rick Herman; L2: 225 (tl), Christy Krames; L4: 230 (b), Stephen Durke/Washington Artists; L6: 234 (br), Leslie Kell; L7: 238 (b), Leslie Kell.

Chapter Twelve: L2: Page 249 (b), Leslie Kell; 250 (b), Mark Heine; 251 (tr), Mark Heine; L4: 257 (tl), Leslie Kell; L5: 258 (bl), Mark Heine; REV: 265 (tr), Marty Roper/Planet Rep.

Chapter Thirteen: L2: Page 274 (br), Leslie Kell; 275 (t), Leslie Kell; L4: 278 (bl), Leslie Kell; L5: 281 (t), Stephen Durke/Washington Artists; 282 (b), Christy Krames; L7: 287 (t), Mark Heine.

Chapter Fourteen: L1: Page 300 (b), Argosy; L2: 302 (b), Stephen Durke/Washington Artists; L4: 313 (t), Argosy; REV: 317 (tr), Leslie Kell.

Chapter Fifteen: L2: Page 324 (bl), (br), Christy Krames; 326 (br), Leslie Kell; L3: 328 (bl), Christy Krames; L4: 330 (bl), Christy Krames; L5: 332 (bl), Christy Krames; L6: 334 (bl), Christy Krames; L7: 336 (bl), Christy Krames; L8: 338 (bl), Christy Krames; L9: 340 (bl), (br), Christy Krames; REV: 343 (tr), Leslie Kell.

Chapter Sixteen: L2: Page 350 (b), Christy Krames; L3: 354 (b), Christy Krames; 355 (t), Christy Krames; L4: 358 (b), Christy Krames; REV: 369 (tr), Leslie Kell; FEA: 371 Laura Bailie.

Chapter Seventeen: L2: Page 378 (b), Argosy; 379 (tl), (tr), Mark Heine; L3: 382 (t), Leslie Kell; L4: 386 (tl), (tr), Stephen Durke/Washington Artists; 387 (tl), (tr), Stephen Durke/Washington Artists; L6: 393 (cl), Argosy; L7: 396 (b), Marcia Hartsock/The Medical Art Company; 397 (t), Marcia Hartsock/The Medical Art Company; REV: 403 (tr), Leslie Kell.

Appendix: 406 (c), Argosy; 407 (cl), (bl), (cr), Rick Herman; 411 (c), Rick Herman; 413 (br), Argosy; 418 (tl), (tr), Christy Krames; 419 (tl), (br), Christy Krames; 420 (tl), (tr), Christy Krames; 421 (tl), (tr), Christy Krames.

Photography

Cover: Gary Russ/HRW.

Table of Contents: v, Index Stock Imagery; vi (t), Peter Van Steen/HRW; (b), Victoria Smith/HRW; vii (t), Sam Dudgeon/HRW; (b), Jim Cummins/Getty Images/FPG International; viii (t), Bill Bachmann/The Image Works; (b), Sam Dudgeon/HRW; ix (tl), David Young-Wolff/PhotoEdit; (bl), Thom DeSanto Photography, Inc./StockFood; (br), John Kelly/Getty Images/Stone; x (tl,tr), Sam Dudgeon/HRW; (bl), Image Copyright 2004 PhotoDisc, Inc.; xi (t), Dennis Curran/Index Stock; (c), David Young-Wolff/PhotoEdit; (b), Catrina Genovese/Index Stock; xii (t), Image Copyright 2004 PhotoDisc, Inc.; (b), Michael Newman/PhotoEdit; xiii (t), David Young-Wolff/PhotoEdit; (b), Myrleen Ferguson Cate/PhotoEdit; xiv (t), Mary Kate Denny/PhotoEdit; (b), Image Copyright 2004 PhotoDisc, Inc.; xv (t), Yoav Levy/Phototake; (b), Kwame Zikomo/Superstock; xvi (t), Index Stock/Steve Stroud; (bl), E. Dygas/Getty Images/FPG International; (br), Mark Reinstein/Index Stock; xvii (t), Image Copyright 2004 PhotoDisc, Inc.; (b), Damien Lovegrove/SPL/Photo Researchers, Inc.; xviii (t), Peter Van Steen/HRW; (b), A. Davidhazy/Custom Medical Stock Photo; xix (t), Paul Windsor/Getty Images/FPG International; (bl), Gavin Wickham; Eye Ubiquitous/Corbis; (br), Microworks/Phototake; xx (t,bl), David Young-Wolff/PhotoEdit; (br), Duomo/Corbis; xxi (t), Sam Dudgeon/HRW; (bl), Bob Daemmrich/The Image Works; xxii (t), Victoria Smith/HRW; (c), Sam Dudgeon/HRW; (b), PhotoSpin, Inc.; xxiii, Network Productions/Index Stock; xv, Victoria Smith/HRW.

Chapter One: 2-3, SW Productions/Index Stock Imagery, Inc.; L1: 4, Sean Cayton/The Image Works; 5, Dana White/PhotoEdit; 6, Paul A. Souders/Corbis; 7, Victoria Smith/HRW; L2: 8, Dick Luria/Getty Images/FPG International; 9, AP Photo/Steve Frischling; L3: 10, Victoria Smith/HRW; 11, David Young-Wolff/PhotoEdit; L4: 12 (all), Peter Van Steen/HRW; 14,

Photography *(continued)*

Rachel Epstein/PhotoEdit; 15, Jennie Woodcock; Reflections Photolibrary/Corbis; FEA: 18, Gibson Photography; 19, Jose Luis Pelaez, Inc./Corbis.

Chapter Two: 20-21, Denis Felix/Getty Images/FPG International; L1: 23, Bob Mitchell/Corbis; L2: 25, Sam Dudgeon/HRW; 26, Sam Dudgeon/HRW; 27, David Young-Wolff; L3: 28, Jonathan Nourok/PhotoEdit; 29, Ghislain & Marie David de Lossy/Getty Images/The Image Bank; 31, Amy E. Conn/AP/Wide World Photos; L4: 32, Jim Cummins/Getty Images/FPG International; 33, Image Copyright 2004 PhotoDisc, Inc.; 35, Mary Kate Denny/PhotoEdit; L5: 36, Mug Shots/Corbis Stock Market; 37 (l), Mark Humphrey, AP Staff; (r), Mark J. Terrill, AP Staff; L6: 38, David Madison/Getty Images/Stone; 39 (all), Peter Van Steen/HRW; L7: 40, Cleve Bryant/PhotoEdit; 41, David Young-Wolff/PhotoEdit; FEA: 46, LWA-Dann Tardif/Corbis; 47, Armen Kachaturian/Comstock.

Chapter Three: 48-49, Maria Taglienti/Getty Images/The Image Bank; L1: 50, Corbis Images/PictureQuest; L2: 54, Index Stock/Table Mesa Prod.; 55 (all), Victoria Smith/HRW; L3: 56, Tom Stewart/Corbis Stock Market; 57, Tom Stewart/Corbis; 59, Bill Bachmann/The Image Works; FEA: 63, David Young-Wolff/PhotoEdit.

Chapter Four: 64-65, Richard Hutchings/Corbis; L1: 66, Terje Rakke/Getty Images/The Image Bank; 67, A. Ramey/PhotoEdit; L2: 69, Image Stock/Omni Photo Communications Inc.; 71, Tom Prettyman/PhotoEdit; L3: 72 (l), Dennis MacDonald/PhotoEdit; (r), Sylvain Grandadam/Getty Images/Stone; 73, Index Stock/Ellen Skye; L4: 74, David Young-Wolff/PhotoEdit; 75, John Langford/HRW; L5: 76, Steve Smith/Getty Images/FPG International; 77, Bob Rowan; Progressive Image/Corbis; 78 (all), Sam Dudgeon/HRW; 79 (all), Sam Dudgeon/HRW; L6: 80, Shelby Thorner/David Madison; L7: 82, Mark E. Gibson/Gibson Stock Photography; 83, Dana White/PhotoEdit; 84, Spencer Grant/PhotoEdit; 86, David Young-Wolff/PhotoEdit; 87, Steve Bly/Getty Images/Stone; FEA: 90, Victoria Smith/HRW; 91, Tony Freeman/PhotoEdit.

Chapter Five: 92-93, Getty Images/The Image Bank; L1: 94 (all), Peter Van Steen/HRW; 95 (b), Corbis Images/HRW; (c), Image Copyright 2004 PhotoDisc, Inc./HRW; (bl), Image Copyright 2004 PhotoDisc, Inc.; (tr,tl), Sam Dudgeon/HRW; 96, Index Stock/Lonnie Duka; 97, David Young-Wolff/PhotoEdit; L2: 98, Don Couch/HRW; 99 (t), Thom DeSanto Photography, Inc./StockFood; (c), Steven Mark Needham/FoodPix; (b), Brian Hagiwara/Getty Images/FoodPix; 100 (c), PhotoSpin, Inc.; (br,tl,cl,cr,t), Image Copyright (c)2004 PhotoDisc, Inc./HRW; (bl,cl), Corbis Images/HRW; Richard Hutchings; L3: 103, John Kelly/Getty Images/Stone; 105, Victoria Smith/HRW; L4: 106 (tr), Index Stock/Roberto Santos; (tl), Thomas Eckerle/Getty Images/FoodPix; (bc), Eisenhut & Mayer/Getty Images/FoodPix; 108 (all), Peter Van Steen/HRW; 109 (l), John Langford/HRW; (r), Victoria Smith/HRW; FEA: 113, Myrleen Ferguson Cate/PhotoEdit.

Chapter Six: 114-15, James Muldowney/Getty Images/Stone; L1: 116,117, Image Copyright 2004 PhotoDisc, Inc.; L2: 118 (l), Camille/Getty Images/FPG International; (c), Anne-Marie Weber/Getty Images/FPG International; (r), Lawrence Manning/Corbis; L3: 120, Peter Van Steen/HRW; 123, Mary Kate Denny/PhotoEdit; L4: 124, Sam Dudgeon/HRW; 126 (all), Sam Dugeon/HRW; 127, Robert Brenner/PhotoEdit; FEA: 130 (t,b), Burke/Triolo Productions/FoodPix; (c), Brian Hagiwara/FoodPix; 131, Chuck Savage/Corbis.

Chapter Seven: 132-33, E. Dygas/Getty Images/FPG International; L1: 134, Mary Kate Denny/PhotoEdit; 136, Davis Barber/PhotoEdit; L2: 138, Jack Hollingsworth/Corbis; 139, Burstein Collection/Corbis; L3: 140, Sam Dudgeon/HRW; 141, Index Stock/Dennis Curran; 142, Index Stock/Catrina Genovese; 143, David Young-Wolff/PhotoEdit; L4: 144, Bruce Ayres/Getty Images/Stone; 145, David Kelly Crow/PhotoEdit; 146, Hulton Archive/Getty Images; 147, Image Copyright 2004 PhotoDisc, Inc.; L5: 148, Image Copyright 2004

PhotoDisc, Inc.; 149, Image 100/Royalty-Free/Corbis; 150, Tom Stewart/Corbis Stock Market; 151, Dennis MacDonald/PhotoEdit; FEA: 154, David Young-Wolff/PhotoEdit.

Chapter Eight: 156-57 Kelly/Corbis; L1: 158 (l), Mary Kate Denny/PhotoEdit; (r), Will Hart/PhotoEdit; 159 (l), Michael Newman/PhotoEdit; (r), Tony Freeman/PhotoEdit;160, PhotoDisc, Inc.; L2: 162, Russell Dian/HRW; L3: 164, David Young-Wolff/PhotoEdit; L4: 167 (c), David Young-Wolff/PhotoEdit; (t), Jonathan Nourok/PhotoEdit; (b), David Young-Wolff/PhotoEdit; FEA: 173, Ian Shaw/Getty Images/Stone.

Chapter Nine: 174-75, David M. Grossman/Photo Researchers, Inc.; L1: 176, JILL SABELLA/Getty Images/FPG International; 177, Mark Gibson; 178 (l), Victoria Smith/HRW; (r), Sam Dudgeon/HRW; 179, David Young-Wolff/PhotoEdit; L2: 180, Bob Daemmrich/Bob Daemmrich Photo, Inc.; 181, Myrleen Ferguson Cate/PhotoEdit; 183, Mary Kate Denny/PhotoEdit; L3: 184, Index Stock/Jeff Greenberg; 185, Syracuse Newspapers/The Image Works; L4: 186, David Young-Wolff/PhotoEdit; 188, Zigy Kaluzny/Getty Images/Stone; 189, Index Stock/SW Production; L5: 190, David Young-Wolff/PhotoEdit; FEA: 194, Kwame Zikomo/SuperStock.

Chapter Ten: 196-97, SW Productions/Index Stock Imagery, Inc.; L1: 198, Index Stock/SW Production; 199, Image Copyright 2004 PhotoDisc, Inc.; 201, Mug Shots/CorbisStock Market; L2: 203 (all), Sam Dudgeon/HRW; 205 (all), Peter Van Steen/HRW; L3: 207, Mary Kate Denny/PhotoEdit; L4: 208, Sam Dudgeon/HRW; 210, Mary Kate Denny/PhotoEdit; 211, Michael Newman/PhotoEdit; L5: 212, David Young-Wolff/PhotoEdit; 213, Image Copyright 2004 PhotoDisc, Inc.; FEA: 216, Mark Richards/PhotoEdit; 217, Mary Kate Denny/PhotoEdit.

Chapter Eleven: 218-19, Joe McBride/Getty Images/Stone; L1: 221, Bill Aron/PhotoEdit; 222, Peter Van Steen/HRW; 223, Index Stock/Doug Mazell; L2: 224, Spencer Grant/PhotoEdit; 225, Moredun Scientific/Photo

Researchers; 226 (b), AP Photo/ Eric Paul Erickson; (tl), Siebert/ Custom Medical Stock Photo; (tr), SIU BioMed/Custom Medical Stock Photo; 227, Yoav Levy/Phototake; L3: 228, Index Stock/Brian Drake; 229, Ron Chapple/Getty Images/ FPG International; L4: 231, Victoria Smith/HRW; L5: 233, Corbis Stock Market; L6: 235, Victoria Smith/HRW; 236, Bob Child/AP/Wide World Photos; 237, David Young-Wolff/PhotoEdit; L7: 239, Kwame Zikomo/Superstock; FEA: 242, Peter Van Steen/HRW; 243, Image Copyright 2004 PhotoDisc, Inc.

Chapter Twelve: 244-45, Corbis Images/HRW; L1: 246, Tony Arruza/Corbis; 247, E. Dygas/Getty Images/FPG International; L2: 248, Index Stock/David Davis; L3: 52, David Young-Wolff/PhotoEdit; 253, Image Copyright 2004 PhotoDisc, Inc.; 254, Rachel Epstein/PhotoEdit; 255, George Steinmetz; L4: 256, Index Stock/ Mark Reinstein; L5: 259, Spencer Grant/PhotoEdit; L6: 260, Index Stock/SW Production; 261, Chuck Savage/Corbis; L7: 262, Myrleen Ferguson Cate/PhotoEdit; 263, Index Stock/Steve Stroud; FEA: 266, Victoria Smith/HRW; 267, EyeWire.

Chapter Thirteen: 268-69, David Young-Wolff/PhotoEdit; L1: 270, Victoria Smith/HRW; 271 (t), Jonathan Nourok/PhotoEdit; (b), Image Copyright 2004 PhotoDisc, Inc./HRW; 272, Damien Lovegrove/SPL/Photo Researchers, Inc.; 273, Victoria Smith/HRW; L3: 276, Walter Hodges/Getty Images/ Stone; 277, Michael P. Gadomski/ Photo Researchers; L4: 278, Mike Siluk/The Image Works; 279, Jeff Greenberg/PhotoEdit; L5: 280, Image Copyright 2004 PhotoDisc, Inc.; 282, Victoria Smith/HRW; 283, Paul Conklin/PhotoEdit; L6: 285, Peter Van Steen/HRW; L7: 286, Henry Diltz/Corbis; L8: 288, H. Schleichkorn/Custom Medical Stock Photo; 289, Tom Stewart/ Corbis; L9: 290, Network Productions/Index Stock; 291, Skjold Photographs; 294, Index Stock/Dave Ryan; FEA: 296,

PUSH/Index Stock; 297, Eric Horan/Index Stock.

Chapter Fourteen: 298-99, Bob Daemmrich/Stock Boston; L1: 301, Ghislain & Marie David de Lossy/ Getty Images/The Image Bank; L2: 303 (l), DR Marazzi Science Photo Library; (r), Barts Medical Library/ Phototake; 304 (l), Sam Dudgeon/ HRW; (r), Barts Medical Library/ Phototake; 305 (l), Corbis; (r), Bettmann/Corbis; L3: 306 (l), CDC/Photo Researchers, Inc.; (r), Kwangshin Kim/Photo Researchers, Inc.; 308, Peter Van Steen/HRW; 309, Michael Newman/PhotoEdit; L4: 310, Victoria Smith/HRW; 312, AP Photo/Amy Sancetta; L5: 314, T.Bannor/Custom Medical Stock Photo; 315, A. Davidhazy/Custom Medical Stock Photo; FEA: 318 (t), Image Copyright 2004 PhotoDisc, Inc.; (b), EyeWire; 319, Will Hart/PhotoEdit.

Chapter Fifteen: 320-21, Kindra Clineff/Index Stock Imagery, Inc.; L2: 324, Sam Dudgeon/HRW; 325, Lester V. Bergman/Corbis; 326 (all), Custom Medical Stock Photo; 327 (tr), Microworks/Phototake; (tl), Sam Dudgeon/HRW; (l), Microworks/Phototake; L3: 328 (l), Sam Dudgeon/HRW; (c), Clark Overton/Phototake; (r), Custom Medical Stock Photo; 329, Mary Steinbacher/PhotoEdit; L4: 330 (r), Collection CNRI/Phototake; (l), Sam Dudgeon/HRW; L5: 332, Sam Dudgeon/HRW; 333, Paul Windsor/Getty Images/FPG International; L6: 334 (l), Sam Dudgeon/HRW; (r), Eye Of Science/Photo Researchers; 335, Salisbury District Hospital/Photo Researchers; L7: 336 (l), Sam Dudgeon/HRW; (c), Lester V. Bergman/Corbis; (r), Siebert/ Custom Medical Stock Photo; 337, Jay Daniel/Photo 20-20/ PictureQuest; L8: 338 (l), Sam Dudgeon/HRW; 338 (c,r), P. Motta/Photo Researchers; L9: 341, Gavin Wickham/Eye Ubiquitous/ Corbis; FEA: 344, Gabriela Medina/SuperStock; 345, Mary Kate Denny/PhotoEdit.

Chapter Sixteen: 346-47, Richard Hutching/Photo Researchers; L1: 348 (br, bl), Michael Newman/

PhotoEdit; (bc), Skjold Photographs; 349, Courtesy Mary Wages; L2: 351, C.N.R.I./ Phototake; 353, Duomo/Corbis; L3: 357, Will Hart/PhotoEdit; L4: 358, Sam Dudgeon/HRW; L5: 360, EURELIOS/Phototake; 361 (t), Lennart Nilsson; (c), Claude Edelmann/Photo Reseachers; (b), Lennart Nilsson/Albert Bonniers Forlag AB, A CHILD IS BORN; 362 (tl), Courtesy Leigh Ann Garcia; (tr), David Young-Wolff/ PhotoEdit; 363 (tl), Painet Inc./Cleo Freelance Photography; (tr), Tom Stewart/Corbis; L6: 364, 365, 366, 367, David Young-Wolff/ PhotoEdit; FEA: 370, Image Copyright 2004 PhotoDisc, Inc.; 371, Victoria Smith/HRW.

Chapter Seventeen: 372-73, Stephen Simpson/Getty Images/FPG International; L1: 375, Sam Dudgeon/HRW; 376, West Stock; 377, Spencer Ainsley/The Image Works; L3: 380, Dana White/ PhotoEdit; 381, Index Stock/Don Romero; 383, Tom Stewart/Corbis Stock Market; L4: 384, Richard Hutchings/PhotoEdit; 385, Bob Daemmrich/The Image Works; L5: 388, Roger Ressmeyer/Corbis; 390, Chris Todd/Getty Images; 391, Peter Van Steen/HRW; L6: 392, Peter Van Steen/HRW; L7: 394, Watson/Custom Medical Stock Photo; 395 (all), Peter Van Steen/HRW; L8: 398, Peter Van Steen/HRW; 400, SPL/Photo Researchers, Inc.; 401, G. Brad Lewis/Getty Images/Stone; FEA: 404, Victoria Smith/HRW; 405, Lonnie Duka/Index Stock.

Appendix: 410, Victoria Smith/HRW; 411 (tr), Nathan Bilow/Getty Images; (cr), David Young-Wolff/PhotoEdit; (br), Davis Barber/PhotoEdit; (tl), Mark Gibson Photography; 412, Terje Rakke/Getty Images/The Image Bank; 414, Peter Van Steen/HRW; 415, 416, Mary Kate Denny/ PhotoEdit; 417, Victoria Smith/ HRW.

Models are for illustrative purposes only. Models do not directly promote, represent, or condone what is written within the text of the book, and are not ill.